PROGRESS IN CLINICAL AND BIOLOGICAL RESEARCH

RECENT TITLES

Please contact the publisher for information about previous titles in this series.

CELLULAR ENDOCRINOLOGY
Hormonal Control of
Embryonic and Cellular
Differentiation

CELLULAR ENDOCRINOLOGY
Hormonal Control of Embryonic and Cellular Differentiation

Proceedings of the First International Symposium on Cellular Endocrinology
Held in Lake Placid, New York, August 12–16, 1985

Editors

Ginette Serrero
Jun Hayashi
W. Alton Jones Cell Science Center, Inc.
Lake Placid, New York

ALAN R. LISS, INC. • NEW YORK

Address all Inquiries to the Publisher
Alan R. Liss, Inc., 41 East 11th Street, New York, NY 10003

Library of Congress Cataloging-in-Publication Data

International Symposium of Cellular Endocrinology
(1st : 1985 : Lake Placid, N.Y.)
Cellular endocrinology.

(Progress in clinical and biological research; 226)
Includes bibliographies and index.
1. Cell differentiation—Congresses. 2. Developmental
cytology—Congresses. 3. Embryology—Congresses.
4. Hormones—Physiological effect—Congresses.
I. Serrero, Ginette. II. Hayashi, Jun. III. Title.
IV. Series: Progress in clinical and biological research;
v. 226. [DNLM: 1. Cell Differentiation—drug effects—
congresses. 2. Embryo—drug effects—congresses.
3. Hormones—physiology—congresses. W1 PR668E v. 226/
WK 102 I6087 1985c]
QL971.I58 1985   574.87'612   86-20092
ISBN 0-8451-5076-6

Contents

Contributors

Eileen D. Adamson, La Jolla Cancer Research Foundation, La Jolla, CA 92037 **[159]**

Francesco S. Ambesi-Impiombato, Centro di Endocrinologia ed Oncologia Sperimentale del CNR c/o Dipartimento di Biologia e Patologia Cellulare e Molecolare, II Policlinico, 80131 Naples, Italy **[277]**

Juan Arechaga, Department of Pathology, University of Colorado Health Sciences Center, Denver, CO 80262 **[67]**

M. Asashima, Department of Biology, Yokohama City University, Yokohama 236, Japan **[55]**

Gerald D. Aurbach, Section on Endocrine Regulation, Metabolic Diseases Branch, National Institute of Arthritis, Diabetes, and Digestive and Kidney Diseases, National Institutes of Health, Bethesda, MD 20892 **[265]**

Uriel Barkai, Roche Institute of Molecular Biology, Roche Research Center, Nutley, NJ 07110 **[205]**

John C. Bell, Departments of Medicine and Biology, University of Ottawa, Ottawa K1H 8M5, Canada **[175]**

Jochen Born, Institut für Molekularbiologie und Biochemie, Freie Universität Berlin, D-1000 Berlin 33, Federal Republic of Germany **[11]**

Eugenie L. Boutin, Department of Anatomy, University of Wisconsin, Madison, WI 53706 **[103]**

Maria Luisa Brandi, Section on Endocrine Regulation, Metabolic Diseases Branch, National Institute of Arthritis, Diabetes, and Digestive and Kidney Diseases, National Institutes of Health, Bethesda, MD 20892 **[265]**

Theodore R. Breitman, Laboratory of Biological Chemistry, National Cancer Institute, Bethesda, MD 20205 **[215]**

Sarah A. Bruce, Division of Biophysics, School of Hygiene and Public Health, The Johns Hopkins University, Baltimore, MD 21205 **[245]**

Wilson H. Burgess, Department of Cell Biology, Biotechnology Research Center, Rockville, MD 20850 **[361]**

Jose Campione-Piccardo, Departments of Medicine and Biology, University of Ottawa, Ottawa K1H 8M5, Canada **[175]**

Jill L. Carrington, Department of Anatomy, University of Wisconsin, Madison, WI 53706 **[103]**

The numbers in brackets are the opening page numbers of the contributors' articles.

xi

A.B. Chapman, Department of Pharmacology, Stanford University School of Medicine, Stanford, CA 94305 **[433]**

Haing Choi, Department of Connective Tissue and Orthopedics, Albert Einstein College of Medicine, Bronx, NY 10461 **[333]**

Tseng Mi-Pai Chuang, Laboratory of Embryonic Differentiation, Shanghai Institute of Cell Biology, Academia Sinica, Shanghai, Peoples Republic of China **[35]**

Kathleen S. Cook, Dana-Farber Cancer Institute and Department of Pharmacology, Harvard Medical School, Boston, MA 02115 **[445]**

Hayden G. Coon, Laboratory of Genetics, National Cancer Institute, National Institutes of Health, Bethesda, MD 20892 **[265]**

Kathryn L. Crossin, Department of Developmental and Molecular Biology, The Rockefeller University, New York, NY 10021 **[81]**

Scott F. Deamond, Division of Biophysics, School of Hygiene and Public Health, The Johns Hopkins University, Baltimore, MD 21205 **[245]**

Jean-Loup Duband, Institut d'Embryologie du CNRS et du Collège de France, F-94130 Nogent sur Marne, France **[127]**

Gerald M. Edelman, Department of Developmental and Molecular Biology, The Rockefeller University, New York, NY 10021 **[81]**

Goro Eguchi, Department of Developmental Biology, National Institute for Basic Biology, Myodaijicho, Okazaki, Japan **[307]**

Peter Ekblom, Max-Planck-Institut für Entwicklungsbiologie und Friedrich-Miescher-Laboratorium der Max-Planck-Gesellschaft, D-7400 Tübingen, Federal Republic of Germany **[147]**

John F. Fallon, Department of Anatomy, University of Wisconsin, Madison, WI 53706 **[103]**

Susan Fedak, Section on Endocrine Regulation, Metabolic Diseases Branch, National Institute of Arthritis, Diabetes, and Digestive and Kidney Diseases, National Institutes of Health, Bethesda, MD 20892 **[265]**

Lorraine A. Fitzpatrick, Section on Endocrine Regulation, Metabolic Diseases Branch, National Institute of Arthritis, Diabetes, and Digestive and Kidney Diseases, National Institutes of Health, Bethesda, MD 20892 **[265]**

Joanna Floros, Department of Pediatrics, Harvard Medical School, Boston, MA 02115 **[141]**

Irving B. Fritz, Banting and Best Department of Medical Research, University of Toronto, Toronto, Ontario M5G 1L6, Canada **[371]**

Mishiyasu Fujita, Department of Molecular Pharmacology, Albert Einstein College of Medicine, Bronx, NY 10461 **[333]**

Jane S. Geduspan, Department of Zoology, University of Tennessee, Knoxville, TN 37996 **[115]**

Edward S. Golub, Department of Biological Sciences, Purdue University, West Lafayette, IN 47907 **[235]**

Horst Grunz, Department of Zoophysiology, FB 9 (Biology), University GHS of Essen, D-4300 Essen 1, Federal Republic of Germany **[45]**

Mary Lou Gubler, Roche Institute of Molecular Biology, Roche Research Center, Nutley, NJ 07110 [205]

Lorraine J. Gudas, Department of Pharmacology, Harvard Medical School and Dana-Farber Cancer Institute, Boston, MA 02115 [181]

K. Hashimota, Department of Biology, Yokohama City University, Yokohama 236, Japan [55]

Jun Hayashi, W. Alton Jones Cell Science Center, Inc., Lake Placid, NY 12946 [xvii]

Hiromichi Hemmi, Laboratory of Biological Chemistry, National Cancer Institute, Bethesda, MD 20205 [215]

Elliot Hertzberg, Department of Biochemistry, Baylor University, Houston, TX 77030 [333]

Peter Hoppe, Institut für Molekularbiologie und Biochemie, Freie Universität Berlin, D-1000 Berlin 33, Federal Republic of Germany [11]

Clayton R. Hunt, Dana-Farber Cancer Institute and Department of Pharmacology, Harvard Medical School, Boston, MA 02115 [445]

Masue Imaizumi, Laboratory of Biological Chemistry, National Cancer Institute, Bethesda, MD 20205 [215]

Jutta Janeczek, Institut für Molekularbiologie und Biochemie, Freie Universität Berlin, D-1000 Berlin 33, Federal Republic of Germany [11]

Tina F. Jaskoll, Graduate Program in Craniofacial Biology and Department of Biological Sciences, School of Dentistry, University of Southern California, Los Angeles, CA 90089-0191 [93]

Douglas M. Jefferson, Department of Molecular Pharmacology, Albert Einstein College of Medicine, Bronx, NY 10461 [333]

Peter A. Jones, USC Comprehensive Cancer Center, Los Angeles, CA 90033 [391]

Elissavet Kardami, Department of Zoology, University of California, Berkeley, CA 94720 [287]

D.M. Knight, Department of Pharmacology, Stanford University School of Medicine, Stanford, CA 94305 [433]

Jeffrey A. MacCabe, Department of Zoology, University of Tennessee, Knoxville, TN 37996 [115]

Mary MacDougall, Graduate Program in Craniofacial Biology and Department of Biological Sciences, School of Dentistry, University of Southern California, Los Angeles, CA 90089-0191 [93]

Thomas Maciag, Department of Cell Biology, Biotechnology Research Center, Rockville, MD 20850 [361]

M.A. Mancini, Department of Biological Sciences, Oakland University, Rochester, MI 48063 [401]

T. Matsunaga, Department of Biology, Yokohama City University, Yokohama 236, Japan [55]

Micheal W. McBurney, Departments of Medicine and Biology, University of Ottawa, Ottawa K1H 8M5, Canada [175]

Lesley A. Michalowsky, USC Comprehensive Cancer Center, Los Angeles, CA 90033 [391]

A.A. Moscona, Department of Molecular Genetics and Cell Biology, The University of Chicago, Cummings Life Science Center, Chicago, IL 60637 [297]

A.C. Nag, Department of Biological Sciences, Oakland University, Rochester, MI 48063 [401]

H. Nakano, Department of Biology, Yokohama City University, Yokohama 236, Japan [55]

Shuji Nakano, Division of Biophysics, School of Hygiene and Public Health, The Johns Hopkins University, Baltimore, MD 21205 [245]

Toshimitsu Okeda, Division of Biophysics, School of Hygiene and Public Health, The Johns Hopkins University, Baltimore, MD 21205 [245]

Teresita Pagan, Department of Biological Sciences, Purdue University, West Lafayette, IN 47907 [235]

G. Barry Pierce, Department of Pathology, University of Colorado Health Sciences Center, Denver, CO 80262 [67]

Martin Post, Department of Pediatrics, Harvard Medical School, Boston, MA 02115 [141]

Lola M. Reid, Department of Molecular Pharmacology and Department of Microbiology and Immunology, Albert Einstein College of Medicine, Bronx, NY 10461 [333]

G.M. Ringold, Department of Pharmacology, Stanford University School of Medicine, Stanford, CA 94305 [433]

Werner Risau, Max-Planck-Institut für Entwicklungsbiologie und Friedrich-Miescher-Laboratorium der Max-Planck-Gesellschaft, D-7400 Tübingen, Federal Republic of Germany [147]

Sylvie Rocher, Institut d'Embryologie du CNRS et du Collège de France, F-94130 Nogent sur Marne, France [127]

Larry C. Rosenberg, Department of Connective Tissue and Orthopedics, Albert Einstein College of Medicine, Bronx, NY 10461 [333]

A.K. Roy, Department of Biological Sciences, Oakland University, Rochester, MI 48063 [401]

Ali M. Saboori, Division of Biophysics, School of Hygiene and Public Health, The Johns Hopkins University, Baltimore, MD 21205 [245]

Juan Saez, Department of Neurosciences, Albert Einstein College of Medicine, Bronx, NY 10461 [333]

F.H. Sarkar, Department of Biological Sciences, Oakland University, Rochester, MI 48063 [401]

G. Sato, W. Alton Jones Cell Science Center, Inc., Lake Placid, NY 12946 [xvii]

Walter Schwarz, Institut für Molekularbiologie und Biochemie, Freie Universität Berlin, D-1000 Berlin 33, Federal Republic of Germany [11]

Ginette Serrero, W. Alton Jones Cell Science Center, Inc., Lake Placid, NY 12946 [xvii, 191]

Jerry W. Shay, Department of Cell Biology, University of Texas Southwestern Medical School, Dallas, TX 75235 [417]

Michael I. Sherman, Roche Institute of Molecular Biology, Roche Research Center, Nutley, NJ 07110 [205]

K. Shimada, Department of Biology, Yokohama City University, Yokohama 236, Japan [55]

Harold C. Slavkin, Graduate Program in Craniofacial Biology and Department of Biological Sciences, School of Dentistry, University of Southern California, Los Angeles, CA 90089-0191 **[93]**

Barry T. Smith, Department of Pediatrics, Harvard Medical School, Boston, MA 02115 **[141]**

Steven C. Smith, Departments of Medicine and Biology, University of Ottawa, Ottawa K1H 8M5, Canada **[175]**

Bruce M. Spiegelman, Dana-Farber Cancer Institute and Department of Pharmacology, Harvard Medical School, Boston, MA 02115 **[445]**

David C. Spray, Department of Neurosciences, Albert Einstein College of Medicine, Bronx, NY 10461 **[333]**

Leroy C. Stevens, The Jackson Laboratory, Bar Harbor, ME 04609 **[7]**

Richard C. Strohman, Department of Zoology, University of California, Berkeley, CA 94720 **[287]**

Jean Paul Thiery, Institut d'Embryologie du CNRS et du Collège de France, F-94130 Nogent sur Marne, France **[127]**

Heinz Tiedemann, Institut für Molekularbiologie und Biochemie, Freie Universität Berlin, D-1000 Berlin 33, Federal Republic of Germany **[11]**

Hildegard Tiedemann, Institut für Molekularbiologie und Biochemie, Freie Universität Berlin, D-1000 Berlin 33, Federal Republic of Germany **[11,25]**

F.M. Torti, Department of Pharmacology, Stanford University School of Medicine, Stanford, CA 94305 **[433]**

Philip L. Townes, Department of Pediatrics, University of Massachusetts Medical Center, Worcester, MA 01605 **[3]**

Donatella Tramontano, Centro di Endocrinologia ed Oncologia Sperimentale del CNR c/o Dipartimento di Biologia e Patologia Cellulare e Molecolare, II Policlinico, 80131 Naples, Italy **[277]**

Paul O.P. Ts'o, Division of Biophysics, School of Hygiene and Public Health, The Johns Hopkins University, Baltimore, MD 21205 **[245]**

Hiroaki Ueo, Division of Biophysics, School of Hygiene and Public Health, The Johns Hopkins University, Baltimore, MD 21205 **[245]**

Bianca M. Veneziani, Centro di Endocrinologia ed Oncologia Sperimentale del CNR c/o Dipartimento di Biologia e Patologia Cellulare e Molecolare, II Policlinico, 80131 Naples, Italy **[277]**

Sho-Ya Wang, Department of Pharmacology, Harvard Medical School and Dana-Farber Cancer Institute, Boston, MA 02115 **[181]**

Robert S. Wells, Department of Pathology, University of Colorado Health Sciences Center, Denver, CO 80262 **[67]**

Mike J. Whitcutt, W. Alton Jones Cell Science Center, Lake Placid, NY 12946 **[319]**

Woodring E. Wright, Department of Cell Biology, University of Texas Southwestern Medical School, Dallas, TX 75235 **[455]**

Reen Wu, Department of Anatomy, School of Veterinary Medicine, University of California, Davis, CA 95616 **[319]**

Kenneth M. Yamada, Laboratory of Molecular Biology, National Cancer Institute, Bethesda, MD 20205 **[127]**

Yasushi Yokogawa, Division of Biophysics, School of Hygiene and Public Health, The Johns Hopkins University, Baltimore, MD 21205 **[245]**

Margarita Zeichner-David, Graduate Program in Craniofacial Biology and Department of Biological Sciences, School of Dentistry, University of Southern California, Los Angeles, CA 90089-0191 **[93]**

Preface

The differentiation events occurring during development are highly coordinated in time and space. Such coordination depends on transmitted signals either via cell-cell, cell-matrix interactions or diffusible factors. The existence of embryonic diffusible inducers has been the object of the work of early embryologists. The transplantation of the dorsal lip of the blastopore of the newt gastrula embryo into presumptive lateral or ventral position of the host gastrular embryo has been shown to initiate an additional embryonic morphogenesis at the site of transplantation resulting in the formation of sham tadpoles. This classical experiment by Spemann and Mangold has indicated that the cells in the dorsal lip of the blastopore have the ability to initiate by themselves, a series of programmed morphogenesis steps and also to induce primary neural structures from the presumptive ectoderms of an embryo. Because of their ability to induce the harmonious primary embryonic structures in the early embryos, this region—the dorsal lip of the blastopore—has been named "organization center-organizer."

The early experiments on the organizer have revealed that the inductive and the morphogenetic effect of organizer did not require the cellular structural integrity of the organizer: viz; 1) A total destruction of the organizer by physical means did not diminish its activity; 2) the organizer still retained its activity after heat treatment (40°C, 5 min) and ethanol denaturation (96% E t OH, 3 min). Subsequent experiments carried out by Holtfreter and Chuang have shown the existence of inducers differing in regional inductive specificities, i.e. archencephalic, deuterencephalic and spino-caudal inductions. These works and that of others led to the conclusion that the factors involved in the primary induction must be multiple. In fact, it was shown that two major factors—neuralizing (N) and mesodermalizing (M) factors—were involved in the induction of the primary head-tail axis of the embryos (for review, see Saxen, L. and S. Toivonen, 1962; Nakamura and Toivonen, 1978). Although a partial isolation and characterization of M-factor had been carried out by Yamada and co-worker in the 50's, these studies encountered problems due to the complexity of embryological phenomena and the paucity of tissue that made biochemical analysis difficult. It would appear that optimism faded in the midst of the excitement over the birth of molecular biology and modern cell biology.

During this time, technical advances were being made in cell culture. These were: (1) the development of systematic methods for culturing hormone-dependent cell lines which retained in culture many of their important specialized functions and their hormonal responsiveness. This was first done with tumors and later with normal tissues; (2) the elucidation of the nature of the hormones and factors present in the fluids that sustain cellular function outside the body;

and (3) the replacement of serum in culture media with defined components such as hormones, growth factors, basement membrane components, etc. (for a review on these three points see Sato, 1975; Barnes and Sato, 1980). This led to the realization that the hormonal regulation of growth and differentiation was much more complex than previously thought and involved a host of novel factors which could not be discovered by classical animal experimentation.

We are now aware that the classical concept of endocrinology is no longer adequate to explain cellular growth and differentiation. Autocrine and paracrine control of various cellular events have been proposed and to some extent have been proven. It has been shown that not only the cells from specialized endocrine organs but also from unrelated tissues can synthesize and secrete hormones. Thus, it is quite possible that both autocrine and paracrine control, in addition to endocrine control, play an important role in the peripheral tissue maintenance and in the embryonic development at the stage in which no endocrine organ is present. In fact, it has been shown by various investigators that cells derived from germ cell tumors (embryonal carcinoma cells) produce several factors including fibronectin, IGF-like molecules, transferrin, PDGF-like molecule, TGF-like molecules, insulin-related molecule calcitonin and parathyroid hormones. The important question for both developmental biologists and cell biologists is "are any of these hormones and factors in anyway related to the embryonic inducers?" The resurgence of interest in these questions has made it timely and desirable to organize a symposium which concentrated on these aspects of developmental and cell biology and which provided a forum for the direct exchange of knowledge and experience between embryologists and cell and molecular biologists. It is only appropriate that this meeting be dedicated to one of the original pioneers in the study of the organizer, Dr. Johannes Holtfreter.

It is hoped that the future will be one of fruitful interactions between embryology, cellular and molecular biology to solve these basic and complex developmental questions.

J. Hayashi
G. Sato
G. Serrero

References

Barnes, D. and G. Sato (1980). Serum-free culture: A unifying approach. Cell 22:649–655.

Nakamura, O. and S. Toivonen, eds. (1978) Organizer—A milestone of half-century from Spemann. Elsevier, North-Holland.

Sato, G. (1975). The role of serum in cell culture. *In:* Biochemical Action of Hormones, III. G. Litwick, ed. Academic Press, New York, pp. 391–396.

Saxen, L. and S. Toivonen (1962). Primary Embryonic Induction. Logos Press, London.

INTRODUCTION: TRIBUTE TO JOHANNES HOLTFRETER

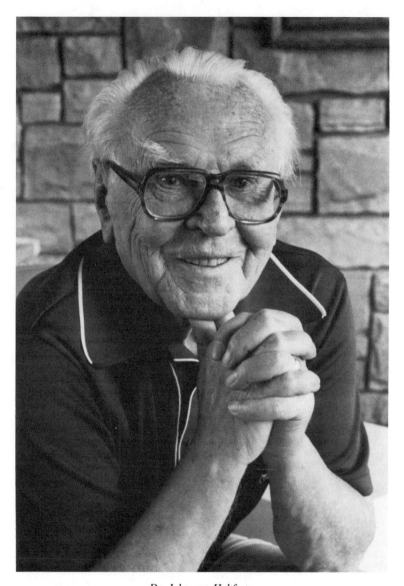

Dr. Johannes Holtfreter

Cellular Endocrinology: Hormonal Control of Embryonic
and Cellular Differentiation, pages 3–6
© 1986 Alan R. Liss, Inc.

Reflections on Johannes Holtfreter

Philip L. Townes
Department of Pediatrics
University of Massachusetts Medical Center

Worcester, MA   01605

I am most pleased to have the opportunity to join you
in honoring my good friend and mentor Johannes Holtfreter.
As I began to seriously consider the possible content of
my remarks, I realized that my reflections on Dr. Holtfreter
are primarily of events of almost 40 years ago. Turning my
mind back to that period, I began to realize the enormity of
the differences in how research in experimental embryology
is and was conducted. Many of the biological phenomena
that were studied by Holtfreter and his contemporaries
continue to be subjects of very active investigation, as
is amply evident in the program of this symposium, but the
methods of analysis are now far more sophisticated. In the
short time available, I will attempt to briefly review some
of the highlights of Dr. Holtfreter's long and distinguished
career,
    On completion of his doctoral studies with Hans
Spemann (1924) Holtfreter studied at the Statzione Zoologica
Napoli, then traveled throughout Italy as an itinerant
portrait artist where he earned the title "Giovanni il
Pittore" before his stint as marine biologist responsible
for oyster culture at Helgoland. His four post-doctoral
"Wanderjahren" were completed by a period of travel in
Finland and return to home in Griefswald where his plans
to become a school teacher were halted by an unexpected
offer of appointment as assistant to Otto Mangold at the
prestigious Kaiser Wilhelm Institute in Berlin-Dahlen. At
the Institute (1928 - 1923) Holtfreter introduced sterile
technique and his balanced salt solution which permitted
for the first time, relatively long term culture of amphibian embryos and explants. The critical importance of the

the improved culture methods may be appreciated by noting that the classic Spemann-Mangold publication (1924) was based on only the five blastoporal lip implants that survived to tail-bud stage from the hundreds that were lost to infection.

The sterile technique and the Holtfreter solution permitted study of embryonic induction, regulation, cell differentiation, morphogenetic cell movements and analysis of organizer phenomenon. The vitalistic concept of the organizer advanced by Spemann was severely challenged by Holtfreter's observations that tissues killed by physical or chemical treatment retained inductive capacity and that neuralizing agents were present in almost all tissues examined. Holtfreter later showed that neural induction occurred in gastrula ectoderm after brief exposure to Ca++ free solutions or even to distilled water. These experiments led to the concept that sub-lethal cytolysis could trigger autoinduction and the emphasis shifted from inducer or organizer to the competence of the reacting system. The challenge then as now is to understand competence in molecular terms. That challenge is well reflected in the many exciting studies being reported at this symposium. The shift in emphasis did not deter investigators from their search for the chemical constitution of inducing agents; it continues to the present time.

From the Kaiser Wilhelm Institute, Holtfreter went to the Institute of Zoölogy at Munich which was then headed by the renowned Karl von Frisch. In 1939, Holtfreter fled from Germany to the laboratory of Joseph Needham at Cambridge. Tragically, Holtfreter was later sent to Canada and interned as an enemy alien for two years before release and appointment at McGill University (1942) and then at Rochester (1946) where he has remained to the present time as Tracy H. Harris Professor Emeritus of Zoölogy.

I arrived in Rochester in 1948 as a new graduate student with interest in experimental embryology having been stimulated by courses taken with the late Leigh Hoadley at Harvard. Although it was after the dawning of the nuclear age, Holtfreter's laboratory was, by current standards incredibly primitive. The major tools of the day were dissecting and compound microscopes, Bunsen burners, glass rods for making dissecting needles, a few Ehrlenmeyer flasks and beakers and castor dishes for culture of embryos and explants. The laboratory did not have an electronic pH meter. Adjustments of pH of culture solutions were made by adding indicator dyes to aliquots of solutions and comparing the developed colors to standards kept in sealed glass ampules.

Dr. Holtfreter worked tirelessly for endless hours at his microscope performing delicate microsurgical manipulations and carefully recording his observations in the form of beautiful drawings and extensive notations. He had no research associates or assistants. Technical assistance was limited to a part-time undergraduate student who fed the axolotls and other amphibians and maintained the aquaria. The Department of Biology had but one histology technician who prepared slides from paraffin blocks for all faculty members. Secretarial service for the entire department was also provided by a single individual.

As there were no laboratory assistants, the graduate students were all expected to devote long hours to their research. Holtfreter expected almost total commitment to research, but his expectations of others did not exceed the demands he placed on himself. Informality, congeniality and mutuality of interest were the main themes in the labs of Holtfreter and his graduate students which at that time included Leroy C. Stevens (also participant at Symposium), Alex Haggis, Morris Smithberg and myself. Each student had his own office/laboratory and each student generally had daily dialogue with their mentor. Although Holtfreter was sometimes perceived as being somewhat autocratic, to those who knew him better, he was an inspiring teacher, a helpful colleague and a loyal friend. Investigators from all over the world regularly sent reprints to Dr. Holtfreter and his large collection was always available to everyone. His intimate knowledge of the literature was most impressive, seemingly able to quote and recall details of thousands of publications.

On comparing the research laboratory of that period with the present, the most striking difference seems to be the personal involvement of the investigator in the actual performance of the study. Holtfreter always did his own research without benefit of assistants. There was an undiluted one-to-one relationship between science and scientist. On review of the scientific program of this outstanding symposium, one notes many "Holtfreterian" themes in the subjects and topics being presented. Indeed, many of the questions, principles and concepts to be discussed here were defined and investigated by Dr. Holtfreter. Today, they are being successfully investigated by the tools of molecular biology. I know that Hiroko and Hans Holtfreter are pleased to be here and to learn of your new findings. It is for me

a very great privilege and honor to join you in honoring
them..

Cellular Endocrinology: Hormonal Control of Embryonic
and Cellular Differentiation, page 7
© 1986 Alan R. Liss, Inc.

A Tribute to Professor J. F. K. Holtfreter

Leroy C. Stevens
The Jackson Laboratory
Bar Harbor, Maine 04609

I began my graduate work at the University of Rochester
in 1947 while Prof. Curt Stern was chairman of the Biology
Department. Shortly after my arrival, Dr. Stern invited Dr.
Holtfreter, who had been interned in Canada during the war,
to join his Department. I took a seminar course in Experimental Embryology given by Dr. Holtfreter which I found more
fascinating than any other course I'd taken. I changed my
major from vertebrate zoology to experimental embryology and
Dr. Holtfreter accepted me as one of his students. Working
with Holtfreter was an invaluable intellectual experience.
It was most enjoyable to hear the many personal anecdotes
that involved other giants in the field of embryology and
made it seem so much alive. It was a treat to read his
papers that contained his beautiful drawings and sketches
that illustrated his discoveries much better than any photo-
graphs could have. Holtfreter was personally involved with
his students, and it was a great pleasure to be exposed to
his vast knowledge and extertise in science, art, and literature. I shall always treasure my association with him, and
I am deeply grateful to him for that unique experience. It
is with pleasure that I salute Holtfreter's distinguished
career.

Section 1. FACTORS IN EMBRYOGENESIS

Cellular Endocrinology: Hormonal Control of Embryonic
and Cellular Differentiation, pages 11–24
© 1986 Alan R. Liss, Inc.

INFORMATIVE MOLECULES AND INDUCTION IN EARLY EMBRYOGENESIS

Jutta Janeczek, Jochen Born, Peter Hoppe, Walter
Schwarz, Hildegard Tiedemann and Heinz Tiedemann
Institut für Molekularbiologie und Biochemie,
Freie Universität Berlin, Arnimallee 22,
D-1000 Berlin 33, FR Germany

In the amphibian oocyte a dorso-ventral and an animal-
vegetal polarity is established when after fertilization a
cytoplasmic streaming occurs. The dorsal side is located
opposite to the random point of sperm entry (Gerhart et al.,
1981). The animal-vegetal polarity is easily recognized by
the distribution of embryonic pigment in the egg cortex. It
is likely that substances which are involved in the control
of differentiation in later stages are also distributed in
the egg in a special pattern. When the egg is constricted
into a dorsal and a ventral part, the dorsal part forms as
Spemann (1938) has shown a complete embryo with an axis system. These results have recently been extended by more re-
fined techniques (Grunz, 1977; Gimlich and Gerhart, 1984).
These and other experiments suggest that a certain pattern
of substances is established in the fertilized egg. Some of
these substances are present in a complex inactive state.
They become activated at a certain time of development and
in a certain region of the embryo.

CHEMICAL NATURE OF INDUCING FACTORS

The search for chemical substances with inducing activity began in the thirties but soon did lead to results
which were difficult to interpret. It was not until the fif-
ties that mesoderm inducing extracts were obtained by Yamada
(1958, 1961) from guinea pig bone marrow which preferentially induces trunk and tail structures (Toivonen, 1953) and by
Tiedemann and Tiedemann (1956a) from 9-11 day chicken embryos
which induce trunk and tail as well neural tissues. Both pre-

parations proved to be proteins. For the separation of the chicken factor from nucleic acids we developed the hot phenol procedure (i.e. extraction with phenol at 60 °C; Tiedemann and Tiedemann, 1956b). Most of the neural inducing activity is separated from the mesoderm inducing activity at this step. The chicken factor was further purified by a number of steps including combined gel electrophoresis/size exclusion chromatography on Sephadex G 100 and isoelectric focusing. The most highly purified fraction focusing at about pH 8 still contained several proteins.

The final purification was achieved by size exclusion and reversed phase HPLC. The fraction with the highest inducing activity from the size exclusion column (M_r 13,000) was on line adsorbed to a reversed phase microbore column and eluted with a propanol/formic acid gradient. Reversed phase rechromatography of the active fraction gives a symmetric peak. The factor is completely inactivated after reduction with mercaptoethanol or thioglycolic acid or by reductive methylation with formaldehyde and $NaBH_4$ and is thereby split into peptides of about half the original molecular mass. Dimers are formed in 6 M urea or when dodecylsulfate is added. The yield of highly purified factor (about 40 pMol/ 1000 g chicken embryos) is small. The factor is enriched 10^5 - 10^6 times. The amino terminal groups may be blocked and could not yet be determined (Born et al., 1985). The highly purified factor induces endodermal as well mesodermal organs depending on its concentration in the test (pg. 5).

A factor with a similar activity has been detected in the presumptive endoderm of amphibian embryos. The mesoderm inducing activity of <u>homogenates</u> from eggs and early embryos is however very low. This may be due to the much higher neural inducing activity of the homogenate which covers up the vegetalizing activity. The partially purified factor from early Xenopus embryos is probably a larger molecule than the chicken factor (Faulhaber, 1970).

A higher mesoderm inducing activity is found in the endoplasmic (microsomal) membranes and the 100,000xg supernatant from hatched Xenopus embryos (Janeczek et al., 1984a). The localization corresponds to the subcellular localization of the vegetalizing factor in 9-11 day chicken embryos (Tiedemann et al., 1962). Whether the factor in early embryos is biosynthetically related to the factor in later stages of development is not yet known.

Neural inducing factors have recently been isolated from subcellular fractions of Xenopus oocyte and gastrula homogenates. A high inducing activity has been found in a heterogeneous population of RNP-particles (18-27S), which were prepared from the microsomal fraction by treatment with EDTA and centrifugation on step-wise sucrose gradients. Ribosomal subunits do not induce. The factor is not released from the RNP-particles by treatment with buffer of higher ionic strength (0.5 M KCl). This suggest that the factor is not artificially associated to the particles by non-specific ionic bonds (Janeczek et al., 1984b). Treatment with a very small amount of RNase (0.1 µg/ml, 30 min, 4 °C) disintegrates the RNP-particles and releases the factor, as was shown by gradient centrifugation. Further degradation of the RNA moiety with pancreatic RNase leads to the precipitation of (hydrophobic) proteins including the neuralizing factor. The inducing activity of the precipitated protein is diminished. Separation of the protein moiety from the RNA by isopycnic centrifugation in CsCl gradients or extraction with phenol leads also to a decrease of inducing activity of the protein. This is probably due to the very low solubility of the factor. But a chemical modification is not excluded. Degradation with proteolytic enzymes (proteinase K, trypsin or pepsin) abolishes the inducing activity of Xenopus RNP-particles (Janeczek et al., 1984b) as well RNP from other sources (Hayashi, 1958). RNA extracted from RNP-particles or whole embryos (Kocher-Becker and Tiedemann, 1968) does not induce. This shows that the factor is protein in nature.

The neuralizing factor from gastrula RNP-particles has been further purified by hydrophobic chromatography on ε-aminopentylagarose. The purified factor contains very little RNA. Other methods (chromatography on DEAE-sephadex or oligo (dT)-agarose) did not give satisfactory separations.

The neuralizing factor from RNP-particles is a basic protein. The factor elutes from size exclusion HPLC columns at an apparent $M_r > 70,000$ and as a broad band with a maximum at an apparent $M_r \sim 40,000$ (Si 300 Diol, Serva, Heidelberg; eluent 75% formic acid). But the molecular weight is difficult to determine because of degradation during the isolation and reversible adsorption to the gel matrix.

The neuralizing factor which was extracted and partially purified from the small microsomal vesicles and the factor from the high speed supernatant are in contrast to the

factor from the RNP-particles acidic proteins (I.P. ∼ 5.5).
The 100,000xg supernatant contains glycoconjugates in high
concentration. They prevent an efficient fractionation by
size exclusion chromatography on Sephadex or Sephacryl co-
lumns even at high ionic strength (as was also observed with
extracts from other sources; Spiro, 1973). Size exclusion
HPLC under conditions where the protein and protein-carbohy-
drate interactions are reduced gives a better separation.
The factor from gastrula high speed supernatant elutes from

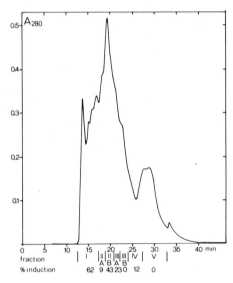

Figure 1. SE-HPLC of Xeno-
pus gastrula 100,000xg su-
pernatant prepared without
protease inhibitors (∼ 4 mg
reduced protein). Column:
Si 300 Diol 5 μm (Serva,
Heidelberg), 8x500 mm.
Elution: 50% formic at
20 °C, 0.6 ml/min.
Abscissa: % forehead induc-
tions with eye.

HPLC columns in 50% formic acid at several size classes at
M_r *10,000-16,000,* M_r *35,000-50,000 and* M_r *>130,000 (Fig. 1).*
It is not yet known whether the very large molecules are
large precursors or whether the factor is tightly bound to
a large structural protein. The factor molecules of smaller
size are in part formed by proteolytic cleavage during the
isolation precedure. Addition of the protease inhibitors $[\alpha_2]$
macroglobulin and leupeptin leads to a shift to the higher
size classes. But the processing of precursor molecules to
smaller molecules is probably a process which also occurs in
the embryo. When the factor was extracted immediately after
homogenization of Xenopus gastrulae with diluted acetic acid

under conditions where any proteolysis is prevented and fractionated by size exclusion chromatography a small percentage
of the factor is eluted in a range from 10,000 to 20,000 Dal-
ton.

The nature of the acidic groups is not yet known. Hydrolysis of the supernatant factor with sulfuric acid under conditions where only sialic acid is released from glycoproteins did not change the isoelectric point. Extraction with
phenol at 60 °C converts a small part of the acidic factor
into a basic protein. It is possible, that a biosynthetic
precursor-product relationship exists between the basic factor in the RNP-particles and the acidic factors in the small
vesicles and the high speed supernatant. The apparent molecular mass of the supernatant factor does not change after
reduction with mercaptoethanol or dithioerythrol. The neuralizing factor remains fully active. Contaminating proteins
are however shifted to molecules of smaller size, so that
the large sized neuralizing factor can be separated from
other proteins. Further purification by SDS-polyacrylamide
electrophoresis is in progress.

PATTERN FORMATION AND MECHANISM OF ACTION

Besides the neuralizing factor and the vegetalizing factor additional factors are involved in the determination of
the organ pattern. These factors, which take part in the interaction between the primarily induced anlagen, are however
less well characterized. The vegetalizing factor from chicken
embryos as the factor isolated by Yamada induce at high concentrations endoderm. At a somewhat lower concentration in
addition ventral mesodermal tissues as pronephric tubules,
endothel and blood cells and at a still lower concentration
dorsal mesodermal tissues as myomeres and notochord are induced. A similar shift is observed when the highly purified
factor is mixed without further dilution with a crude protein fraction, which was separated in the course of its purification from the vegetalizing factor (Table 1). The crude
protein fraction which induced some hindhead structures, but
no endoderm or mesodermal tissues is inactivated by proteolytic enzymes (Asahi et al., 1979). This suggests that an
additional factor, which is protein in nature, is involved.
Dissociation-reassociation experiments after induction of
ectoderm with the vegetalizing factor did lead Grunz and
Minuth to similar conclusions. Endodermal tissues as liver

Table 1. Histological examination of the tissues induced by the highly purified vegetalizing factor and a combination of the factor with a crude fraction tested by the
implantation method on Triturus alpestris

Fraction	No.of	induced tissues (%)								
	cases	brain	ear ves.	neur. tube	noto- chord	muscle	renal tubules	blood	coel. epith.	exovagi- nation (endod.)
Crude $(NH_4)_2SO_4$ supernatant	22	77 (1.9)	36	0	0	0	0	0	0	0
Veg. factor +γ-glob. (1+9)	49	0	0	0	7 (1.0)	47 (1.2)	100 (2.5)	33 (2.2)	73 (1.2)	93
Combination of veg. factor with crude sup. (1+9)	24	0	0	15 (1.6)	75 (2.6)	80 (2.6)	100 (2.7)	25 (1.6)	90 (1.3)	17

Figures in brackets refer to the mass of induced tissues. To each induced tissue a
size number (large, 3; medium, 2; small, 1) was assigned. The sum of all size class
numbers was then divided by the number of inductions.

and intestine were formed after dissociation of the induced
ectoderm for about 20 h to prevent secondary interactions
(Minuth and Grunz, 1980). It is likely that also in the normal amphibian embryogenesis mesoderm is induced by the endoderm. It was shown by Hildegard Tiedemann that gastrula endoderm induces tails (cit. in Tiedemann, 1975). Nakamura and
coworkers (Nakamura and Takasaki, 1970; Nakamura et al.,
1971), Nieuwkoop and coworkers (Nieuwkoop and Ubbels, 1972;
Boterenbrood and Nieuwkoop, 1973) and Asashima (1975) investigated the inducing capacity of the endoderm and the
formation of the mesoderm in detail. Nieuwkoop found that
dorsal endoderm of blastula stages induces dorsal mesodermal
structures whereas the ventral endoderm induces ventral mesodermal tissues. It is however not definitively known whether
under all conditions where mesodermal tissues are induced
endoderm is induced first. To answer this question differentiation markers for the early identification of endoderm
would be needed.

The segregation of the neural anlage depends likewise
on secondary interactions. The neuralizing factor induces
forebrain. Hindbrain and spinal cord are induced when neuralizing inducers are mixed in different proportions with vegetalizing inducers. The mesoderm which is induced by the diluted vegetalizing factor transforms the neural anlage,
which is induced by the neuralizing factor, to hindbrain or

neural tube (Toivonen and Saxén, 1968; Tiedemann and Tiedemann, 1964). Generally different organs are not induced by
different threshold concentrations of one and the same factor but by the interaction of different factors and different anlagen.

It is a critical question for the inducing mechanisms,
whether the factors act on the plasma membrane or whether
they must be taken up by the cells to exert their inducing
activity. The answer to this question is different for different factors. When the vegetalizing factor is covalently
bound to BrCN-sepharose or BrCN-sephadex particles, which
can not be taken up by the ectoderm cells, the inducing activity is greatly diminished (Tiedemann and Born, 1978 s. Born
et al., 1980; Table 2). This is also true under conditions
where the factor is bound to the particles with only one

Table 2. Inducing activity of a partially purified vegetalizing fraction, vegetalizing fraction mixed with Sepharose or covalently bound
to Sepharose

Fraction	No. of cases	Posi-tive	induced region (%)			
			trunk/ tail	hind-head	fore-head	neural (not specified)
Crude veg. fraction (inducer control)	83	87	84	10	0	0
Veg. fraction (2.5 mg) mixed with Seph. (40 mg)	23	61	56	13	0	0
Veg. fraction (2 mg) bound to Seph. (40 mg)	75	55	0	5	26	24

binding site so that trapping of the bound factor in an inactive conformation is prevented. This suggests that the
vegetalizing factor must be taken up by the competent ectoderm cells. Enzymatic degradation of the dextran matrix of
the sephadex particles leads to a complete recovery of active factor.

When crude preparations from chicken embryos which contain some neuralizing besides the vegetalizing factor were
bound to BrCN-sepharose the activity of the neuralizing factor was not diminished. This was the first hint that the neuralizing factor acts at the cell surface. Recently we have

covalently bound the neuralizing factors from Xenopus gastru-la supernatant and from the RNP-particles to BrCN-sepharose (Table 3). The supernatant factor as well the factor from

Table 3. *Inducing activity of neuralizing factors from Xenopus 100,000xg supernatant, Xenopus RNP-particles and of these fractions covalently bound to BrCN-sepharose, tested by the implantation method on Triturus alpestris*

Fraction	No. of cases	Posi-tive (%)	L	M	S	fore-head	neural (not spec.)	not spec. (%)
				Size of ind. (%)			Ind. region (%)	
Neural ind. from 100,000xg supernatant (control)								
not diluted	59	43	8	15	20	29	3	11
Neural ind. from 100,000xg supernat. bound to BrCN-seph.								
3.3 mg prot./20 mg seph.	29	72	0	4	58	34	0	38
3.3 mg prot./20 mg seph.*	31	65	0	4	61	43	0	22
3.5 mg prot./20 mg seph.	27	70	0	8	62	52	4	14
3.5 mg prot./20 mg seph.*	28	82	0	0	82	64	0	18
Neural ind. from ribonucleoprot. particles (control)								
1 pt. RNP prot. + 1 pt. γ-globulin	35	51	0	14	37	14	26	11
Neural ind. from ribonucleoprot. particles bound to BrCN-sepharose								
0.43 mg prot./20 mg seph.	32	41	0	3	38	19	10	12
1.2 mg prot./20 mg seph.	25	92	12	36	44	56	5	31

cross linked sepharose

RNP-particles retained their full activity despite the fact that the two proteins have different molecular properties, the supernatant factor being an acidic protein, the particle factor a basic protein. This suggests that both factors have similar structural domains which are responsible for their neural inducing activity. Non-inducing proteins bound to BrCN-sepharose do not evoke any induction. - It seems to be possible that neuralizing factor which is synthesized early in development and stored in cytoplasmic RNP-particles is in part modified in Golgi vesicles, then transported to the plasma membrane and exported from the inducing tissue, the mesodermal archenteron roof. Experiments to prove or dis-prove this hypothesis are in progress.

Proteins, which are bound to BrCN-sepharose are slowly released by non-enzymatic and by enzymatic processes. The amount of factor which is released is however small. The in-

ducing activity is therefore not due to neuralizing factor
which is released from the particles.

THE PHYSIOLOGICAL SIGNIFICANCE OF INDUCING FACTORS IN THE
NORMAL DEVELOPMENT OF EMBRYOS

     It is generally accepted that tissue differentiation
depends on the expression of different sets of genes. These
genes are probably regulated by different sets of proteins.
It was shown that in the ectoderm an intrinsic program for
the synthesis of nuclear proteins is running down. This program is changed when the ectoderm is induced to develop into
other tissues (Minuth et al., 1981). It is possible that the
vegetalizing factor, which must be taken up by the ectoderm
cells, acts at the chromatin level. The vegetalizing factor
binds tightly to DNA. But an association with sequence specific DNA has not yet been proven. Such experiments would
require cloned regulatory genes. The neuralizing factor on
the other hand acts on the plasma membrane of ectoderm cells.
This is reflected by the localization of the factors in embryos. A factor similar to the vegetalizing factor is already prelocated in the presumptive endoderm (s. pg. 6).
The neuralizing factor is on the other hand exported from
the mesodermal archenteron roof and induces the neural plate
in the overlying dorsal ectoderm. Some neural inducing activity has been found in phenol extracted protein isolated
from the extracellular space between the inducing mesoderm
and the induced early neural plate in accordance with this
hypothesis. The material isolated from the extracellular
space does not contain RNA and hence it is not contaminated
with cellular material (John et al., 1983).

     Other experiments also suggest that the neuralizing fac-
tor, which is synthesized and stored in earlier stages, is
in part exported from the inducing mesoderm. Several years
ago we have incubated the isolated dorsal blastoporal lips
with actinomycin D ($\sim$ 3 h 2.5 µg/ml) then with Holtfreter
solution and finally treated with ethanol (Tiedemann et al.,
1967). After these treatments the inducing activity was not
diminished as compared to the controls without actinomycin D
incubation (45% of all inductions were forehead inductions).
The inducing activity of the intact blastoporal lips which
were treated in the same way with actinomycin D and Holtfreter solution, but not with ethanol was however greatly diminished (8% of all inductions were small forehead inductions;

χ^2 test: $P < 0.02$). This is to be expected when the export of
neural inducing factor from the blastoporal lip depends on
the synthesis of new mRNA's which in turn are needed for the
synthesis of components of the export machinery. For the synthesis of the factor itself newly synthesized mRNA is however
not needed, because the factor is already synthesized and
stored in earlier stages of development.

Neural induction involves two different processes. (1)
The differentiation of ectoderm to neural tissues is initiated. (2) The induced ectoderm acquires neural inducing activity as was already discovered in the twenties (Mangold and
Spemann, 1927; Tiedemann-Waechter, 1960). The biological significance of this "autoinduction" may be the induction of
ectoderm cells which are not or not at the right time reached by the inducing signal from the archenteron roof. This
reminds on the so called autocrine secretion where growth
factors are secreted from transformed cells to further stimulate their own growth. The inducing factors do however not
primarily stimulate the mitotic rate in the induced tissues,
but change their developmental pathway.

It is known since the thirties (Holtfreter, 1934) that
gastrula ectoderm, which has no inducing activity contains
neural inducing factors in a masked, inactive form. The
masked factor in the ectoderm is partially activated by
freezing and fully activated by treatment of the ectoderm
with ethanol. Hence it must be in a labile association with
cell constituents which probably involve cytoskeletal elements (John et al., 1984).

Neural induction leads to an activation of the masked
inducers in the ectoderm as was shown by Grunz and Hildegard
Tiedemann. Table 4 shows that the neural inducing activity
of the high speed sediment (which contains the RNP-particles
as well the small vesicles) from neural plate homogenates is
much higher than the inducing activity of the sediment from
uninduced ectoderm. The neural inducing activity of the high
speed supernatant from ectoderm homogenates is very low, but
the neural plate supernatant has a significant inducing activity. This is consistent with the hypothesis that the masked
factor in the ectoderm is activated and exported upon induction.

Taken together the experiments suggest that the neuralizing factors which have been found in amphibian eggs and

Table 4. Inducing activity of the 100,000xg sediment and the 100,000xg supernatant from homogenates of gastrula ectoderm or of neural plates (Triturus alpestris)

Source	No. of cases	Posi- tive (%)	Size of ind. (%)			Ind. region (%)		not spec. (%)
			L	M	S	fore- head	neural (not spec.)	
Sed. Ectoderm*	66	42	5	6	31	5[+]	2	35
Sed. Neural plate*	63	67	15	18	34	38[+]	11	18
Sup. Ectoderm	71	27	0	0	27	1[+]	11	15
Sup. Neural plate	34	27	0	0	27	12[+]	12	3

*The sediment was prepared under sterile conditions and directly tested without freezing or ethanol treatment.

[+]Statistical significance of difference of Sed. Ectoderm to Sed. Neural plate $X^2=21.92$, $P <0.001$; difference Sup. Ectoderm to Sed. Neural plate $X^2=5.44$, $P <0.02$.

embryos are involved in the physiological process of neural induction. To prove this hypothesis we are preparing mono- clonal and polyclonal antibodies to neural inducers to test whether they impair neural plate formation after injection into fertilized eggs.

The signals which are generated on the plasma membrane of the induced cells and which lead to the activation of the masked factor, as well the chain of signals which leads to an activation of genes in the induced cells are unknown. So far there is no evidence that the factor in ectodermal RNP- particles is involved in the transfer of signals from the plasma membrane to nuclear chromatin. Cyclic nucleotides or their mono- and dibutyrylderivatives in a concentration range of 10^{-3} M to 10^{-8} M and the Ca-ionophore A 23187 were tested, but did not lead to neural or mesodermal induction (Grunz and Tiedemann, 1977; Siegel et al., 1985). This does not mean that cyclic nucleotides or Ca^{++} are not involved in the induction process, but they are certainly not rate- limiting. Ca^{++} may be needed for the binding of the neuraliz- ing factor to the plasma membrane or other events, because a small excess of EDTA in neuralizing fractions abolishes their inducing activity completely.

Davids has shown in our laboratory that phosphoproteins appear in a membrane fraction isolated from neurulae. It is however not yet known whether the phosphorylation of proteins is directly involved in the signal chain of neural induction. A modification of plasma membrane-cytoskeletal interactions or the release of unknown substances from the plasma membrane or the endocytosis of certain membrane constituents could also be of importance.

To mention future prospectives, the cloning of the vegetalizing and neuralizing factors could greatly facilitate further experiments on their chemical structure and mechanism of action. This can be done with the vegetalizing factor, but needs further purification of the neuralizing factor. In addition immunological procedures will help to unravel the signal chains in tissue determination.

Supported by Deutsche Forschungsgemeinschaft and Fonds der Chemischen Industrie.

REFERENCES

Asahi K-i, Born J, Tiedemann H, Tiedemann H (1979). Formation of mesodermal pattern by secondary inducing interactions. Wilhelm Roux's Archives 187:231-244.
Asashima M (1975). Inducing effects of presumptive endoderm of successive stages in Triturus alpestris. Wilhelm Roux's Archives 177:301-308.
Born J, Grunz H, Tiedemann H, Tiedemann H (1980). Biological activity of the vegetalizing factor: Decrease after coupling to polysaccharide matrix and enzymatic recovery of active factor. Wilhelm Roux's Archives 189:47-56.
Born J, Hoppe P, Tiedemann H, Tiedemann H (1985). An embryonic inducing factor: Isolation by HPL-chromatography and chemical properties. Biol Chem Hoppe-Seyler 366:729-735.
Boterenbrood EC, Nieuwkoop PD (1973). The formation of the mesoderm in urodelean amphibian. V. Its regional induction by the endoderm. Wilhelm Roux's Archives 173:319-332.
Faulhaber I (1970). Anreicherung des vegetalisierenden Induktionsfaktors aus der Gastrula des Krallenfrosches (Xenopus laevis) und Abgrenzung des Molekulargewichtsbereiches durch Gradientenzentrifugation. Hoppe-Seyler's Z Physiol Chem 351:588-594.
Gerhart J, Ubbels G, Black S, Hara K, Kirschner M (1981). A reinvestigation of the role of the grey crescent in axis formation in Xenopus laevis. Nature (London) 292:511-516.
Gimlich RL, Gerhart J (1984). Early cellular interactions promote embryonic axis formation in Xenopus laevis. Dev Biol 104:117-130.
Grunz H (1977). Differentiation of the four animal and the four vegetal blastomeres of the eight-cell-stage of Tri-

turus alpestris. Wilhelm Roux's Archives 181:267-277.

Grunz H, Tiedemann H (1977). Influence of cyclic nucleotides on amphibian ectoderm. Wilhelm Roux's Archives 181:261-265.

Hayashi Y (1958). The effects of pepsin and trypsin on the inductive ability of pentose nucleoprotein from guinea pig liver. Embryologia 4:33-53.

Holtfreter J (1934). Der Einfluß thermischer, mechanischer und chemischer Eingriffe auf die Induktionsfähigkeit von Tritonkeimteilen. Wilhelm Roux's Archives 132:225-306.

Janeczek J, Born J, John M, Scharschmidt M, Tiedemann H, Tiedemann H (1984b). Ribonucleoprotein particles from Xenopus eggs and embryos. Eur J Biochem 140:257-264.

Janeczek J, John M, Born J, Tiedemann H, Tiedemann H (1984a). Inducing activity of subcellular fractions from amphibian embryos. Wilhelm Roux's Archives 193:1-12.

John M, Janeczek J, Born J, Hoppe P, Tiedemann H, Tiedemann H (1983). Neural induction in amphibians. Transmission of a neuralizing factor. Wilhelm Roux's Archives 192:45-47.

John M, Born J, Tiedemann H, Tiedemann H (1984). Activation of a neuralizing factor in amphibian ectoderm. Wilhelm Roux's Archives 193:13-18.

Kocher-Becker U, Tiedemann H (1968). Untersuchungen am Amphibienektoderm zur Frage der Induktionsfähigkeit von Nucleinsäuren. Wilhelm Roux's Archives 160:375-400.

Mangold O, Spemann H (1927). Über Induktion von Medullarplatte durch Medullarplatte im jüngeren Keim, ein Beispiel homoögenetischer oder assimilatorischer Induktion. Wilhelm Roux's Archives 111:341-422.

Minuth M, Grunz H (1980). The formation of mesodermal derivatives after induction with vegetalizing factor depends on secondary cell interactions. Cell Differentiation 9: 229-238.

Minuth W, Minuth M, Tiedemann H (1981). Changes in the electrophoretic pattern of nuclear proteins from non-induced and induced embryonic ectoderm. IRCS Medical Science 9:36.

Nakamura O, Takasaki H (1970). Further studies on the differentiation capacity of the dorsal marginal zone in the morula of Triturus pyrrhogaster. Proc Japan Acad 46:546-551.

Nakamura O, Takasaki H, Ishihara M (1971). Formation of the organizer from combinations of presumptive ectoderm and endoderm. I. Proc Japan Acad 47:313-318.

Nieuwkoop PD, Ubbels GA (1972). The formation of the mesoderm in urodelean amphibians. IV. Qualitative evidence for the purely "ectodermal" origin of the entire mesoderm and of the pharyngeal endoderm. Wilhelm Roux's Archives 169: 185-199.

Siegel G, Grunz H, Grundmann U, Tiedemann H, Tiedemann H (1985). Embryonic induction and cation concentrations in amphibian embryos. Cell Differentiation in press.

Spemann H (1938). "Embryonic Development and Induction." New Haven: Yale Univ. Press.

Spiro RG (1973). Glycoproteins. In Anfinsen CB, Edsall JT, Richards FM (eds): "Adv. Protein Chem 27," New York: Academic Press, pp 349-467.

Tiedemann-Waechter H (1960). Die Selbstdifferenzierungsfähigkeit und Induktionsfähigkeit medianer und lateraler Teile der Rumpfmedullarplatte bei Urodelen. Wilhelm Roux's Archives 152:303-338.

Tiedemann H (1975). Substances with morphogenetic activity in differentiation of vertebrates. In Weber R (ed): "Biochemistry of animal development vol. III", New York: Academic Press pg 276.

Tiedemann H, Tiedemann H (1956a). Versuche zur chemischen Kennzeichnung von embryonalen Induktionsstoffen. Hoppe-Seyler's Z Physiol Chem 306:7-32.

Tiedemann H, Tiedemann H (1956b). Isolierung von Ribonucleinsäure und Nucleotiden aus Embryonalextrakt und Leber und ihr Verhalten im Induktionsversuch. Hoppe-Seyler's Z Physiol Chem 306:132-142.

Tiedemann H, Tiedemann H (1964). Das Induktionsvermögen gereinigter Induktionsfaktoren im Kombinationsversuch. Rev Suisse de Zool 71:117-137.

Tiedemann H, Born J, Tiedemann H (1967). Embryonale Induktion und Hemmung der Ribonukleinsäuresynthese durch Actinomycin D. Z Naturforsch 22b:649-659.

Tiedemann H, Kesselring K, Becker U, Tiedemann H (1962). Über die Induktionsfähigkeit von Mikrosomen- und Zellkernfraktion aus Embryonen und Leber von Hühnern. Dev Biol 4: 214-241.

Toivonen S (1953). Bone-marrow of the guinea-pig as a mesodermal inductor in implantation experiments with embryos of Triturus. J Embryol exp Morph 1:97-104.

Toivonen S, Saxén L (1968). Morphogenetic interactions of presumptive neural and mesodermal cells mixed in different ratios. Science 159:539-540.

Yamada T (1958). Induction of specific differentiation by samples of proteins and nucleoproteins in the isolated ectoderm of Triturus gastrulae. Experientia 14:81-87.

Yamada T (1961). A chemical approach to the problem of the organizer. In Abercrombie M, Brachet J (eds): "Adv. in Morphogenesis 1", New York: Academic Press, pp 1-53.

Cellular Endocrinology: Hormonal Control of Embryonic
and Cellular Differentiation, pages 25–34

TEST OF EMBRYONIC INDUCING FACTORS: ADVANTAGES AND DIS-
ADVANTAGES OF DIFFERENT PROCEDURES

Hildegard Tiedemann

Institut für Molekularbiologie und Biochemie,
Freie Universität Berlin, Arnimallee 22,
D-1000 Berlin 33, FR Germany

Amphibian eggs and embryos have been widely used to investigate the determination and differentiation processes in
vertebrates. They can easily be handled because they develop
independently of the maternal organism. During the first
cleaving steps distinct cytoplasmic areas of the egg become
distributed to different cells. After a number of cell divisions the blastocoele cavity is formed which separates the
presumptive ectoderm in the animal half from the endoderm in
the vegetal half. The "marginal zone" between endoderm and
ectoderm becomes mesoderm.

At the beginning of gastrulation the blastopore is formed at the vegetal side and through it endoderm and mesoderm
invaginate into the embryo whereas the ectoderm enlarges
("epibolic movement") and at the end of gastrulation covers
the whole embryo. The dorsal mesoderm forms the archenteron
roof from which originate notochord and myotomes, whereas
the ventral mesoderm develops into renal tubules, blood and
endothelia.

During gastrulation the neural plate, the primordium of
the neural system is induced in the dorsal ectoderm by the
underlying mesodermal "archenteron roof". The neural anlage
segregates into the archencephalon with eyes (and noses),
the deuterencephalon (with ear vesicles) and the neural tube.
Deuterencephalon and neural tube develop when the neural anlage is transformed by secondary interactions with the surrounding mesoderm.

The ectoderm is still omnipotent up to the early gastru-

la stage. It is determined to form epidermis-like cells
(Grunz, 1973) but its pathway of differentiation can still
be changed by the addition of the appropriate inducing factors. The effect of inducing factors can therefore been tested on gastrula ectoderm.

   Three different methods have been developed for the
test of inducing factors. The first method, the so called implantation method (Fig. 1A), was devised by Otto Mangold

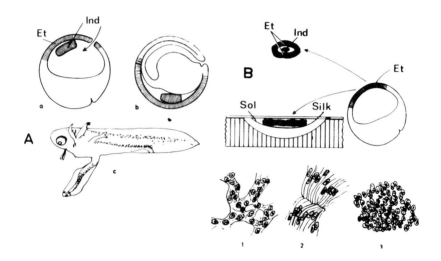

Figure 1. Test methods for inducing factors. A implantation
method: inducing factor Ind implanted into blastocoele of
early gastrula (a), in contact with belly epidermis Et (b),
induces trunk and tail (c); B (above) sandwich method: inducer Ind wrapped in two pieces of gastrula ectoderm Et; (below) tissue culture method: gastrula ectoderm Et cultured in
salt or inducing solution Sol, covered with silk; result
without inducing factor cuboidal cells (1), with vegetalizing factor muscle cells etc. (2), with neuralizing factor
neural tissue (3). (From 33 Colloquium Mosbach 1982 Biochemistry of differentiation and morphogenesis. Berlin-Heidelberg:
Springer.)

(1923). He implanted a piece of tissue through a slit in the

ectoderm into the blastocoele cavity of an early gastrula.
Through the gastrulation movements the implanted tissue is
brought into contact with the ventral ectoderm which later
on becomes the epidermis of the belly. This method has widely been used to test particulate subcellular fractions from
homogenates as well purified inducing factors. Purified factors can be tested in different dilutions, when the inducing
fraction is mixed with a non-inducing protein in different
proportions. The total amount of protein must be the same in
all tests (~ 2 mg). The protein mixtures are precipitated
with ethanol/ether, washed and dried on a suction pump. For
implantation pieces of equal size are cut with glass or tungsten needles. For dilution we use mostly γ-globulin dialysed
from 6 M urea as a non-inducing protein because its consi-
stency in the dried pellet is especially suitable for implantation. After 14 days the inductions on the belly of the host
larvae are inspected under the dissection microscope. The regional quality of the inductions can easily be determined
when eyes and noses (forehead or archencephalic inductions,
Fig. 2), ear vesicles (hindhead or deuterencephalic induction, Fig. 3) or trunk and tail with myomeres and fin
(Fig. 4) are induced. Other organs can be recognized by histological examination.

Whether the inductions are more cranially or more cau-
dally located in the host has no influence on the induced
tissues when purified inducing factors are tested. With crude
substances a small influence of the host region may be observed. The implantation method provides a nearly complete
physiological environment for the ectoderm cells which may
be induced. The blastocoele fluid is reconstituted after the
operation. As will be discussed, certain constituents of the
blastocoele fluid seem to be needed for the structural.inte-
grity of the plasma membrane of the reacting cells.

When endoderm is induced it combines easily with the
host endoderm in the neighbourhood. It can therefore only be
shown as induction when before the operation the ventral ectoderm of the host is exchanged against labelled ectoderm of
another embryo. By this method it was shown (Kocher-Becker,
1974) that the highly purified vegetalizing factor from
chicken embryos actually induces endoderm. The induction of
a larger part of the host's ectoderm to mesoderm and endoderm has a dramatic effect on gastrulation. At first gastrulation proceeds normally, mesoderm and endoderm invaginate
through the blastopore, but after about 12-24 h the host en-

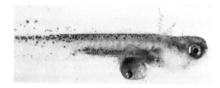

Figure 2. Archencephalic (forehead) induction with eye on the belly of a Triturus alpestris larva.

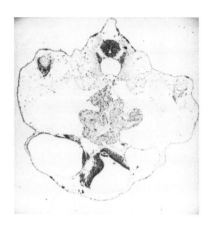

Figure 3. Histological section through a deuterencephalic (hindhead) induction with rhombencephalon and two ear vesicles (limb region).

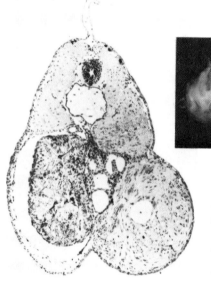

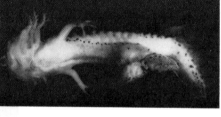

Figure 4 a. Trunc and tail induction on the belly of a Triturus alpestris larva. b. Histological section through a trunk induction with notochord and myomeres.

doderm migrates out of the blastopore and spreads over the
induced ectoderm as an unicellular or multicellular layer
(Fig. 5; Kocher-Becker et al., 1965). The moving force for

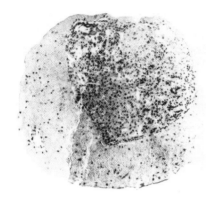

Figure 5. Histological section
through an exovagination larva after implantation of purified vegetalizing factor: multicellular outer layer of induced and host endoderm, inside mostly renal tubules and
muscles.

this exovagination (which should not be confused with the so
called exogastrulation) is a change of cell affinities. Townes and Holtfreter (1955) have observed that endodermal and
ectodermal cells do not adhere but endodermal and mesodermal
cells strongly adhere to each other. The change of cell affinities is probably due to a change of the pattern of cell
surface glycoproteins as a result of the induction process.

The implantation method has been applied to Triturus
and Ambystoma embryos. The method is however not suitable
for Xenopus gastrulae because the topographical situation of
the tissues in Xenopus is somewhat different. Implantation
of a pellet can lead to splitting of the axis system.

The differentiation of neural tissues is more easily
evoked in Ambystoma ectoderm as compared to Triturus ectoderm.
The rate of neural inductions is therefore higher when crude
fractions which contain neuralizing factor are tested in Ambystoma. But the purified vegetalizing factor induces only
mesodermal tissues in both species. Proteins which have no
inducing activity in Triturus like γ-globulin, ovalbumin and
many other proteins do also not induce Ambystoma ectoderm.

The second method which can be used for the test of in-

ducing substances was developed by Holtfreter (1933). Two
pieces of ectoderm are isolated from early gastrulae. Tissue fragments or pellets which contain inducing factors are
then enveloped in the two isolated pieces of ectoderm like
a sandwich (Fig. 1B, above). This procedure is therefore
known as the sandwich method. When the vegetalizing factor
is tested the method gives the same results as the implantation method. Endodermal tissues as liver and intestine could
be identified when the sandwiches were raised for very long
periods. The differentiation of the different endodermal organs depends on an interaction with mesenchyme as was shown
by Okada (1960). Induction with highly purified vegetalizing
factor in high concentrations does therefore not lead to the
differentiation of distinct endodermal organs because no mesenchyme is induced. The identification of endoderm especially in the first days after induction would be greatly facili-
tated when a biochemical marker for endoderm would be available.

Neural inducing fractions have a lower activity when
they are tested by the sandwich method as compared to the implantation method. A similar observation has been made by
Chuang (1939) many years ago. Whether this has mechanical
reasons (i.e. incomplete contact of inducer and ectoderm) or
whether other factors play a role is not yet known.

The two methods are supplemented by tissue culture methods (Fig. 1B, below). Isolated ectoderm tends to curl up
and then becomes inaccessible to inducing substances. The
curling up can be prevented by covering the ectoderm with a
piece of silk, filter paper or a nylon sheet (Becker et al.,
1959; Yamada and Takata, 1961). These methods allow to test
low molecular substances which are soluble in buffer solution
as well macromolecules in solution. Mesodermal tissues as
striated muscle and notochord and flat layers of neural tissue can be induced by appropriate inducers.

A problem which we face with this method is autoneuralization. Holtfreter (1947) has shown that the neuralizing factor which is already present in gastrula ectoderm in a masked,
biologically inactive form can be activated by short treatment of ectoderm at pH below 5.0 or above 9.0. This treatment
(or short treatment with substances injurious to cells) leads
to neural differentiation of the ectoderm without the addition of external factors. Ectoderm of Ambystoma is especially
sensitive to autoneuralization (Table 1). It forms neural

Table 1. Differentiation of gastrula ectoderm explanted in Flickinger solution* a) Ectoderm from Ambystoma mexicanum

No. of explants	atypical epidermis (%)	neural tissue**			neuroid*** (%)	mesen- chyme (%)	melano- phores (%)
		50-30%	30-10%	<10%			
46	17	2	28	20	33	33	13
31	64		13		23	0	0
13	31		15		54	0	0

b) Ectoderm from Triturus alpestris

50	98	0	0	0	0	2	0
11	100	0	0	0	0	0	0

* $NaCl$ 58 mM, KCl 1 mM, $NaHCO_3$ 2.4 mM, Na_2HPO_4 1 mM, KH_2PO_4 0.2 mM, $CaCl_2$ 0.5 mM, $MgSO_4$ 1 mM, gentamycin 50 mg/l, penicillin 100.000 IU/l, streptomycin 100 mg/l, pH adjusted to 7.35

** percentage of the total cell mass of the explant

*** clusters of neural cells without typical organ structure

tissues after explantation in a buffered saline solution as was observed by Barth (1941) and confirmed by Holtfreter (1944). Ectoderm of Triturus torosus (Holtfreter, 1944), Triturus pyrrhogaster or Triturus alpestris do not show auto-neuralization under exactly the same conditions.

Recently we have investigated whether changes in the composition of the buffer solution may lead to an autoneuralization of the ectoderm of Triturus alpestris. Unexpectedly autoneuralization was observed when in the Flickinger solution (Flickinger, 1949) which we use as a medium, the bicarbonate buffer was replaced by Hepes (Table 2). The degree of

Table 2. Neural differentiation of gastrula ectoderm of Triturus alpestris explanted in different media

Culture medium	No. of cases	Expl. with neural diff. (%)	part of explant diff. to neural tissue			
			50%	50-20%	20-10%	<10%
Flickinger-Bicarb.	31	0	0	0	0	0
Flickinger-Bicarb. (1.5 x conc.)	24	84	17	28	20	17
Flickinger-Hepes	34	62	10	11	17	24
L 15 (0.5 x conc.)	11	9	0	9	0	0

autoneuralization shows however variations with different charges of Hepes and it is not known whether Hepes or contaminating substances are responsible for the autoneuralization. Altura et al. (1980) have shown that Hepes and other organic buffer substances attenuate induced contractions of vascular and smooth muscle. Their experiments suggest that the exchangeability and transmembrane movement of Ca^{2+} is inhibited (Turlapaty et al., 1979). Whether these effects are related to autoneuralization is however not known.

The most dramatic effect has an 1.5 fold increase of the NaCl and KCl concentrations of the Flickinger solution (from 58 to 87 mM NaCl and 1.0 to 1.5 mM KCl). Large parts of the explanted Triturus ectoderm differentiate to neural tissue. In contrast an 1.5 fold increase of Ca^{++} and Mg^{++} does not lead to autoneuralization. The autoneuralization could be caused by an increase of the NaCl concentration in the cells or by a structural change in the plasma membrane of ectoderm cells. A transient 4-fold increase of the intracellular Na^+ concentration after treatment of ectoderm with quabain or treatment of ectoderm with the Na^+/K^+-ionophore gramacidin did not evoke neural differentiation (Siegel et al., 1985). It is more likely that the interaction of membrane constituents is modified and that this modification triggers a chain of signals which finally leads to neural differentiation.

The Na^+ concentration in the blastocoele fluid was determined by Slack et al. (1973) to about 100 mM Na^+. This corresponds to the Flickinger solution with the increased Na^+ concentration causing autoneuralisation. But the blastocoele fluid which is in direct contact with the ectoderm does not evoke any inductions. The blastocoele fluid contains, as we have recently shown, besides ions other components including glycoconjugates. It is well known that glycoconjugates (and glycoproteins) interact in different ways with plasma membranes (review: Aplin and Hughes, 1982). Such an interaction may be necessary for the structural integrity of the membranes and prevent autoneuralization. - The transmembrane distribution of Cl^- has not yet been studied.

At a NaCl concentration of 58 mM (Flickinger solution) with bicarbonate as buffer substance autoneuralization does not or only to a very small extent occur in Triturus ectoderm. Diluted Leibowitz medium (L 15) which contains in addition to salts amino acids and vitamins shows also little autoneuralization. *In these media substances can be tested for inducing activity (s. pg. 7). It has been shown by this method that substances with M_r <10,000 obtained by ultrafiltration from a Xenopus homogenate have no inducing activity. Neural inducing substances are only found in the fraction with M_r > 10,000. The neurotransmitters acetylcholine, 5-hydroxytryptamine and arterenol ($5x10^{-5}$ M each) as well the head activator of Hydra ($3x10^{-4}$ M; Bodenmüller and Schaller, 1981) have no inducing activity.*

The three test methods supplement each other so that the limits of the single method can be compensated if a substance is tested by more than one method. The optimal condition for the tissue culture test should further be explored to make the test as sensitive as possible.

Supported by Deutsche Forschungsgemeinschaft and Fonds der Chemischen Industrie.

REFERENCES

Altura BM, Altura BT, Carella A, Turlapaty PDMV (1980). Adverse effects of artificial buffers on contractile responses of arterial and venous smooth muscle. Brit J Pharmac 69:207-214.

Aplin ID, Hughes RC (1982). Complex carbohydrates of the extracellular matrix. Structures, interactions and biological roles. Biochim Biophys Acta 694:375-418.

Barth LG (1941). Neural differentiation without Organizer. J exp Zool 87: 371.

Becker U, Tiedemann H, Tiedemann H (1959). Versuche zur Determination von embryonalem Amphibiengewebe durch Induktionsstoffe in Lösung. Z Naturforsch 14b:608-609

Bodenmüller H, Schaller HC (1981). Conserved amino acid sequence of a neuropeptide, the head activator, from coelenterates to humans. Nature 293:579-580.

Chuang HH (1939). Induktionsleistungen von frischen und gekochten Organteilen (Niere, Leber) nach ihrer Verpflanzung in Explantate und verschiedene Wirtsregionen von Tritonkeimen. Wilhelm Roux's Archives 139:556-638.

Flickinger RA (1949). A study of the metabolism of amphibian neural crest cells during their migration and pigmentation in vitro. J exp Zool 112:465-484.

Grunz H (1973). The ultrastructure of amphibian ectoderm treated with an inductor or with actinomycin D. Wilhelm

Roux's Archives 173:283-293.

Holtfreter J (1933). *Nachweis der Induktionsfähigkeit abgetöteter Keimteile. Roux' Arch Entw Mech 127:584-633.*

Holtfreter J (1944). *Neural differentiation of ectoderm
through exposure to saline solution. J exp Zool 95:307-343.*

Holtfreter J (1947). *Neural induction in explants which have
passed through a sublethal cytolysis. J exp Zool 106:197-
222.*

Kocher-Becker U, Tiedemann H, Tiedemann H (1965). *Exovagination of newt endoderm: cell affinities altered by the mesodermal inducing factor. Science 147:167-169.*

Kocher-Becker U (1974). *Habilitationsschrift, Universität
Ulm (Bundesrepublik Deutschland).*

Mangold O (1923). *Transplantationsversuche zur Frage der
Spezifität und der Bildung der Keimblätter. Arch mikr
Anat and Entw Mech 100:198-301.*

Okada TS (1960). *Epithelio-mesenchymal relationships in the
regional differentiation of the digestive tract in the
Amphibian embryo. Roux' Arch Entw Mech 152:1-21.*

Siegel G, Grunz H, Grundmann U, Tiedemann H, Tiedemann H
(1985). *Embryonic induction and cation concentrations in
amphibian embryos. Cell Differentiation: in press.*

Slack C, Warner AE, Warren RL (1973). *The distribution of
sodium and potassium in amphibian embryos during early
development. J Physiol 232:297-312.*

Townes P, Holtfreter J (1955). *Directed movements and selective adhesion of embryonic amphibian cells. J exp Zool
128:53-120.*

Turlapaty PDMV, Altura BT, Altura BM (1979). *Tris(hydroxy-
methyl)aminomethane inhibits calcium uptake in vascular
smooth muscle. Biochim Biophys Acta 551:459-462.*

Yamada T, Takata K (1961). *A technique for testing macromo-
lecular samples in solution for morphogenetic effects on
the isolated ectoderm of the amphibian gastrula. Dev Biol
3:411-423.*

Cellular Endocrinology: Hormonal Control of Embryonic
and Cellular Differentiation, pages 35–44
© 1986 Alan R. Liss, Inc.

ON THE CELLULAR COMMUNICATION OF AMPHIBIAN EMBRYOGENESIS

Tseng Mi-Pai Chuang

Laboratory of Embryonic Differentiation, Shanghai
Institute of Cell Biology, Academia Sinica, 320
Yo-Yang Road, Shanghai, China.

Since the discovery of the organizer phenomenon by
Spemann, the transmission problem has attracted much attention (Toivonen, 1979). It has been shown that the transmission is of two main types: one involves the transmission
of signal substance at a distance while the other requires
the direct contact between adjacent cells. For the latter
case, from the recent accumulated knowledge about the cell
junctions, gap junctions should be considered first.

Gap junctions are also known as communicating junctions
and they are permeable to molecules about 1000 Daltons,
thereby coupling cells both electrically and metabolically.
They are found in almost all animal cell types, in excitable
as well as in non-excitable cells, in adult as well as in
embryonic cells. The early occurrence of gap junctions in
embryonic cells has led to the suggestion that they may play
important role in mediating intercellular transfer of signals
during embryonic development. The recent findings of Warner,
Guthrie and Gilula (1984) has provided the first experimental
evidences that the blockage of the junctional communication
interferes normal embryogenesis.

According to Nieuwkoop (1973) and Nakamura (1978) that
the organizing capacity of the organizer was not inherent
in itself but was acquired under the influence from the
vegetal cells. Do gap junctions play the role in the transmission from the vegetal cells?

Microinjection experiments were carried out with Xenopus embryos to see whether antibodies against gap junction

protien will interfere with the communication between the vegetal cells and the cells adjacent to them.

32-cell stage were chosen because our previous observations have shown that gap junctions occur on the lateral membrane of cells of this stage (Tseng, in press). The injections were made at the dorsal side into the blastomere left to the midplane either of the vegetal-most tier (VII_1) or into the blastomere of the tier next to the vegetal-most (VI_1) as shown in the accompanying diagram.

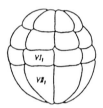

A 32-cell embryo showing the site of injection

The antibodies we used were from Prof. Klaus Willecke of University of Essen, Fed. Republic of Germany. We used both polyclonal and monoclonal antibodies. The polyclonal antibody is an anti-26K-protien from mouse liver gap junctions and the monoclonal is a rat monoclonal antibody against purified mouse liver gap junctions. By immunofluorescence microscopy of the monoclonal antibody, discrete spots on opposed membranes were detected in mouse liver, but for the Xenopus liver, with much higher concentration of the antibody, the fluorescent zones appear to be continuous lines along the opposed plasma membranes of neighbouring cells or in diffused pattern. Some cross reactivity seems to exist between the mouse liver gap junctions and those of Xenopus.

The results were summarized in the following table.

TABLE 1   Results of the injection experments

Material injected	Site of injection	Number of embryos injected	Embryos with asymmetrical sense organs			Embryos with no asymmetry
			Nose	Eye	Otocyst	
Monoclonal antibody	VI_1	49	10	16	10	24
	VII_1	16	1	6	2	8
Polyclonal antibody	VI_1	16	3	7		7
	VII_1	12	4	8	3	4
Control IgG	VI_1	11				11
	VII_1	6				6

For the two series of monoclonal antibody injections, about 50% (25/49 for VI_1 and 8/16 for VII_1) of the injected embryos showed asymmetry of the sense organs with defects at the injected side (Figs. 1-3). For the polyclonal series the effect on the sense organs is almost the same as that of the monoclonal (Fig.4), but the percentages of defect seemed to be higher (9/16 for VI_1 and 8/12 for VII_1). In the two control series, all the injected embryos did not show any assymmetry in the sense organs.

The defects in the sense organs observed at the injected side seemed to indicate the gap junctional communication plays important role in the transmission from the vegetal cells.

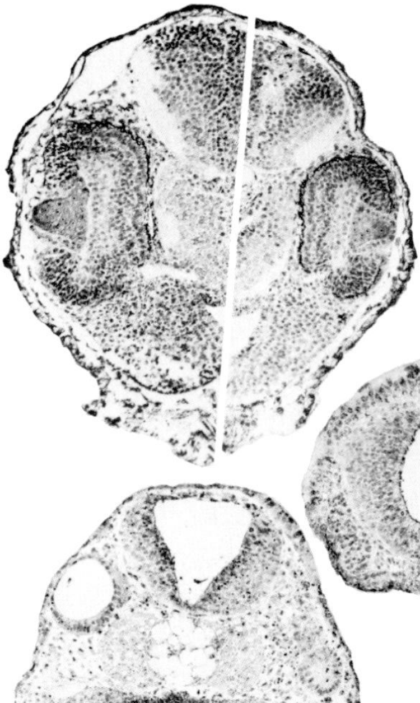

Figs. 1-3. Sections from embryos injected with the monoclonal antibody.

Fig. 1. When the median section of each of the two eyes were compared, the eye at the injected side is evidently smaller than the other one.

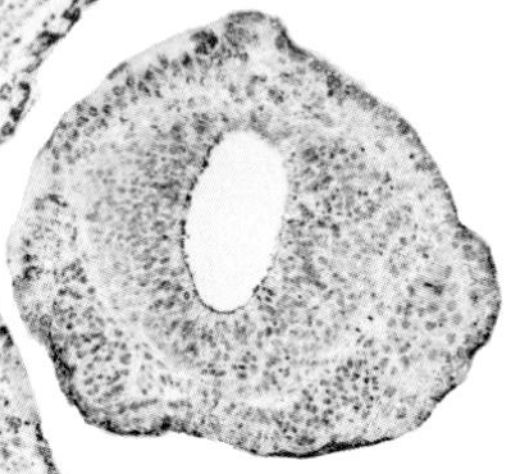

Fig.2. At the injected side the nasal pit is absent and the nasal placode is smaller than that of the other side.

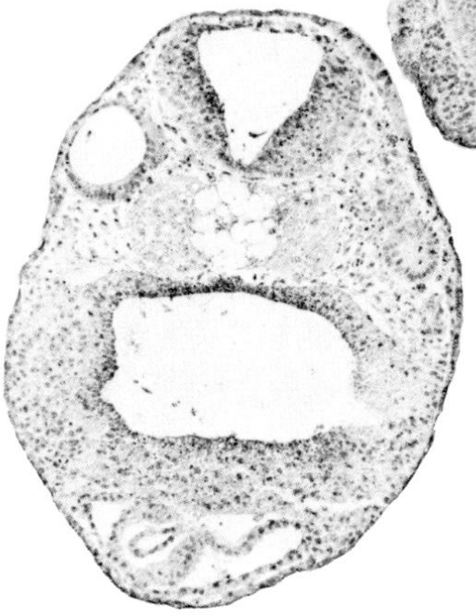

Fig. 3. The otocyst at the injected side was impeded from developing into a normal one as that of the other side.

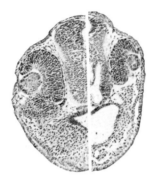

Fig. 4. In the embryo injected with the polyclonal antibody, the difference in sizes of the median sections of the eyes of the two sides is evident.

The presence of gap junctions was not only verified at the early cleavage stages, they were also observed in the later embryonic stages in the reactive cells. We have carried out electron microscopical observations of freeze-etching replicas of some embryonic material of Cynops orientalis, a species of newts commonly found in the districts near Shanghai. Two experimental systems have been chosen. First, neuroepithelium cells were extirpated from early and mid-neurula when the inductive action of the underlying chorda-mesoderm has practically accomplished. Second, ectoderm explants from early gastrula were treated with the crude extract of guinea pig bone marrow (BME), a well known abnormal mesoderm inductor. For the control of these two series freeze-etching replicas of ectoderm cells of early gastrula were observed for the gap junctions at a stage before the induction has been initiated.

In neuroepithelium cells of early as well as mid-neurula, gap junctions occurred beneath the apical belt of the tight junctions. The intimate topographical relationship between these two junctions has attracted our attention (Tseng and Wang, 1984). They were found directly connected to the free endings of the sealing strands of tight junctions (Fig. 5) or surrounded on all sides by the sealing strands (Fig. 6-7). Sometimes the demarkation between the two junctions is difficult to be made (Fig. 8). They vary in sizes. Some were large and others may be composed of not more than a hundred connexons. Scattered particles were often found in the vicinity of the junctions (Fig. 1) and they were of similiar size as the connexons of the gap junc-

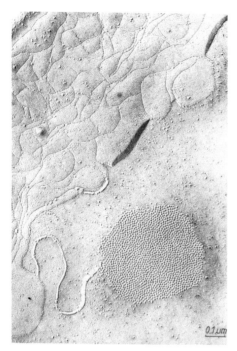

Fig. 5. Freeze-etching replica of a neuroepithelium
cell of early neurula. Scattered paricles were seen at
the site of connection of
the gap junction with the
free ending of the sealing
strand.

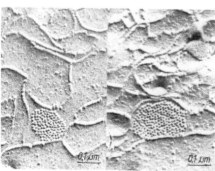

Fig. 6-7. Freeze-etching
replicas of two portions
of a single neuroepithelium
cell of mid-neurula. Both
of the gap junctions are
surrounded at all sides by
the sealing strands.

tions, but whether they were motivated toward or away from
the junctions could not be discriminated. Anyway, they appear to be in a dynamic state.

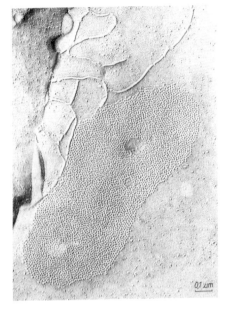

Fig. 8. Freeze-etching replica of a neuroepithelium cell of early neurula. The gap junction is in close contact with the tight junction but no sealing strand can be found at the upper left corner of the gap junction.

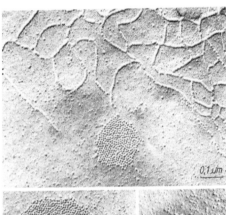

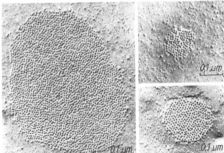

Fig. 9-12. Freeze-etching replicas of ectoderm cells treated with crude BME.

Fig. 9. A gap junction is situated near the tight junction.

Figs. 10-12. Gap junctions are of different sizes.

For the ectoderm explants treated with the crude extract of guinea pig bone marrow, gap junctions were usually
found in the lateral membrane sometimes they may be observed near the tight junctions (Fig. 9). Their sizes vary from
0.30 to 0.01 μm^2 (Figs. 10-12).

In the control series, gap junctions of the ectoderm
cells of early gastrula usually occurred at a distance from
the tight junction (Fig. 13). No direct connection of whatever type between these two junctions has ever been observed.
Most of them were small in size (<0.05 μm^2), composed of den-
sely arranged connexons (Figs. 14-18).

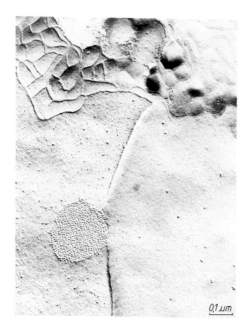

Fig. 13. Freeze-etching
replica of an ectoderm
cell of early gastrula.

0,1 μm

The density of the connexons of the gap junctions of
all the above series were measured by the Mop-videoplan
image analysis system. (Table 2). The statistical differences between each of the first three series and the series
of ectoderm cells of early gastrula were examined with the
Student t test. The differences of the two series of neuroepithelium cells and the control were found to be highly

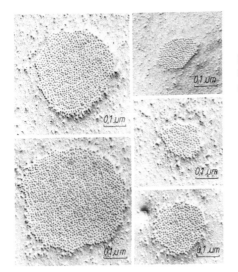

Figs. 14-18. Gap junctions of ectoderm cells of early gastrula.

significant while the difference between the ectoderm cells treated with the crude BME and that of the control was significant.

TABLE 2   Packing density of connexons of gap junctions

| | Neuroepithelium cells | | Ectoderm explants treated | Ectoderm cells of |
| | early neurula | mid neurula | with crude BME | early gastrula |
	n=5	n=5	n=6	n=5
	7244	5798	9353	13213
	7345	6310	9338	14657
	7493	6364	9705	12080
Connexons per square μm	7570	5777	8764	10414
	7316	6744	9799	10349
			9777	
Mean value	7394	6199	9456	12142
Standard deviation	134	411	396	1849
Standard error of mean	60	184	162	827
P	$\leqslant 0,001$	$< 0,001$	$< 0,01$	

From the above, it can be seen that the connexons of ectoderm cells of early gastrula are arranged more tightly in a more or less regular array, while those after neural induction are arranged loosely and more irregularly. The gap junctions before and after induction are different not only in their dynamic states but also in the arrangement of the connexons as indicated by the packing density. Viable explanations offered by Bennett and Goodenough (1978) and Peracchia (1980) hold that the contractions of the connexon on lattice are directly related to the opening and closing of the junctional channels of adjacent cells. Our observations on the correlations between the morphological changes of gap junctions and the transition between coupled and uncoupled stages of the embryonic epithelia (Chuang-Tseng et al. 1982) support this concept.

So, gap junctions are present between ectoderm cells both before and after induction, but in the latter case they are found in a more dynamic state. After the cessation of the induction process what can be the function of gap junctions? The experimental evidence from some different approach seem to indicate that communications between the reacting cells are indispensable. The gastrula ectoderm is heterogenous with respect to phases of the cell cycle. Experiments in which the gastrula ectoderm cells were synchronized and induced at different phases revealed that the S phase is the most sensitive to react to the inductive stimulus. In this case tha gap junctions might act to insure a uniform response of the reacting cells. Certainly more data should be accumulated to evaluate the functional activity of the gap junctions.

REFERENCES

Bennett MVL, Goodenough DA (1978). Gap junctions, electrotonic coupling and intercellular communication. Neurosci Res Progr Bull 16:373-486.
Chuang-Tseng MP, Chuang HH, Sandri C, Akert K (1982). Gap junctions and impulse propagation in embryonic epithelium of amphibia. Cell Tissue Res 225:249-258.
Gao H, Chuang HH (1984). The cell cycle and competence of ectodermal cells of early gastrula of Cynops orientalis III. The reactivity of ectoderm cells at different phases. Acta Biol Exp Sinica 17:255-267.
Nakamura O (1978). Epigenetic formation of the organizer.

In Nakamura O, Toivonen S (eds):"Organizer--A milestone of a half-century from Spemann" Elsevier / North-Holland, Amsterdam, pp 179-220.

Nieuwkoop PD (1973). The "organization center" of amphibian embryo: Its origin, spatial organization, and morphogenetic action. Advan Morphog 10:1-39.

Peracchia C (1980). Structural correlates of gap junction permeation. Int Rev Cytol 66:81-146.

Toivonen S (1979). Transmission problem in primary induction. Differentiation 15:177-181.

Tseng MP, Wang XM (1984). Cell junctions and neural tube formation in Cynops orientalis. Acta Biol EXp Sinica 17: 219-243.

Tseng MP, Wang XM (in press). Polarization of tight junction during the process of its formation. Scientia Sinica (Series B)

Warner AE,Guthrie SC, Gilula NB (1984). Antibodies to gap-junctional protein selectively disrupt junctional communication in the early amphibian embryo. Nature 311: 127-131.

Cellular Endocrinology: Hormonal Control of Embryonic
and Cellular Differentiation, pages 45–54
© 1986 Alan R. Liss, Inc.

NEW ASPECTS OF EARLY EMBRYONIC INDUCTION IN AMPHIBIANS

Horst Grunz
Department of Zoophysiology,FB 9(Biologie),
University GHS of Essen, 4300 Essen 1, FRG

Although there exist a lot of informations about the morphological processes in amphibian development, many steps in
the chain of events during primary embryonic induction and
differentiation especially at the molecular level are still
unclear. Since there are now available different modern
techniques, experiments are in progress in some laboratories
to answer unsolved questions.
The classic experiment of Spemann and Mangold (1924), which
showed that a certain part of the embryo acts as an
"organizer", raised the question about the chemical nature
and mechanism of action of morphogenetic factors. The interest of research on early embryonic induction and differentiation to day concentrates mainly on the topics as follows:
1.The localisation of morphogenetic factors in the inducing
tissue 2.The isolation and chemical characterization of
morphogenetic factors 3. the transfer of inducing factors
from the inducing tissue (chordamesoderm) to the ectodermal
target cells 4.The interaction of inducing factors with receptors on the plasmamembrane of the ectodermal target
cells 5. the further intracellular events within the target
cells including specific gene expression as a result of induction. There are available a lot of data on the isolation
and characterization of morphogenetic factors.a vegetalizing
factor could be purified to homogeneity and recently also
crude factors with neuralizing activity (Tiedemann,1982;
Tiedemann, 1984). Our interest has been focussed mainly on
the mechanism of action of vegetalizing and neuralizing
factor(s).The inducing factors can be tested in different
ways:by the implantation technique after Mangold, the sand-
wich-technique after Holtfreter, the moist chamber-technique

after Becker(cited by Tiedemann,1982) or by the filter-
platelet-method(Grunz, 1972).The data on the isolation and
the specificity of action of vegetalizing factor were
published in detail elsewhere (Born et al.,1980; Tiedemann,
1982; Grunz,1984,1985).Therefore I like to summarize the
main data only.the vegetalizing factor exerts the following
effects in competent amphibian ectoderm:1.ectoderm, which is
not finally determined in the early gastrula, will be
triggered by vegetalizing factor to differentiate into endodermal and mesodermal derivatives.the pattern of the induced
tissue depends on the concentration and incubation time of
vegetalizing factor (Grunz, 1983). Short incubation with low
concentrations of inducing factor results in the formation
of blood cells, longer incubation time or/and higher concentration of vegetalizing factor evoke the differentiation of
notochord and somites, 2. vegetalizing factor causes a
change of the cell affinity (Grunz, 1972), 3. the change of
the surface architecture (Grunz et al., 1975), 4. the change
of the charge of the plasmamembrane (Grunz and Staubach,
1979a). The pattern of induced structures depends on the
initial cell mass and secondary cell interactions (Grunz,
1979; Asahi et al.,1979; Minuth and Grunz, 1980).
Of interest is the molecular mechanism of action of the
vegetalizing factor. By binding of the vegetalizing factor
to polysaccharide matrixes could be shown that this factor
apparently must be internalized to exert its biological
activity (Born et al, 1980). On the other hand neuralizing
factors apparently interact with specific receptors on the
plasmamembrane, since a factor with neuralizing activity was
still active after immobilization by binding to sepharose
beads (Born et al., 1980). Further evidence for the interaction of neuralizing factors with receptors of the plasmamembrane of ectodermal target cells was received from experiments with Concanavalin A (Takata et al., 1981, 1984;
Grunz 1984,1985). Con A, a plant lectin, which binds to
α-D-glucoside and α-D-mannoside-residues of glycoproteins
of the plasmamembrane, induces also in competent ectoderm of
Xenopus laevis archencephalic brain structures(Grunz, 1985).
The Con A must be present in the culture medium for at least
3 hours in Cynops pyrrhogaster (Takata et al.,1984) and
about 1 hour in Xenopus laevis to evoke neural structures.
Using Xenopus ectoderm, consisting of two layers, which can
be seperated mechanically by fine glass needles, we could
show that the superficial ectoderm layer in contrast to the
inner ectoderm layers does not differentiate into neural
structures after treatment with Con A (Grunz, 1985). There

exist close relationships between the neural reaction of the two ectoderm layers and the bindung of Con A to the plasmamembrane. By studies with gold-Con A together with Dr.Tacke in my laboratory we could show that the outer ectoderm layer binds substantially less lectin than the inner layer. Apparently a relative low amount of Con A-receptors are present on the plasmamembrane of the superficial ectodermal layer. These results together with informations about the fate (internalization by receptor-mediated endocytosis and lysosomal degradation) of the gold-Con A-complex will be published in detail elsewhere (Tacke and Grunz, 1986). In normogenesis the outer neuroectodermal layer of anurans forms the ependymal part of the brain only (cited in Asahima and Grunz,1983). The main parts of the brain develop from the inner neuroectoderm layer of the medullary plate. This view could be further supported by our experiments removing the whole outer neuroectoderm of the medullary plate of an early neurula. Those neurulae develop into nearly normal embryos (Fig.1A-D).

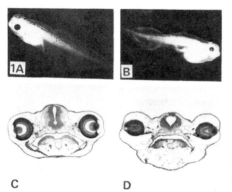

C   D

Fig.1A Normal Xenopus larva
Fig.1B Larva,which developed from an early neurula after removal of the outer neuroectoderm layer of the medullary plate. The forebrain is more compact in comparison with a normal larva and there are malformations in the neural part of the eye(see Fig.1D)
Fig.1C Section of an normal embryo in the eye area.
Fig.1D Section of the embryo, shown in Fig.1A. The eye-cup has not developed into the typical form.

The poor reaction of the outer ectoderm layer to neuralizing stimuli could be correlated with the fact that in normogenesis this layer in contrast to the inner neuroectodermal layer does not come into contact with the inducing stimulus of the chordamesoderm. However, under special experimental conditions,i.e. superficial ectoderm in close contact with chordamesoderm, archencephalic brain structures were formed (Grunz,1985). This raises the question, if the cell contact between inducing and reacting tissue is a must in normogenesis. Transfilter experiments of Saxen and Toivonen have shown that under in vitro conditions apparently diffusible

factors migrate from the inducing to the reacting tissue
(Saxen 1961,Toivonen, 1979). However, these results do not
exclude the posssibility that this migration takes place in
areas of close cell-to-cell contacts in normogenesis (Grunz
and Staubach, 1979b). Since the inner ectodermal layer in
Xenopus acts like a barrier between inducing chordamesoderm
and superficial ectoderm layer, it can be assumed that
neuralizing factors are not transmitted over long distances
and do not cross several cell layers to reach the target
cells. Experiments together with Dr.Tacke show that archencephalic brain structures are formed by competent ectoderm,
when chordamesoderm has established close cell-to-cell
contacts to the ectodermal target cells after an incubation
time of about 3 hours. When the chordamesoderm is removed
within this period, no neural induction takes place.
A further phenomenon, which could be correlated with the
amount of receptors on the plasmamembrane, is the loss of
competence of the ectoderm during gastrulation (Grunz,1970).
It could be shown by gold-Con A that late gastrula ectoderm,
which has lost its competence to react on inducing factors,
does not contain a smaller amount of receptor sites for ConA
than early gastrula ectoderm(Tacke and Grunz, submitted).
These results support the view that the loss of competence
is not caused by a reduction of specific receptors on the
plasmamembrane but depends on intracellular mechanisms.
Apparently an autonomous intrinsic programm is running down
at the transcriptional or/and translational level including
regulation factors protein in nature.
In this context it should be pointed out that we do not
support the view that ions or cyclic nucleotides play any
role as primary signals initiating the inducing processes.
Treatment with cyclic nucleotides did not evoke neural inductions in competent ectoderm of Triturus alpestris (Grunz
and Tiedemann,1977) and of Xenopus laevis(Grunz, 1985).This
also holds true for ectoderm after the increase of the
intracellular calcium concentration by calciumionophore
A 23187(Grunz, 1985). Furthermore during the primary phase
of induction we could not observe significant changes of the
sodium- and potassium- concentration (comparison of induced
and non induced ectoderm)(Siegel et al., 1985). On the other
hand calciumionophore A 23187 influences the pattern of induced mesodermal and neural differentiations. High intracellular calcium concentrations, caused by the treatment of
ectoderm with calciumionophore A 23187, could result in the
closure of gap junctions and in turn an interruption of cell
communication, which are thought to be responsible for

specific pattern formation. Pattern formation is apparently correlated with secondary cell interactions (Grunz, 1979; Asahi et al.,1979; Minuth and Grunz,1980). That gap junctions presumeably play an important role in early embryogenesis could be shown by injection of antibodies to gap junction protein into early amphibian embryos (8-cell-stage)(Warner et al., 1984). Warner and colleagues fond an asymmetric development of the head area. We also injected two different antibodies (monoclonal anti-mouse-26K-gap junction protein and affinity purified antibody - on a protein A-column -, prepared by the group of Dr.Willecke, Institute of Cell Biology, University of Essen) into one blastomere of 2-or 4-cell-stages of Xenopus laevis(50 cases per series). However, we did not observe any effect neither in the control series (50 nl rabbit IgG, concentration 1-5 mg/ml) nor in the experimental series (50 nl monoclonal anti-26K or affinity-purified anti-26K, concentration 1-5 mg/ml). Further experiments must be carried out to explain the negative results received in our laboratory.

In our lab there are now experiments in progress, which try also the "opposite" method. Together with Dr.Schweiger and Dr.Koop, Ladenburg/Heidelberg we recently were successful to fuse two or three single amphibian ectoderm cells by electrofusion. This technique is very promising for the study of gen expression in hybrid cells in respect to nuclear/cytoplasmic interactions of animal and vegetal blastomeres of early cleavage stages.
Also recent basic experiments should be mentioned. Karin Buiting in our laboratory could show by systematic studies that also the routine technique for the removal of the jelly coat of Xenopus embryos by cysteine is a critical step. The speed of the degradation of the jelly coat by cysteine depends on the pH, the temperature, the strenght of agitation and the number of eggs per vessel. When early gastrulae are treated with cysteine-Holtfreter-solution longer than necessary (8 min. at 20°C), the embryos develop into larvae with malformations in the head area (missing forebrain, no eyes, microcephaly,etc.). Probably the superficial cells of the embryo and in turn the morpho-genetic movements during gastrulation are severely affected after non optimal treatment with the cysteine-solution. Although we use a standard technique in our laboratory, we remove the jelly coat with cysteine-Holtfreter-solution always by stereomicroscopic control.
The activity of our laboratory has not only concentrated on

the ectodermal target cells, but also recently on the inducing activity of the upper blastopore lip. Similar to the
ectoderm also the upper blastopore lip, which after invagination stimulates the overlaying neuroectoderm to form the
central nervous system,consists of two distinct cell layers.
After invagination only the inner layer comes into contact
with the inner layer of overlaying neuroectoderm, while the
former outer layer of the blastopore lip is facing to the
blastocoel.The superficial layer can be separated mechanically from the inner layer by fine glass needles.
Ulrich Koch in our laboratory has combined superficial or
inner layers of upper blastopore lip of early gastrulae and
competent ectoderm. Preliminary results indicate that also
the superficial layer is able to induce neural structures in
compentent ectoderm (but in a less extent than the inner
layer), although in normogenesis it does not come into
contact with the ectodermal target cells. Furthermore he
could show that the inner blastopore layer of early gastrula
induces spinocaudal structures, while the same layer induces
archencephalic brain structures, when kept for 15 hours in
vitro prior to its combination with early gastrula ectoderm.
This corresponds to the shift in the inducing capacity of
whole dorsal blastopore lip of urodelean species, which does
not contain two distinct cell layers(Okada and Takaya,1942).
Further experiments are in progress to receive very exact
data on the inducing activity of the different layers of the
upper blastopore lip before and after their aging in vitro.
Apparently in the dorsal blastopore lip an intrinsic program
is running down. The result is a shift in the inducing
capacity. Winfried van Ackeren in our lab has started intensive studies to find out, if significant differences
exist in the protein pattern between dorsal blastopore
lip of early gastrula and blastopore lip after aging for 18
hours at 11°C in vitro. Dorsal blastopore lips (both layers;
dorsal blastopore lip of early gastrulae and blastopore lip
after 18h aging) were incubated for 3h in culture medium,
containing ^{35}S-methionine (Amersham, 250 μCi/ml, specific
activity 1255 Ci/mmol). Proteins were isolated and then
separated by isoelectrofocussing (1.dimension) and SDS-PAA-
gelelectophoresis. The labeled proteins, representing the
newly synthesized polypeptides, were detected by fluorography. The preliminary results are promising. Several spots
could be identified, representing proteins which are present
in gels of early or aged blastopore lip, respectively
(Fig. 2A, 2B).

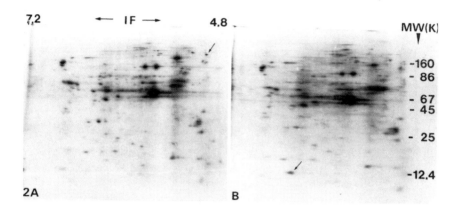

Fig.2A Protein pattern of upper blastopore lips of early gastrulae (both ectodermal layers), labeled with ³⁵ S-methionine for 3 hours prior to the electrophoretic preparations (7 blastopore lips were used for the analysis).

Fig.2B Protein pattern of upper blastopore lips (both ecto-dermal layers) cultured in Flickinger-solution for 18 hours at 11°C prior to the exposure to ³⁵ S-methionine for 3 hours, followed by the electrophoretic preparations. (7 blastopore lips were used for the analysis).

Arrows indicate the differences between the "young" and "aged" blastopore lip.Isofocussing (1.dimension:pH 4.8-7.2), SDS-PAGE (2. dimension), followed by fluorography.

The assumption is of course too speculative that these diff-erences in the protein pattern represent neuralizing factor(s). However, it should be mentioned that such differ-ences could not be found between early gastrula ectoderm and ectoderm after culture in vitro for 18 hours. Further ex-periments are in progress to identify possible differences in the protein pattern of superficial and inner cell layer of dorsal Xenopus blastopore lip of early gastrulae and blastopore lip after a culture in vitro for 18 hours.

Conclusions

Summarizing we can postulate the following chain of events
during early embryonic induction: Neuralizing factors
could be associated with nucleoprotein particles in the
inducing chordamesoderm as recently could be shown by the
group of Tiedemann. It can be assumed that it is released
by exocytotic processes into the intercellular gap between
chordamesoderm and reacting neuroectoderm. After migration
perhaps especially in the zones of close cell-to-cell
contacts between inducing and target tissue the inducer will
interact with specific receptors on the plasmamembrane of
the target cells. The further events within the ectodermal
target cells are still unknown. However, it can be postulated that the induced cells themselves in secondary steps
will liberate also inducing factors by exocytosis and will
stimulate neighbouring non induced cells, since it is known
that factors with neuralizing and mesodermalizing activity
are present in ectodermal cells in a masked form. Finally I
like to point out that we could not find any indication for
neuralizing effects triggered by cAMP or its derivatives,
calciumionophore A 23187 or shifts in the ionic intracellular concentration. In our oppinion those factors cannot be
considered as primary signals for the early embryonic
induction.

The investigations were supported by the Deutsche
Forschungsgemeinschaft (Schwerpunkt: "Steuerung der Differ-
enzierung von ein- und wenigzelligen eukaryontischen System-
en") and in part by a grant of the University of Essen).

References

Asahi K J, Born J, Tiedemann H, Tiedemann H (1979) Formation
    of mesodermal pattern by secondary inducing interactions.
    Wilhelm Roux's Archives 187, 231-244.

Asashima M, Grunz H (1983) Effects of inducers on inner and
    outer gastrula ectoderm layers of Xenopus laevis.
    Differentiation 23 , 157-159

Born J, Grunz H, Tiedemann H, Tiedemann H (1980) Biological
    activity of the vegetalizing factor: Decrease after
    coupling to polysaccharide matrix and enzymatic recovery
    of active factor. Wilhelm Roux's Archives 189, 47-56.

Grunz H (1970) Abhängigkeit der Kompetenz des Amphibien-Ektoderms von der Proteinsynthese. Wilhelm Roux's Archives 165, 91-102.

Grunz H (1972) Einfluß von Inhibitoren der RNS- und Protein-Synthese und Induktoren auf die Zellaffinität von Amphibiengewebe. Wilhelm Roux's Archives 169, 41-55.

Grunz H (1979) Change of the differentiation pattern of amphibian ectoderm after the increase of the initial cell mass. Wilhelm Roux's Archives 187, 49-57.

Grunz H (1983) Change in the differentiation pattern of Xenopus laevis ectoderm by variation of the incubation time and concentration of vegetalizing factor. Wilhelm Roux's Archives 192, 130-137.

Grunz H (1984) Early embryonic induction: The ectodermal target cells.In Duprat A M, Kato M, Weber M (eds): "The role of cell interactions in early neurogenesis", Plenum Press, Ser.A, Life Sciences, Vol.77, pp. 21-38

GRUNZ,H.(1985a) Effect of concanavalin A and vegetalizing factor on the outer and inner ectoderm layers of early gastrulae of Xenopus laevis after treatment with cytochalasin B. Cell Differentiation 16 , 83-92

Grunz H (1985b) Information transfer during embryonic induction in amphibians (in press, JEEM)

Grunz H, Staubach J(1979a) Change of the surface charge of ectodermal cells after induction. Wilhelm Roux's Archives 186, 77-80.

Grunz H, Staubach J(1979b) Cell contacts between the chorda-mesoderm and the overlying neuroectoderm (presumptive central nervous system) during the period of primary embryonic induction in amphibians. Differentiation 14, 59-65.

Grunz H, Multier A M, Herbst R, Arkenberg G (1975) The differentiation of isolated Amphibian ectoderm with or without treatment of an inductor. A scanning electron microscope study. Wilhelm Roux's Archives 178, 277-284.

Grunz H, Tiedemann H (1977) Influence of cyclic nucleotides on amphibian ectoderm. Wilhelm Roux's Archives 181,261-332

Minuth M, Grunz H (1980) The formation of mesodermal derivatives after induction with vegetalizing factor depends on secondary cell interactions. Cell Differentiation 9, 229-238.

Okada Yo K, Takaya H (1942) Further studies upon the regional differentiation of the inductive capacity of the organizer. Proc. Imp. Acad.(Tokyo) 18, 514-519.

Saxen L (1961) Transfilter neural induction of amphibian ectoderm. Dev. Biol. 3, 40-152.

Siegel G, Grunz H, Grundmann U, Tiedemann H, Tiedemann H
(1985) Embryonic induction and cation concentrations
in amphibian embryos (in press, Cell Differentiation)
Spemann H, Mangold, H (1924) Über Induktion von Embryonal-
anlagen durch Implantation artfremder Organisatoren.
Wilhelm Roux's Archives 100, 599-638
Tacke L and Grunz H (1986) Electron microscope study of the
binding of Concanavalin A-gold to superficial and inner
ectoderm layers of Xenopus laevis in correlation to the
neural inducing activity of this lectine (submitted).
Takata K, Yamamoto KY, Ozawa R (1981) Use of lectins as
probes for analyzing embryonic induction. Wilhelm Roux's
Archives 190, 92-96.
Takata K, Yamamoto KY, Takahashi N (1984) A molecular aspect
of neural induction in CYNOPS presumptive ectoderm treated
with lectins.In Duprat A M, Kato M, Weber M (eds): "The
role of cell interactions in early neurogenesis", Plenum
Press, Ser.A, Life Sciences Vol.77, 83-88
Tiedemann H (1982) Signals of cell determination in embryo-
genesis.In Jaenicke L (ed): "Biochemistry of Differentia-
tion and Morphogenesis", Springer Verlag, Berlin,
Heidelberg, pp 275-287(33. Colloquium - Mosbach).
Tiedemann H (1984) Neural embryonic induction. In Duprat
A M, Kato M, Weber M (eds): "The role of cell inter-
actions in early neurogenesis", Plenum Press, Life
Sciences, Vol.77, 89-105.
Toivonen S (1979) Transmission problem in primary induction.
Differentiation 15, 177-181.
Warner AE, Guthrie SC, Gilula NB (1984) Antibodies to gap-
junctional protein selectively disrupt junctional
communication in the early amphibian embryo. Nature 311,
127-131.

Cellular Endocrinology: Hormonal Control of Embryonic
and Cellular Differentiation, pages 55–66
© 1986 Alan R. Liss, Inc.

PURIFICATION OF MESODERMAL INDUCING SUBSTANCE AND PROTEIN
SYNTHESIS USING THIS MATERIAL

Asashima, M., H. Nakano, T. Matsunaga, K.
Hashimota and K. Shimada
Department of Biology, Yokohama City University,
22-2 Seto, Kanazawa-ku, Yokohama 236, Japan

INTRODUCTION

The blastopore lip region of the amphibian gastrula
has the capacity to organize an entire second embryonic
axis when grafted into the ventral side of a recipient gastrula or inserted into the blastocoel (Spemann and Mangold,
1924; Mangold, 1923). It has been thought that the morphogenetic factors contained in this region play a part in
the control of embryonic differentiation. Many investigators have tried to isolate inducing substances or morphogenetic factors from amphibian embryos as well as from
other animal tissues such as chick embryo extracts (Born
et al., 1972), bone marrow (Toivonen and Saxén, 1957),
liver and kidney (Hayashi, 1956; Yamada, 1962), and so
on. Kawakami et al. (1976, 1978) showed that materials
extracted from carp swimbladders have very high mesodermal-
inducing activity. The swimbladder consists of relatively
homogeneous cells and it seems that it is effective to
isolate the inducing substances from this material. The
inducing substances contained in this material are stable
under heat treatment. After defining the characteristics
and chemical properties of inducing substances, we can use
them as a tool for pursuing the cell differentiation of
early embryonic development.

In the present study, we have attempted to isolate mesodermal-inducing substances from the swimbladder by biochemical methods such as extraction with 8 M urea, isoelectrofocusing, and affinity with Con A Sepharose. We then examined the effects of addition of the inducing substances on
the protein content of the presumptive ectoderm of the

gastrula.

MATERIALS AND METHODS

Purification steps: Swimbladders of adult crucian carp
(Carassius auratus) were used as the starting material for
this experiment.   After removal, the swimbladders were
fixed in 90% ethanol and stored in a refrigerator at -30
°C until use. Five grams wet weight of swimbladder were
cut into small pieces on ice, and then washed three times
with Holtfreter's solution (pH 7.2). To this was added
180 ml of 8 M urea. They were then homogenized and extracted with urea by a Homoblender. The homogenate was then
centrifuged at 18,000 g for 30 min. The supernatant was
collected, and 40 ml of 8 M urea was added to the sediment.
The sediment was homogenized and centrifuged using the
same method. This procedure was repeated once again. These
supernatants (crude solution) were collected together
and used for further purification.

Isoelectric focusing was carried out with crude solution
after extraction with 8 M urea (Vesterberg and Svensson,
1966; Geithe et al., 1970). The ampholine concentration
was 2% in all experiments. The buffer column was stabilized
by a sucrose density gradient (25% sucrose at the bottom
to 4% at the top). The sample solution containing 20 mg of
protein was prepared by dilution of the supernatant. The
top of the column was the cathode (sodium hydroxide),and
the bottom was the anode (phosphoric acid). Electricfocus-
ing was performed at 3-4 W for 50-60 hours at 4°C. The samples were eluted for 2 hours using a fraction collector.
Each tube contained 2.0 ml of solution. After fractionation the pH and the absorption at 280 nm were measured.
From the elution pattern, the fractions were divided into
five parts, from A to E. Each part was collected and tested for its biological activity.

Affinity method with Con A Sepharose was performed as
follows (Aspberg and Porath, 1970; Kennedy and Rosevear,
1973) : Concanavalin A covalently bound to Sepharose 4B
was suspended in 0.1 M acetate buffer, pH 6.0, containing
1 M NaCl, 1mM MnCl$_2$, 1 mM MgCl$_2$, 1mM CaCl$_2$and 0.01%
Merthiolate. About 15 ml of adsorbent gel was packed into
a 100ml flask (batch method). The adsorbent was washed
with 20 mM HEPES buffer, pH 7.5, containing 0.5 M NaCl,
1 mM CaCl$_2$and 1mM MnCl$_2$(basic buffer). This buffer was

filtrated before use. Samples were suspended in 30 ml of
basic buffer and applied to the adsorbent. After 90 min.,
the solution was eluted (Frac. 1). The adsorbent was
washed continuously with the following buffers to elute 4
more fractions; basic buffer containing 0.2 M methyl-
mannoside(Frac. 2), basic buffer containing 0.5 M methyl-
mannoside(Frac. 3), 0.1 M Tris-HCl buffer, pH 8.5,contain-
ing 0.5 M NaCl (Frac. 4), 0.1 M acetic acid buffer,
pH 4.5,containg 0.5 M NaCl (Frac. 5).

Biological test and histological examination: An aliquot
of sample fractions prepared at each biochemical step,i.e.,
after crude extraction with 8 M urea, after isoelectric focusing, and after the affinity method, were dialysed in
tubes (Seamless cellulose) against distilled water (10
liters X 10 times) at 4 °C for two days. After dialysis,
the samples were lyophilized and precipitated with ice-
cold 66% ethanol. The samples were then dried for
biological testing. The inducing activity of each sample
was examined on early gastrula (stage 11) of newt,
Cynops pyrrhogaster,by the sandwich method(Holtfreter,
1933). The sandwich explants were cultured in Holtfreter
solution (pH 7.2) with antibiotics for 14 days at 20 °C.
Gamma globulin was used as a control experimental material.
After culturing, the explants were embedded in paraffin,
sectioned at 8 μm and stained with hematoxylin-eosin for
histological observation.

Gel-electrophoresis: Protein concentration was estimated
by Folin phenol reagent (Lowry et al.,1951). Sugar was
measured by anthrone reagent (Morris, 1948). One-dimensional (1-D) slab gel electrophoresis (Laemmli, 1970)
was done to check the purity of the fractions in the process of the biochemical steps. The separation gel was made
up of 10% acrylamide, 0.375M Tris-HCl (pH 8.8), and 0.1%
sodium dodecyl sulphate (SDS). After running of the sample , the gel was stained with Coomassie Brilliant blue.
Changes in two-dimensional (2-D) gel protein content patterns of explants with or without inducer were examined.
Proteins were separated by the 2-D gel electrophoresis
method (O'Farrell, 1975). The first-dimension gel was an
isoelectrofocusing gel of 3.5% acrylamide, 8M urea, ampholine (LKB, pH 3.5-10) and NP-40. The pH gradient of the
first-dimension gel was found to be approximately 5.5-8.5.
In the second dimension, a concentration of 10% acrylamide
was used. Four sandwich explants with or without inducer
were homogenized with 0.2 ml of lysis buffer and were
centrifuged at 5000 rpm for 30 min. 50 μl of the superna-

tant were routinely loaded on each gel. That volume of supernatant contains approximately one sandwich explant equivalent. The gels were stained with ammoniacal silver solution (Oakley et al., 1980).

RESULTS

Inducing activity after urea extraction and isoelectric focusing: As a control explant, ectoderm alone showed no differentiation at all. In another control explant, ectoderm with γ-globulin showed an atypical epithelium cell mass, and did not induce other tissues in 12 cases.

Extracted samples from carp swimbladders with 8 M urea had high percentages of inducing activities in 14 out of 15 cases (93.3%). Six out of 15 cases showed obvious trunk and tail formation with pigment from the external view. This extracted fraction showed high mesodermal-inducing activities accompanied with muscle (73.3%), notochord (80.0%), renal tubules (20.0%) and mesenchyme cells (66.7%). Though neural tissues were observed in three out of 15 cases(20.0%), other neural organs such as brain and eye were never observed. Blood cells and coelemic epithelium were induced at 20.0 percentage (3 cases).

After electric focusing, the elution patterns of pH gradient and absorbance at 280 nm were determined, as shown in Fig.1. About seven peaks were observed in absorbance at 280 nm. Based on the absorption pattern, the fractions were divided into five parts, from A to E. Part A was the acidic area from pH 2.0 to 4.8. Part B was from pH 4.8 to 6.0. Part C was from pH 6.0 to 7.0. Part D was from pH 7.0 to 9.0, and part E was from pH 9.0 to 12. In parts C and D, there were high mesodermal-inducing substances (Fig.2). Notochord was observed in parts C and D at 66.7% and 82.6%, respectively. Muscle was induced in 13 out of 18 cases (72.2%) in part C, and 15 out of 23 cases (65.2%) in D part. Renal tubules and mesenchyme cells were induced at 61.1% and 77.8%, respectively, in part C and at 66.9% and 100%, respectively, in part D. Though brain structures were induced at low percentages, unspecified neural tissues were induced at the relatively high rates of 38.9% and 47.8% in parts C and D, respectively. In part B, there was high absorption at 280 nm, but

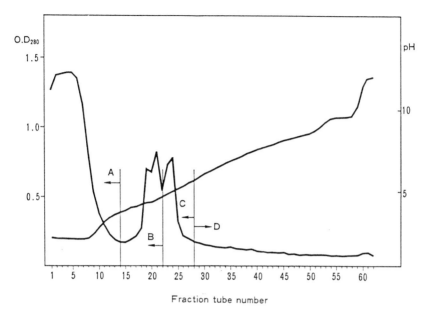

Figure 1. Isoelectric focusing of inducing substances extracted by 8 M urea. Abscissa, fraction tube number. Left ordinate, O.D.280 nm. Right ordinate, pH. Following the elution pattern, the samples were divided into five.

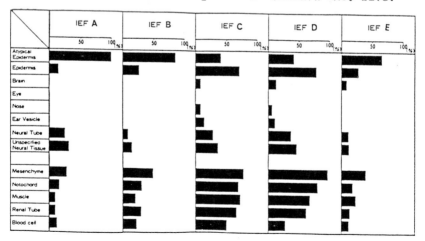

Figure 2. Differentiation of the ectoderm induced by the fractions after isoelectric focusing.

inducing activity was not as high as that in parts C and
D. Low inducing activities of mesoderm and neural tissues
were also observed in parts A and E.
Inducing activity after affinity method:Inducing activity
after the affinity method with Con A Sepharose 4B is shown
in Fig.3. The applied samples used in the methods were
parts C and D after isoelectric focusing. Five fractions
(from Frac.1 to Frac.5) were isolated from them by the
affinity method. Substances contained in Frac. 1 had
very high mesodermal-inducing activity. In this fraction,
muscles were induced in 16 out of 26 cases (61.5%), but
in other fractions muscles were observed at a low rate of
less than 5 percent. In fraction 1, mesenchyme,notochord,
renal tubules and coelomic epithelium were induced at
80.8%, 53.8%, 26.9% and 30.8%, respectively. This fraction
had low neural-inducing activity. The other fractions,
from Frac. 2 to 5, had low mesodermal-inducing activity.
Fraction 5 had relatively high neural inducing activity at
33.3%. In fraction 1, there were 520 µg of protein and
230 µg of sugar.

Fractions

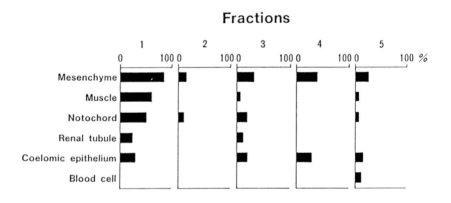

Figure 3. Inducing activity of the substances fractionated
by the affinity method on Con A Sepharose 4B.

1-Dimension slab gel electrophoresis: To check the purity
of the fractions prepared in the biochemical steps, 1-D
slab gel electrophoresis (10% acrylamide and 0.1% SDS)
was employed. The gels stained with 0.05% Coomassie

Brilliant BR are shown in Fig.4. As standard marker
proteins, albumin bovine (M.W. 66,000), albumin egg (M.W.
45,000), trypsinogen (M.W.24,000), β-lactoglogulin (M.
W. 18,400) and lysozyme (M.W. 14,300) were used. Crude
solution extracted with 8 M urea shows more than 45 bands,
and C and D fractions after isoelectric focusing contained more than 32 bands. In Frac.1 after affinity method,
four main bands (M.W. 30,700; 29,400; 14,900 and 10,400)
and four minor bands (M.W. 97,100; 63,000; 57,500 and
45,300)were observed. Molecular weights of the bands
were calculated from the standard proteins.

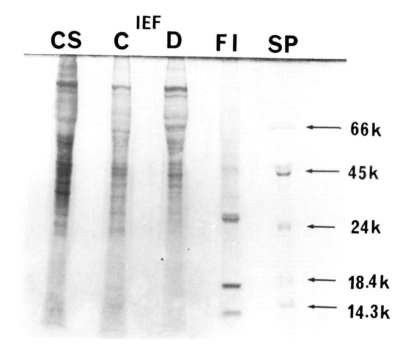

Figure 4. 1-D slab gel electrophoresis of the inducing
substances purified in several biochemical steps. SP,
standard marker proteins; CS, crude solution extracted
with 8 M urea; IEF C and D, Parts C and D after isoelectric focusing; F1, Fraction 1 after affinity method.

Protein synthesis checked by 2-Dimension gel electrophoresis: ·   We attempted a molecular experiment
to see if F1 inducer could induce or activate protein
synthesis in the presumptive ectoderm. F1 sample without

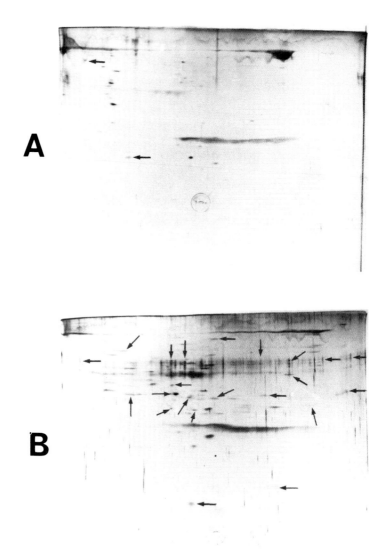

Figure 5. Two-D gel separations of proteins. (A) ectoderm only (control, 0 day culture). (B) ectoderm with F1 inducer (cultured for 14 days). arrows; main newly synthesized proteins compared with control ectoderm explants (cultured for 14 days).

ectoderm showed seven spots on the gel. As a control, the
ectoderm explants without culture(0 day culture) showed
about 40 spots of proteins(Fig. 5A). As another control,
ectoderm explants were cultured for 2 weeks without F1 inducer. The latter control showed about 58 spots in total.
In these control ectoderm explants, some protein spots dis-
appeared(Fig. 5A, arrows) or appeared during the culture.
In the explants with F1 inducer after two weeks culture,
many proteins were present, as seen by more than 82 spots
on the gel(Fig. 5B). Comparison with the three control
experiments showed that F1 induced some new proteins in the
explants(Fig. 5B, arrows). However, some proteins were
also present in the explants which were cultured for 2
weeks without inducer. These proteins were synthesized more
in the explants with F1 inducer. The main muscle proteins,
actin and myosin, were identified by running standard actin
and myosin on the 2-D gel. We also recognized actin by
comparing peptide maps from chymotrypsin digests(Cleveland
et al., 1977). Though the contents of these proteins increased in the explants with F1 inducer, the spots were
already observed in explants cultured for 2 weeks without
inducer.

DISCUSSION

    Holtfreter(1934) proposed that two or more " specific
inducing substances " are involved in the regional induction of embryogenesis. The spinocaudal or mesodermal inductive activity of the Triturus organizer disappears very
quickly after various chemical and physical treatments, but
its neural inductive activity remains even after longer
treatment. For these activities and factors, Saxén and
Toivonen (1961) proposed the two-gradient hypothesis; One
leads to determination of mesodermal structures by mesodermal factors, and the other controls the neuralization of
the ectoderm by a neural factor. Though neural induction
such as that of neural tissues on presumptive ectoderm is
caused by many substances, mesodermal induction such as
that of muscle, notochord and renal tubules is caused only
by limited substances or materials. It is thus useful to
purify and isolate mesodermal-inducing substances as a tool
to analyse or determine the mechanism of cell differentiation in early amphibian development. Though natural mesodermal substances in normal embryos seem to be highly

unstable under heat treatment(Holtfreter, 1933,1934),
mesodermal substances from the swimbladder were highly
stable under such treatment(Kawakami et al., 1976, 1978;
Togashi and Asashima, 1980). It seems to be important to
clarify or understand the mechanism of mesodermal differentiation in the developmental process. It is possible that
the active molecules are unstable in nature in the normal
embryo, but are stable in the swimbladder.

The starting material used in this study is less heterogeneous than chick embryo(Born et al.,1972) which has been
used most for purification of mesodermal inducer. Mesodermal-inducing substances from fish swimbladders were partially fractionated and isolated by biochemical methods.
These substances were extracted with 8 M urea and isoelectric focusing between pH 6 and 9. Fractions C and D, which
had high inducing activity and contained the proteins and
sugars after isoelectric focusing were further fractionated
by the affinity method. The highest inducing activity was
observed in the fraction which was not adsorbed by Con A
Sepharose. Though the crude samples extracted with 8 M urea
showed many bands by gel electrophoresis, there were only
some bands in fraction 1 (F1) after the affinity method
as shown by Coomassie Brilliant blue or silver staining.
Some of these bands corresponded in molecular weight and
pH range to the mesodermal inducer of the chick (Geithe
et al., 1981; Asahi et al., 1982) suggesting that the
active inducers in chick and swimbladder may be similar.
To fully characterize the mesodermal-inducing substances
from swimbladder, we need to further purify these substances and to test their characteristics.

By adding inducing substances, some new proteins were
found and some existing proteins increased in content in
the ectoderm as shown by 2-D gel electrophoresis. Protein
synthesis patterns during early amphibian embryogenesis
were reported in detail (Meuler and Malacinski, 1984).
They observed that during morphogenesis of amphibian
embryos, several additional novel proteins were synthesized
and some proteins detected at earlier stages ceased synthesis. In our experiments, changes of protein spots
patterns with or without inducer during morphogenesis
were also observed.

REFERENCES

Asahi, K.,M. Asashima, H.P. Geithe, J. Born, H. Tiedemann and H. Tiedemann(1982). Radioiodination with ^{125}I and reductive methylation with tritium of a vegetalizing inducer protein. Hoppe-Seyler's Z. Physiol. Chem. 363: 563-571.

Aspberg, K., and J.Porath (1970). Group-specific adsorption of glycoproteins. Acta Chem. Scand., 24:1839-1841.

Born,J., H.P. Geithe, H.Tiedemann, H.Tiedemann and U. Kocher-Becker (1972). Isolation of a vegetalizing inducing factor. Hoppe-Seyler's Z. Physiol.Chem., 353: 1075-1084.

Cleveland, D.W., Fischer, S.G., Kirschner, M.W. and U.K. Laemmli (1977).Peptide mapping by limited proteolysis in sodium dodesyl sulfate and analysis by gel electrophoresis. J. Biol. Chem. 252: 1102-1106.

Geithe, H.P., H. Tiedemann and H. Tiedemann (1970). Electrofocusing of the vegetalizing inducing factor. Biochim. Biophy. Acta, 208: 157-159.

Geithe, H.P., M.Asashima, Asahi, K., J.Born, H.Tiedemann and H. Tiedemann (1981). A vegatalizing inducing factor. Isolation and chemical properties. Biochi. Biophy. Acta, 676: 350-356.

Hayashi, Y. (1956). Morphogenetic effect of pentose nucleoprotein from the liver upon the isolated ectoderm. Embryologia, 2: 145-162.

Holtfreter, J. (1933). Nachweis der Induktionsfähigkeit abgetöteter Keimteile. Isolations-und Transplantationsversuche. Wilhelm Roux' Arch. Entwickl.-Mech.Org. 128: 584-633.

Holtfreter, J. (1934). Über die Verbreitung induzierender Substanzen und ihre Leistungen im Triton-Keim. Wilhelm Roux' Arch.Entwickl.-Mech. Org.132: 307-383.

Kawakami, I. (1976). Fish swimbladder: an excellent mesodermal inductor in primary embryonic induction. J. Embryol. exp. Morphol., 36: 315-320.

Kawakami, I., Sasaki,N., Sata, A., and N. Osako (1978). Vegetalization of presumptive ectoderm of newt gastrulae in a transfilter experiment with fish swimbladder as the inductor. Develop. Growth and Differ., 20: 353-361.

Kennedy, F.J., and A,Rosevear (1973). An assessment of the fractionation of carbohydrates on Concanavalin A-Sepharose 4B by affinity chromatography. J. Chem. Soc., Perkin Trans., I(19) 2041-2046.

Laemmli, U.K. (1970). Cleavage of structural proteins during the assembly of the head of Bacteriophage T4. Nature, 227: 680-685.

Lowry, O.H., N.J. Rosebrough, A.L.Farr and R.J.Randall (1951). Protein measurement with the Folin phenol reagent. J. Biol. Chem., 193: 265-275.

Mangold, O. (1923). Transplantationsversuche zur Frage der Spezifität und der Bildung der Keimblätter. Arch. Mikroskop. Anat. Entwiclungsmech., 100: 193-301.

Meuler, D.C. and G.M. Malacinski (1984). Protein synthesis patterns during early amphibian embryogenesis. In; Malacinski GM and WH Klein (eds). "Molecular aspects of early development". Plenum Press, New york, 267-288.

Morris, D.L. (1948). Quantitative determination of carbohydrates with Dreywood's anthrone reagent. Science, 107: 254-255.

Oakley, B.R., D.R.Kirsch and N.R. Morris (1980). A simplified ultrasensitive silver stain for detecting proteins in polyacrylamide gels. Anal. Biochem., 105: 361-363.

O'Farrell, P. (1975). High resolution 2-D electrophoresis of proteins. J. Biol. Chem. 1250: 4007-4021.

Saxén, L., and S. Toivonen (1961). The two-gradient hypothesis in primary induction. The combined effect of two types of inductors mixed in different ratios. J.Embryol. exp. Morp., 9: 514-533.

Spemann, H. and H. Mangold (1924). Über Induktion von Embryonalanlage durch Implantation artfremder Organisatoren. Roux' Arch. EntwMech. Org.,100: 599-638.

Togashi, S. and M. Asashima (1980). Changes in the electrophoretic mobility of presumptive ectoderm cells treated with mesodermal inducing substances. Develop. Growth and Differ., 22: 797-803.

Toivonen, S., and L. Saxén (1957). Embryonic inductive action of normal and leukemic bone marrow of the rat. J. nat. Cancer Inst., 19: 1095-1104.

Verterberg, O., and H. Svensson (1966). Isoelectric fractionation, analysis and characterization of Ampholytes in natural pH gradient. IV. Further studies on the resolving power in connection with separation of myoglobins. Acta Chem. Scand., 20: 820-834.

Yamada, T., (1962). The inductive phenomenon as a tool for understanding the basic mechanism of differentiation. J. Cell Comp. Physiol., 60: Suppl.1, 49-64.

Cellular Endocrinology: Hormonal Control of Embryonic and Cellular Differentiation, pages 67–77
© 1986 Alan R. Liss, Inc.

EMBRYONIC CONTROL OF CANCER

G. Barry Pierce, M.D., Juan Arechaga, M.D. and
Robert S. Wells, M.D.
Department of Pathology, University of
Colorado Health Sciences Center, 4200
E. Ninth Avenue, Denver, CO 80262 USA

This work was supported in part by a gift from R.J.
Reynolds Industries, Inc., NIH grant CA-35367 and
#CA-36069

INTRODUCTION

The premise behind our work is that irrespective of
the mechanism of carcinogenesis, a neoplastic cell would
behave as a normal cell if placed in the appropriate
embryonic environment. In other words, the mechanism
that causes the differentiation of a cell lineage in the
embryo would cause differentiation of a malignant cell of
that same cell lineage. The result would be the
conversion of a malignant to a normal cell (Pierce,
1983).

Tumor formation of embryonal carcinoma (strain 247),
neuroblastoma (strain C-1300), melanoma (strain B-16),
and leukemia (strain L1210) of the mouse have been
regulated by their appropriate embryonic fields (Pierce,
et al., 1979; Podesta, et al., 1984; Pierce, et al.,
1984; Gootwine, et al., 1982). In addition there is
evidence that adenocarcinoma of the breast may also be
regulated by factors isolated from cells of the milk line
of the appropriate aged embryos (Van Der Haegen, et al.,
unpublished). Each of these is an aneuploid, anaplastic
tumor that has been used experimentally for years.

In the case of embryonal carcinoma and the leukemia
mentioned above the data indicate that the cancer-derived
cells behave as normal cells (Pierce, et al.,
unpublished; Gootwine, et al., 1982).

The mechanism of differentiation is unknown, but it
has been known since the work of Speman and Mangold
(1924) that inducing tissues trigger the process, and
competent cells in a favorable environment then express a
new phenotype in a stable, heritable manner. Having
reiterated this, it is painfully clear that the
mechanisms of differentiation, and of induction in
particular, are unknown. The process of differentiation
has been difficult to study because there are few good
probes available. As will become apparent in this
presentation, malignant cells of the cell lineage in
question are excellent probes of the process of
differentiation.

About 24 hours after fertilization, the ovum of the
mouse divides, a process repeated about every 12 hours.
By three and one-half days the blastocyst stage has been
attained. The blastocyst is a hollow sphere of 52 trophectodermal cells surrounded by an amorphous soft shell,
the zona pellucida. A clump of 12 additional cells, the
inner cell mass is attached to the inner side of the
trophectoderm. The trophectoderm pumps or secretes
blastocele fluid which amounts to about $1 \times 10^{-3} \lambda$. The
origins of the trophectoderm and inner cell mass are
traceable to the 8 cell embryo: One of the cells is
inside, covered by the other seven, and its progeny
become the inner cell mass. The outer cells give rise to
trophectoderm (Tarkowski and Wroblewska, 1967; Barlow, et
al., 1972). Little is known about regulation in the
blastocyst, but Gardner showed that the trophectoderm
overlying the inner cell mass (polar trophectoderm) was
stimulated to divide by the inner cell mass (Gardner,
1972). The polar trophectoderm gives rise to the mural
postmitotic trophectoderm which encloses the blastocele
fluid. Trophectoderm did not contribute cells to the
inner cell mass and the inner cell mass did not
contribute cells to the trophectoderm (Gardner and
Papaioannou, 1975).

If inner cell mass cells are cultivated in vitro,

they spontaneously transform to become embryonal carcinoma cells (Evans and Kaufman, 1981; Martin, 1981). Thus, embryonal carcinoma cells may be viewed as the neoplastic equivalent of inner cell mass cells, even though they may take origin from earlier stages of embryonic developemnt, even from primordial germ cells (Stevens, 1967).

Embryonal carcinoma cells are the multipotential stem cells of teratocarcinomas (Pierce and Dixon, 1959). They, like their normal counterpart, the inner cell mass, are multipotent in the sense that they differentiate into cells of the three primary germ layers (Pierce et al., 1960). In so doing they give rise to the multiplicity of tissues of the teratocarcinoma. In addition cells derived by differentiation of embryonal carcinoma cells are benign and of no danger to the host (Pierce, et al. 1960). These observations and others (Pierce and Wallace, 1971) provided the verification for the idea that the differentiated cells of tumors arise by differentiation and not by dedifferentiation.

Brinster (1974) in studies of injection chimeras wished to determine the ages of blastomeres that could form chimeras. In these experiments some embryonal carcinoma cells were also injected into blastocysts and the injected blastocysts were placed in the uteri of animals made pseudopregnant. Chimeric mice were produced. This observation was confirmed and extended (Papaioannou, et al. 1975; Mintz and Illmensee, 1975) and it quickly became apparent that cancer derived cells colonized most of the tissues of the resulting chimeric embryos. As mentioned, it was known that the cells derived by differentiation of malignant cells were benign (Pierce, et al. 1960). Benign tumor cells do not respond to homeostatic controls. The Brinster experiment proved that cancer-derived cells responded to homeostatic controls, and could therefore be considered to be normal.

How did the blastocyst regulate the embryonal carcinoma cell so that it and its offsprings behaved as normal cells?

To determine the mechanism two assays were developed: the one was dependent upon the ability of the blastocyst to regulate tumor formation (Pierce, et al.

1979), the other the ability of the blastocyst to regulate colony formation of embyronal carcinoma cells in vitro (Wells, 1982). In these assays, embryonal carcinoma cells were injected into blastocysts and the blastocysts were then injected either into the testes of appropriate inbred strains of animals or were placed in tissue culture to test for tumor or colony formation, respectively. It turned out that of three embryonal carcinoma cells tested, two were regulated by the blastocyst (Pierce, et al. 1982). One of the tumors, 247, was chosen as the prototype for the experiments because of its ease of growth in vitro (Lehman, et al. 1974). It turned out that whereas the blastocyst could regulate tumor formation of embryonal carcinoma, it could not regulate L1210 leukemia, B16 melanoma, or sarcoma 180 (Pierce, et al. 1982). Thus it was concluded that the mechanism of regulation had a degree of specificity. 247 cells were also regulated in the colony assay (Wells, 1982).

Cancer cells injected into blastocysts that formed tumors or colonies clearly had not been regulated; but what of cancer cells that did not form tumors or colonies, had they been killed, or induced to differentiate but were incapable of being incorporated into the embryo.

This turned out to be a perplexing technical problem. Embryonal carcinoma cells labeled with polysterine fluorescent beads were injected into blastocysts, which were cultured in vitro. These were embedded in plastic. The fluoresent beads made it possible to step section the blastocysts until the labeled cell was encountered. Then it was sectioned for examination by the electron microscope. The results of the experiment proved inconclusive because the cells had a tendency to release beads, which were engulfed by adjacent cells (unpublished). The impression was gained that most of the 247 cells were incorporated in trophectoderm, very few in the inner cell mass. In confirmation of these studies, embryonal carcinoma cells of glucose phosphate isomerase A were injected into blastocysts of gluocose phosphate isomerase B and no evidences of chimerism could be determined biochemically 72 hours later (Pierce, et al. 1986 in preparation).

It was then decided to repeat the morphologic study using embryonal carcinoma cells that had incorporated tritiated thymidine in their DNA. This proved to be difficult because embryonal carcinoma cells are extremely sensitive to tritiated thymidine, and it was necessary to find an amount small enough not to damage the cells, but large enough to permit autoradiography. Aggregation chimeras were then made using an adaptation of the method originally pioneered by Tarkowsky and Wroblewska (1967). Accordingly, five labeled embryonal carcinoma cells were sandwiched between two 8 cell morulas. After aggregation and incubation, blastocysts developed. These were fixed and imbedded in plastic for electron microscopy. Serial 5 µ thick sections were cut and examined by autoradiography. In confirmation of the impressions gained from the studies just alluded to, few labeled cells have been found in the inner cell mass in comparison to the number found in trophectoderm (Pierce, et al. 1986 in preparation). A final step is required to complete this experiment. The 5 µ thick sections containing the embryonal carcinoma cells will be remounted in plastic and thin sections will be prepared for examination with the electron microscope. This will ensure that the labeled cells are viable and have differentiated. Even though the data presented are incomplete it is possible to state that embryonal carcinoma cells in our assays that do not form tumors are not killed, rather they are incorporated into the blastocyst and are induced to lose the malignant phenotype.

To return to the colony assay: it was observed that Chinese hamster ovary cells when injected into the blastocyst failed to produce colonies at control levels (Pierce, et al. 1984). This apparent regulation seemed unlikely because Chinese hamster ovary cells have no normal counterpart in the blastocyst as does embryonal carcinoma cell. It was postulated that possibly the unique structure of the trophectodermal wall of the blastocele cavity, which precludes passage of macromolecules into and out of the blastocyst, might be responsible for the apparent regulation of the CHO cells. To solve this problem a technique was developed where by fistulas were made in the trophectodermal wall of the blastocyst. These fistulas were kept open with small glass tubes, and blastocele fluid was pumped out of the

blastocyst through them. Whereas embryonal carcinoma
cells were regulated in blastocysts with fistulas,
Chinese hamster ovary cells were not regulated. This
observation was the first clue that there was a
diffusible factor in blastocele fluid that inhibited the
growth of certain cell types (Pierce, et al. 1984). Each
of the components of the blastocyst, fluid, inner cell
mass, and trophectoderm were tested for their ability to
regulate embryonal carcinoma (Pierce, et al. 1984). None
could accomplish the regulation alone. In other words,
when embryonal carcinoma cells were cultured in the
presence of blastocele fluid they were not regulated.
When embryonal carcinoma cells were attached to inner
cell mass by phytohemaglutinin and cultured in vitro they
formed colonies at control levels. When mural
trophectodermal cells were isolated as single cells and
rosetted around embryonal carcinoma cells, and cultured
in tissue culture media, the embryonal carcinoma cells
were not regulated.

Embryonal carcinoma cells were regulated when they
were placed in vesicles of trophectoderm which contained
blastocele fluid (Pierce, et al. 1984). Thus it was
concluded that trophectoderm in the presence of
blastocele fluid regulates the embryonal carcinoma cell.
Unfortunately, the logistics of the system are such, that
it has been impossible to test the regulation of
embryonal carcinoma cells by inner cell mass cells in the
presence of blastocele fluid.

If one accepts the premise that embryonal carcinoma
cells are the malignant counterpart of inner cell mass
cells, then the conclusion must be reached that mural
trophectoderm in the presence of blastocele fluid
regulates inner cell mass. It is known from the
experiments of Gardner and Papaioannou that inner cell
mass also regulates the proliferation of polar trophectoderm which in turn gives rise to mural trophectoderm.

If trophectoderm in the presence of blastocele fluid
regulates inner cell mass and causes it to differentiate
into endoderm, then much has been learned about the
mechanism of induction. Induction requires cell contact
of competent and inducing cells plus an inhibitor of
mitosis that in the case of the blastocyst is soluble.
If these observations and deductions are true, then one

can understand how people came to the conclusion that induction was nonspecific. Administration of the nonspecific stimuli to competent cells would injure them, cause the release of the soluble factor which coupled with contact of competent cells with the inducing tissue would result in the differentiation.

In making these postulates we are aware that much work is required to establish the idea in fact.

We attempted to mass produce blastocele fluid by transforming trophectoderm with SV_{40} virus or by hybridizing the cells to rapidly growing tumor cells. Neither experiment worked. Thus, constrained by the logistics, it was decided to test neuroblastoma in the neurula stage embryo for regulation of tumor formation (Podesta, et al. 1984) and melanoma in the skin of the mouse embryo at the time when normal pigment cells arrive in the skin (Pierce, et al. 1986 in preparation). It turns out that C1300 neuroblastoma cells are regulated in the neural crest migratory route (Podesta, et al. 1984). They are better regulated in the adrenal primordium (Miotto and Wells, submitted 1985). There is no evidence at this time for the existence of a diffusible factor in this system, but there is evidence that neuroblastoma cells are also regulated when put the primordium of the kidney, testis, and liver of the 16 day mouse embryo (Miotto and Wells, submitted 1985). It is to be noted that transforming growth factor beta has been isolated from 17 day old mouse embryos (Moses, et al. 1985), and we wonder if it may play an as yet undetected role in the regulation of the neuroblastoma cells.

In the case of the melanoma, it was necessary to develop techniques with which the mouse embryo could be injected at the appropriate time in utero. To this end a method was developed for injecting mouse embryos in utero. They were injected with 300 melanoma cells in the skin of the back or in the skin of the limb bud. The uterus was closed and the number of tumors that developed in the offspring was determined and compared to the incidence of tumors that occurred when 300 melanoma cells were injected into the skin of newborn mouse embryos. Over 70% of animals injected in the skin of the back at 14 days developed tumors whereas less than 50% developed tumors in the limb buds of animals of the same age

(Pierce et al. 1986 in preparation). Eighty-two percent of newborn animals developed tumors. The conclusion was reached that the skin of the limb bud at the time neural crest-derived pigment céll precursors arrive in it is refractory to the growth of melanoma cells in comparison to the skin of the back (Pierce et al. 1986 in preparation).

Organ cultures were prepared from the skin of the back and from limb buds from 14 day old mouse embryos. A conditioned medium was obtained, which when added to Eagles minimal essential media containing 10% fetal calf serum, regulated the growth of clones of melanoma cells. Clones of melanoma cells in conditioned medium were half the diameter of the experimental ones at 6 days. These data were highly significant. An assay based upon uptake of tritiated thymidine to measure the regulation has been made, and in addition, it limb bud cells were transformed in vitro with SV_{40} virus. Thirty transformed cell lines were obtained and two of these which secrete an inhibitory factor are now being used to characterize the molecule.

Finally, Sachs and his associates in Israel injected leukemia cells into the placentas of 10 day mouse embryos (Gootwine, et al. 1982). The vast majority of these animals died of leukemia, but in two cases animals survived that had circulating leukemia derived leukocytes in their circulation. These cells were identified by the appropriate isoenzyme. Thus, it can be concluded that mouse embryos at 10 days of gestational age were able to regulate all of the leukemia cells. Whether or not the growth factors that have been identified by Sachs (1983), Metcalf (1983), and others in the regulation of leukopoiesis in the adult mouse is operative in this situation or not is not clear.

We reach our adult stature through two processes: cell division and differentiation. When adult stature is attained, these processes are not discarded rather they are used in a fine tuned manner to replace senescent cells in the process of tissue renewal. Thus, it is quite possible that the circulating molecules responsible for embryonic induction may well persist into the adult as regulators in the process of tissue renewal.

From our studies, which are in no way conclusive at this time, we believe that it is possible to use neoplastic cells as uniquely labeled cells capable of probing differentiation. Using this approach there is evidence, in two systems that we have studied, for the presence of a diffusible factor as an important component in the mechanism of differentiation. Such factors may ultimately be shown to be the gene products of so-called oncogenes. It is important to remember that oncogenes were identified in neoplastic tissues (Braun, 1959; Todaro, et al., 1980). Because some of them were inhibitory of growth, great emphasis was placed upon them as possible therapeutic agents. Our approach has been an attempt to bridge developmental biology and neoplasia. We have identified the presence of a growth inhibitor that in conjunction with contact with the normal cell, in one case, can cause malignant cells to behave as benign if not normal cells. Possibly the most unique aspect of the studies is the use of malignant cells as probes of normal development. If the assumptions referred to in this paper are true, then it is clear that differentiation of inner cell mass cells is mediated by an endocrine factor in blastocele fluid that is synthesized by trophectoderm plus cell-cell contact with trophectoderm and/or inner cell mass cells.

REFERENCES

Barlow P, Owen DAJ, Graham C (1972). DNA synthesis in the preimplantation mouse embryo. J Embryol Exp Morph 27:431-445.
Brinster R (1974). The effect of cells transferred into the mouse blastocyst on subsequent development. J Exp Med 140:1049-1056.
Evans MJ, Kaufman MH (1981). Establishment in culture of pluripotential cells from mouse embryos. Nature (Lond) 292:154-156.
Gardner RL (1972). An investigation of inner cell mass and trophoblast tissues following their isolation from the mouse blastocyst. J Embryol Exp Morph 28:279-312.
Gardner RL, Papaioannou VE (1975). Differentiation in the trophectoderm and inner cell mass. In Balls M, Wild AE (eds): "The Early Development of Mammals," London: Cambridge University Press, pp 107-132.
Gootwine E, Webb CG, Sachs L (1982). Participation of myeloid leukaemia cells injected into embryos in

haematopoietic differentiation in adult mice. Nature 299:63-65.

Lehman J, Speers, WC, Swartzendruber, DE, Pierce GB (1974). Neoplastic differentiation: characteristics of cell lines derived from a murine teratocarcinoma. J Cell Physiol 84:13-28.

Martin GR (1981). Isolation of a pluripotential cell line from early mouse embryos cultured in medium conditioned by teratocarcinoma stem cells. Proc Natl Acad Sci USA 78:7634-7638.

Metcalf C (1983). Regulation of self-replication in normal and leukemic stem cells. In DW Golde, PA Marks (eds): "Normal and Neoplastic Hematopoiesis, UCLA Symposia on Molecular and Cellular Biology-New Series, Vol 9, Alan R. Liss, Inc, pp 141-156.

Mintz B, Illmensee K (1975). Normal genetically mosaic mice produced from malignant teratocarcinoma cells. Proc Natl Acad Sci USA 72:3585-3589.

Miotto K, Wells RS (submitted 1985). Widespread inhibition of neuroblastoma cells in the 13 to 17 day mouse embryo. Cancer Research.

Moses HL, Tucker RF, Leof, EB, Coffey RJ, Halper J, Shipley GD (1985). Type B transforming growth factor is a growth stimulator and a growth inhibitor. In J Feranisco, B Ozanne, C Stiles (eds): Cancer Cells, Growth Factors, and Transformation. Cold Spring Harbor Laboratory, pp 65-71.

Papaionnou, VE, McBurney MW, Gardner RL, Evans RL (1975). Fate of teratocarcinoma cells injected into early mouse embryos. Nature (Lond) 258:70-73.

Pierce GB (1983). The cancer cell and its control by the embryo. Rous-Whipple Award Lecture. Am J Path 113:117-124.

Pierce GB, Aguilar D, Hood G, Wells RS (1984). Trophectoderm in control of murine embryonal carcinoma. Cancer Res 44:3987-3996.

Pierce GB, Arechaga J, Jones A, Wells RS (1985 unpublished).

Pierce GB, Dixon FJ (1959). Testicular teratomas. I. The demonstration of teratogenesis by metamorphosis of multipotential cells. Cancer (Phila) 12:573-583.

Pierce GB, Dixon FJ, Jr, Verney EL (1960). Teratocarcinogenic and tissue forming potential of the cell types comprising neoplastic embryoid bodies. Lab Invest 9:583-602.

Pierce GB, Wells, RS (1986 unpublished).

Pierce GB, Lewis SH, Miller G, Moritz E, Miller P (1979).
Tumorigenicity of embryonal carcinoma as an assay to
study control of malignancy by the murine blastocyst.
Proc Natl Acad Sci USA 76:6649-6651.

Pierce GB, Pantazis CG, Caldwell JE, Wells, RS (1982).
Specificity of tumor formation by the blastocysts.
Cancer Res 42:1082-1087.

Pierce GB, Van Der Haegen BA, Graves, KH, Wells, RS (1985
in press). Control of carcinoma by the murine embryo.
In JG Fortner, JE Rhoads (eds): Accomplishments in
Cancer Research 1984.

Pierce GB, Wallace, C (1971). Differentiation of
malignant to benign cells. Cancer Res 31:127-134.

Podesta AH, Mullins J, Pierce GB, Wells RS (1984). The
neurula stage mouse embryo in control of neuroblastoma.
Proc Natl Acad Sci USA 81(23):7608-7611.

Sachs L (1983). Constitutive gene expression and the
uncoupling of controls in leukemia - regulatory
proteins that control growth and differentiation in
normal and leukemic myeloid cells. In DW Golde, PA
Marks (eds): Normal and Neoplastic Hematopoiesis, UCLA
Symposia on Molecular and Cellular Biology-New Series,
Vol 9, Alan R. Liss, Inc. pp 57-86.

Speman H, Mangold H (1924). Wer induktion von
embryonalenanlagen durch implantation artfremden
organizatoren. Arch f Entw-mech 100:599-638.

Stevens LC (1967). Origin of testicular teratomas from
primordial germ cells in mice. J Natl Cancer Inst
38:549-552.

Tarkowski AK, Wroblewska J (1967). Development of
blastomeres of mouse eggs isolated at the 4- and 8-
cell stage. J Embryol Exp Morph 18:155-180.

Todaro GJ, Fryling CM, De Larco JE (1980). Transforming
growth factors produced by certain human tumor cells:
Polypeptides that interact with epidermal growth factor
receptors. Proc Natl Acad Sci 77:5258.

Van Der Haegen B (unpublished).

Wells RS (1982). An in vitro assay for regulation of
embryonal carcinoma by the blastocyst. Cancer Res
42:2736-2741.

Section 2. FACTORS IN ORGANOGENESIS

Cellular Endocrinology: Hormonal Control of Embryonic
and Cellular Differentiation, pages 81–92
© 1986 Alan R. Liss, Inc.

MECHANISMS OF CELL ADHESION IN EPITHELIAL-MESENCHYMAL TRANSFORMATIONS

Kathryn L. Crossin and Gerald M. Edelman

Department of Developmental & Molecular Biology
The Rockefeller University, 1230 York Avenue
New York, New York 10021

Regulative development consists of a number of parallel primary processes that are governed by complex transactions at the cellular level: cell division, cell movement, cell death, cell adhesion and milieu-dependent differentiation or embryonic induction. The first three may be regarded as "driving force" processes and the last two as regulatory processes. Interaction of these primary processes leads to morphogenesis and histogenesis in a series of epigenetic sequences. The dependence of embryonic induction upon epigenetic sequences that involve cell contact and cell position as a function of time poses the key question of morphogenesis: How does a one-dimensional genetic code specify a three-dimensional animal?

In embryonic induction (Jacobson, 1966), cells of different history are brought into contact by a series of morphogenetic movements. The critical selection and timing of gene expression must therefore be correlated with cell movement and the accumulation of collectives of cells. This suggests that regulatory signals must connect the expression of gene products affecting movement to the altered states of a sufficient number of aggregated cells; the changes in these cells must, in turn, affect subsequent gene expression. Thus, epigenetic sequences must not only consist of events coordinated over relatively long times, they must also involve a regulatory control loop ranging across several levels of organization from genes to tissue aggregates back to the same or other genes. Because of the obligate involvement of cell movement and folding of tissue sheets and epithelia in these events, at least part of this regulatory control loop must involve mechanochemical signals (Edelman, 1985a,b).

All of these properties suggest that the molecular aspects of cell adhesion are likely to be involved in the regulatory loop. The recent characterization of cell adhesion molecules (CAMs) provides an opportunity to examine the role of adhesion in epigenetic sequences. So far, three CAMs of different specificity and structure have been isolated and characterized. The first two, L-CAM (liver cell adhesion molecule (Gallin et al., 1983; Cunningham et al., 1984)) and N-CAM (neural cell adhesion molecule (Edelman, 1983)), are called primary CAMs and appear early in embryogenesis on derivatves of multiple germ layers. The third, Ng-CAM (neuron-glia CAM), is a secondary CAM that is not seen in early embryogenesis and that appears only on neuroectodermal derivatives, specifically on postmitotic neurons (Grumet and Edelman, 1984; Grumet et al., 1984; Thiery et al., 1985; Daniloff et al., 1985). The accumulated data prompt the hypothesis that CAMs act as regulators of morphogenetic movements (Edelman, 1984b). They thus act as important links from the 1D code that specifies these molecules to the 3D cell collectives that are central to morphogenesis. While this hypothesis is far from confirmed, and the roles of other molecules such as substrate adhesion molcules (including laminin, fibronectin and collagens) must also be considered (see Edelman, 1985b), data on CAM expression sequences and on CAM perturbation indicate that these molecules have a particularly significant role in the formation of morphogenetic cell collectives.

It has been suggested (Edelman, 1984a; 1985a) that CAMs act to regulate binding via a series of cell surface modulation mechanisms including changes in their prevalence at the cell surface, in their position or polar distribution on cells, and in their chemistry of binding. All of these mechanisms have been shown to occur for one CAM or another at different developmental times.

In this survey, we will review recent evidence indicating (i) that CAMs have definite sequences of expression that correlate strongly with major morphogenetic events related to epithelial-mesenchymal transformations (Thiery et al., 1982; Edelman et al., 1983; Thiery et al., 1984), and (ii) that modulation of their expression at sites of embryonic induction occurs in two distinct modes: in mesenchyme,

N-CAM diminishes at the surface and then reappears; in epithelia, both N-CAM and L-CAM appear together and one or the other subsequently disappears.

The two characterized primary CAMs, N-CAM and L-CAM, are both present at low levels on the chick blastoderm before gastrulation (Fig. 1A,B). As gastrulation occurs in the chick, epiblast cells express both N-CAM and L-CAM (Fig. 1C,D); as they ingress through the primitive streak, the amount of detectable CAMs decreases (Thiery et al., 1982; Edelman et al., 1983; Thiery et al., 1984, 1985; Edelman, 1984a; Crossin et al., 1985), presumably reflecting the fact that they have been down-regulated or masked. As the ingressing cells condense into the mesoblast, they re-express N-CAM. Thus, epiblast cells lose both CAMs as they undergo epithelial-mesechymal transformation and move into the middle layer. Some of the ingressing cells become the chordamesoderm which also stains for N-CAM and subsequently takes part in neural induction.

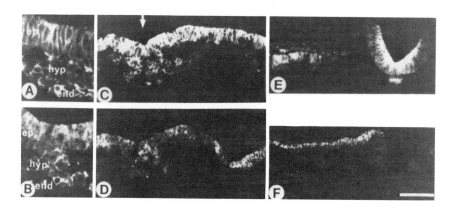

Figure 1. Expression of CAMs in the early embryo. Transverse sections of full primitive streak stage (A,B), head process stage (C,D) or 5 somite chicken embryos (E,F) stained with anti-N-CAM (A,C,E) or anti-L-CAM (B,D,F). Arrow points to the primitive streak. Ep, epiblast, hyp, hypoblast, end, endophyll.

Following gastrulation and coincident with neural induction, there is a marked change in the distribution of the two primary CAMs. An increase in immunofluorescent

N-CAM staining appears in the region of the neural plate and groove as L-CAM staining disappears (Fig. 1E,F). In conjugate fashion, L-CAM staining is enhanced in the surrounding somatic ectoderm as N-CAM staining slowly diminishes. Migration of neural crest cells is also accompanied by down-regulation or masking of cell surface N-CAM (Thiery et al., 1982). Somewhat later, after neurulation, all sites of secondary induction show changes in cell surface prevalence of N-CAM, L-CAM or both (Fig. 2).

At sites of secondary induction, patterns of CAM expression correlate with the apposition of epithelia and mesenchyme prior to their further differentiation. As shown in Table 1 (see Crossin et al., 1985 for detailed examples), the expression sequences of CAMs observed on cells in epithelia and mesenchyme follow two general modes. In mode I, expression of N-CAM (or both CAMs as seen in the epiblast) in mesenchyme decreases to low amounts at the cell surface and then N-CAM is re-expressed. In mode II, one or the other CAM disappears from epithelia initially expressing both CAMs, as seen earliest at neural induction. As a result of the primary processes of development, collectives of cells linked by N-CAM and undergoing modulation mode I are brought into the proximity of collectives of cells linked by L-CAM plus N-CAM or by L-CAM undergoing modulation mode II. Such adjoining cell collectives or CAM couples have been found at all sites of embryonic induction examined. Several examples are presented below.

In the pharynx, for example, the early thyroid epithelium expresses both N-CAM and L-CAM as it is induced by N-CAM positive mesoderm (Fig. 2A,B). Similarly, strongly N-CAM positive mesoderm induces the lung buds from the laryngo-tracheal epithelium which expresses both N-CAM and L-CAM (Fig. 2C,D). More posteriorly, the pancreas is induced from the open anterior intestinal portal by an N-CAM containing mesenchyme (Fig. 2E,F). Later in development, the epithelia of the thyroid and pancreas lose N-CAM and express only L-CAM (Thiery et al., 1984) whereas, in the lung, a population of epithelial cells retains both N-CAM and L-CAM into adulthood (Crossin et al., 1985).

Similar expression sequences have been observed at other sites of secondary induction. The placodes that will give rise to neural structures first express both CAMs but eventually lose L-CAM. The apical ectodermal ridge of the

TABLE 1. Modulation Modes of CAM Expression during Chicken Embryogenesis[a]

Mode I: MESENCHYME	Mode II: EPITHELIA
Ectodermal[b] $N \rightarrow O \rightarrow N$ neural crest	Ectodermal[c] $NL \rightarrow N \;\; (\rightarrow *)$ neural plate $NL \rightarrow L \;\; (\rightarrow *)$ somatic ectoderm
Mesodermal $N \rightarrow O \rightarrow N$ dermis $N \rightarrow O \rightarrow N \rightarrow *$ chondrocytes	Mesodermal $N \rightarrow NL \rightarrow L$ kidney tubules Endodermal $NL \rightarrow L$ thyroid pancreas

[a] Only one example is given; for further examples, see Crossin et al, 1985.
[b] Mode I shows cyclic changes in N-CAM or disappearance. Some of these transitions occur with movement. O represents low levels of CAM; in some cases (*), CAM can be replaced by a differentiation product.
[c] Mode II shows replacement of one CAM by another or disappearance.

limb bud expresses both CAMs as the limb is induced (Thiery et al., 1982, Crossin et al., 1985). Thus, from the time of primary induction, epithelia expressing both N-CAM and L-CAM are induced by N-CAM positive mesodermal tissues. This pattern is seen at sites of secondary induction in the lung and gut derivatives, in the skin (feather), and in the limb bud (Chuong and Edelman, 1985a,b; Crossin et al., 1985). In the kidney, however, the direction appears to be reversed: the L-CAM and N-CAM positive Wolffian duct is the inductor for the N-CAM positive mesonephric mesenchyme (Crossin et al., 1985; Edelman et al., 1983).

The sequences reviewed above indicate that at certain times, one cell can express two CAMs, as first seen for the primary CAMs in blastoderm. In feather formation (described below), and in the induction of pharyngeal and gut append-

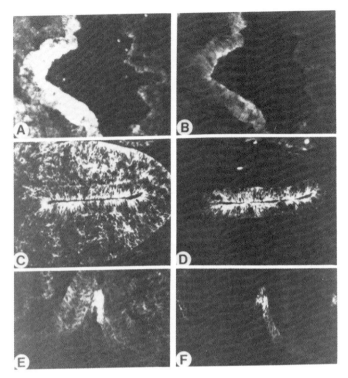

Figure 2. Expression of CAMs in apposed epithelia and mesenchyme. Epithelia of the thyroid rudiment (stage 15) (A,B), laryngotracheal groove (stage 18) (C,D) and pancreatic rudiment (stage 15) (E,F) stain for both N-CAM (A,C,E) and L-CAM (B,D,F) and are adjacent to N-CAM containing mesenchyme (A,C,E).

ages, epithelial cells from ectoderm or endoderm can also express both L-CAM and N-CAM simultaneously; this is also true of kidney mesoderm (Crossin et al., 1985; Chuong and Edelman, 1985a,b). In general, the expressions are dynamic and change so that one or the other CAM disappears during maturation to the adult state (Mode II, Table 1).

Collections of cells linked by L-CAM (or cells expressing both L-CAM and N-CAM) are found adjacent to collectives of cells linked by N-CAM (Table 1) at all sites of secondary embryonic induction so far examined (Crossin et al., 1985). The potential significance of these primary "CAM couples" in morphogenesis is not yet fully understood, but examination of periodic and hierarchically arranged structures such as the feather shows unequivocally that their CAM expression sequences are correlated with other cytodifferentiation events. We shall consider the feather as a particularly compelling example.

The induction of the feather occurs through periodic accumulations in the skin of dermal condensations of mesodermal mesenchyme (Sengel, 1976). Each of these condensations acts upon ectodermal cells to induce placodes. After placode formation, a dermal papilla is formed involving another couple containing mesodermal (N-CAM) and ectodermal (L-CAM) elements. Afterwards, L-CAM positive papillar ectoderm produces collar cells that express both CAMs (Chuong and Edelman, 1985a,b). These cells will provide the basis for the formation of barb ridges and barbule plates through alternating CAM couples ultimately yielding three hierarchical levels of branching: rachis, ramus, and barbules.

There is an extraordinary sequence (Chuong and Edelman, 1985a,b) of CAM couple expression linked first to cell movement and then to cell division in the formation of this hierarchy: (1) Initially, L-linked ectodermal cells are approached by CAM negative mesenchyme cells moving into the vicinity. Just beneath the ectoderm, the mesenchyme cells become N-CAM positive (mode I) and accumulate in lens-shaped aggregates that induce placode formation in the L-CAM linked ectodermal cells (Fig. 3A,B). Later, the L-CAM positive placode cells transiently express N-CAM (mode II). 2) In the formation of the dermal papilla, N-CAM positive mesodermal cells adjoin L-CAM positive ectodermal cells (Fig. 3C,D). At this stage in the highly proliferative collar epithelium, these ectodermal cells express both L-CAM and N-CAM. (3) Derivatives of these cells lose N-CAM while retaining L-CAM as they form barb ridges by division. In the valleys between the ridges, single or small numbers of basilar cells then express N-CAM while losing L-CAM. This mode II process extends cell by cell up each ridge resulting in the formation of the N-CAM positive marginal plate. The net result is alternating barb ridges (L-CAM linked) and marginal plates (N-CAM linked) (Fig. 3E,F). (4) As ridge cells organize into barbule plates linked by L-CAM, a similar process recurs---N-CAM is expressed in cells lying between each of the future barbules resulting in yet another level

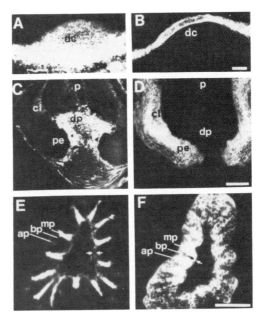

Figure 3. CAM expression in feather morphogenesis. Cells
of the ectodermal placode (A,B) stain for both N-CAM (A) and
L-CAM (B) and are underlain by strongly N-CAM positive (A)
dermal condensations (dc). In the dermal papilla (dp)
(C,D), N-CAM positive cells (C) are surrounded by collar
epithelial cells (cl) expressing both N-CAM (C) and L-CAM
(D). The epithelial papillar ectoderm (pe) expresses only
L-CAM (D). P, pulp. As barbules are formed, cells of the
marginal plate (MP) and axial plate (ap) express both N-CAM
(E) and L-CAM (F) and are separated by L-CAM positive cells
of the barbule plate (BP).

of periodically expressed CAM couples. The net result is a
series of cellular patterns in which cell collectives
expressing L-CAM alternate with those expressing N-CAM at
both the secondary barb level and the tertiary barbule
level. (5) Finally, after further growth of these structures and extension of the barb ridges into rami, the L-CAM
positive cells keratinize and the N-CAM positive cells die
without keratinization. This leaves extracellular N-CAM,
which appears to be reabsorbed or dispersed, leaving alternate spaces between rami and between barbules and yielding
the characteristic feather morphology.

A key feature of this histogenetic CAM expression sequence is periodic CAM modulation in a cycle on particular cells, such as those of inducing mesenchyme. Another important feature is the periodic and successive formation of adjacent N-linked and L-linked cell collectives. Finally, there is a striking association of particular cytodifferentiation events with one or another member of a couple. This association clearly illustrates some modes by which the primary processes of development constituting the driving forces for morphogenesis may be linked to the regulatory processes of adhesion. Morphogenetic movement is coupled to expression of a CAM cycle in mesenchymal cells in the original induction. Cell division is associated with the formation of papillar ectoderm and barb ridge formation. Cell death is linked to the existence of N-linked collectives in barb and barbule formation and it comprises the terminal stages of hierarchical pattern formation in the feather; the conjugate process, cell differentiation, as marked by keratin expression, is linked to prior morphoregulatory CAM differentiation in L-linked cells.

As indicated by this brief survey, in all areas of induction, an epithelial collective of cells linked by L-CAM plus N-CAM (or by L-CAM only) is adjoined by a collective of cells linked by N-CAM alone. Such CAM couples arise either from movement of mesenchymal cells to adjoin epithelia or from differential gene expression and cell division in cells of the same lineage, as seen in the feather. These observations reveal that the primary CAMs are ubiquitous and that the uniform patterns of a small number of CAM expression sequences are repeated in many locales. The evidence suggests that the genes affecting CAM expression (morphoregulatory genes) act independently of and prior to those controlling tissue specific differentiation (historegulatory genes) inasmuch as CAM expression in most induced areas does initially precede the expression of cytodifferentiation products. This is consistent with the observation that the expression of each primary CAM in tissues overlaps several different tissue types as seen in a classical fate map (Edelman et al., 1983).

It is clear from the modulation modes that CAMs play a key role in epithelial-mesenchymal transformation. While the evidence is consistent with the idea that CAMs are directly involved in the regulation of morphogenesis, their causal roles remain to be delineated. This regulator hypo-

thesis (Edelman, 1984b) would be negated if it were found
that CAMs are merely markers that play no causal roles in
the regulation of the expression of primary processes of development. Three lines of evidence suggest that this is not
the case. (i) CAMs have been demonstrated to function
actually as adhesion molecules (Edelman 1983, 1984a, 1985a),
correlative studies (Edelman, 1985a,b) suggest that CAMs
link epithelia (Gallin et al., 1983), and experiments show
that they can be involved in the regulation of morphogenetic
movements (Edelman, 1984a; Grumet et al., 1984). Consistent
with these observations, the expression of primary CAMs in
the feather provides boundaries separating morphogenetically
significant collectives of cells. Such boundaries are
strictly correlated with the expression of different primary
processes in each of the cell collectives comprising a CAM
couple, e.g., differentiation (keratin expression) for
L-linked cells and death for N-linked cells. (ii) Recent
observations indicate that perturbation of early feather
induction in vitro by antibodies to either primary CAM
affects placode formation (W.J. Gallin, C.-M. Chuong, and
G.M. Edelman, unpublished). (iii) Transformation of neural
cell lines by temperature-sensitive mutants of Rous sarcoma
virus shows a loss of surface N-CAM at the permissive temperature followed by loss of adhesion and increased cell motility (Greenberg et al., 1984). Cells at the permissive
temperature can be raised to the non-permissive temperature
and regain surface N-CAM, adhesiveness and histotypic organization. This model allows study of differentiation
events affecting CAM gene expression and may serve as an
analogue for studies of epithelial to mesenchymal transformation.

As exhibited in their expression sequences, and as
indicated by the results of such perturbation experiments,
primary CAMs appear to be mediating factors in epithelial-
mesenchymal transformations, as well as important candidates
for direct involvement in the complex causal chains of
induction.

REFERENCES

Chuong C-M, Edelman GM (1985a). Expression of cell adhesion molecules in embryonic induction: I. Morphogenesis of nestling feathers. J Cell Biol, in press.

Chuong C-M, Edelman GM (1985b). Expression of cell adhesion molecules in embryonic induction: II. Morphogenesis of adult feathers. J Cell Biol, in press.

Crossin KL, Chuong, C-M, Edelman, GM (1985). Expression sequences of cell adhesion molecules. Proc Natl Acad Sci USA, in press.

Cunningham BA, Leutzinger Y, Gallin WJ, Sorkin BC, Edelman GM (1984). Linear organization of the liver cell adhesion molecule L-CAM. Proc Natl Acad Sci USA 81:5787-5791.

Daniloff JK, Chuong C-M, Levi G, Edelman GM (1985). Differentiation distribution of cell adhesion molecules during histogenesis of the chick nervous system. J Neurosci, in press.

Edelman GM (1983). Cell adhesion molecules. Science 219:450-457.

Edelman GM (1984a). Modulation of cell adhesion during induction, histogenesis and perinatal development of the nervous system. Ann Rev Neurosci 7:339-377.

Edelman GM (1984b). Cell adhesion and morphogenesis: The regulator hypothesis. Proc Natl Acad Sci USA 81:1460-1464.

Edelman GM (1985a). Cell adhesion and the molecular processes of morphogenesis. Ann Rev Biochem 54:135-169.

Edelman GM (1985b). Specific cell adhesion in histogenesis and morphogenesis. In Edelman GM, Thiery J-P (eds): "The Cell in Contact," New York: John Wiley & Sons, in press.

Edelman GM, Gallin WJ, Delouvée A, Cunningham BA, Thiery J-P (1983). Early epochal maps of two different cell adhesion molecules. Proc Natl Acad Sci USA 81:4384-4388.

Gallin WJ, Edelman GM, Cunningham BA (1983). Characterization of L-CAM, a major cell adhesion molecule from embryonic liver cells. Proc Natl Acad Sci USA 80:1038-1042.

Greenberg ME, Brackenbury R, Edelman GM (1984). Alteration of neural cell adhesion molecule (N-CAM) expression after neuronal cell transformation by Rous sarcoma virus. Proc Natl Acad Sci USA 81:969-973.

Grumet M, Edelman GM (1984). Heterotypic binding between neuronal membrane vesicles and glial cells is mediated by a specific neuron-glial cell adhesion molecule. J Cell Biol 98:1746-1756.

Grumet M, Hoffman S, Chuong C-M, Edelman GM (1984). Polypeptide components and binding functions of neuron-glia adhesion molecules. Proc Natl Acad Sci USA 81:7989-7993.

Jacobson A (1966). Inductive processes in embryonic development. Science 152:25-34.

Sengel P (1976). "Morphogenesis of Skin." New York: Cambridge Univ. Press.

Thiery J-P, Duband J-L, Rutishauser U, Edelman GM (1982). Cell adhesion molecules in early chick embryogenesis. Proc Natl Acad Sci USA 79:6737-6741.

Thiery J-P, Delouvée A, Grumet M, Edelman GM (1985). Initial appearance and regional distribution of the neuron-glia cell adhesion molecule (Ng-CAM) in the chick embryo. J Cell Biol 100:442-456.

Thiery J-P, Delouvée A, Gallin WJ, Cunningham BA, Edelman GM (1984). Ontogenetic expression of cell adhesion molecules: L-CAM is found in epithelia derived from the three primary germ layers. Dev Biol 102:61-78.

Cellular Endocrinology: Hormonal Control of Embryonic
and Cellular Differentiation, pages 93–102
© 1986 Alan R. Liss, Inc.

HORMONAL AND NON-HORMONAL FEATURES OF SELECTED EPITHELIAL-
MESENCHYMAL INTERACTIONS DURING DEVELOPMENT

Harold C. Slavkin, Tina F. Jaskoll,
Mary MacDougall and Margarita Zeichner-David

Graduate Program in Craniofacial Biology and
Department of Biological Sciences, School of
Dentistry, University of Southern California,
Los Angeles, California 90089-0191.

INTRODUCTION

Following the primary induction processes associated
with neurulation during early embryogenesis, secondary
inductive or epithelial-mesenchymal interactions are described as associated with many examples of organogenesis
such as limb morphogenesis, thyroid, salivary gland,
thymus, heart, mammary, lung and tooth organogenesis (see
reviews by Grobstein, 1967; Saxen et al, 1976; Dhouailly
and Sengel, 1983; Kollar, 1983; Slavkin et al, 1984).

Epithelial-mesenchymal interactions are defined as
tissue interactions which result in profound changes in one
or both of the tissue interactants. More recently,
regional mesenchyme-derived specificity has been implicated
as the instructive source of information for adjacent
epithelial differentiation (see reviews by Kollar, 1983;
Slavkin et al, 1984). However, despite the decades of research attempting to isolate and characterize putative instructive molecules, tissue-specific "morphogens" have not
as yet been characterized and shown to be inductive for
differential gene expression in all responding epithelia.
The nature of intercellular communication associated with
inductive events during embryogenesis has remained a
difficult challenge to developmental biologists in part due
to the numerous and confounding variables related to
experimentation.

The recent advent of serumless and chemically-defined
medium culture conditions has provided a fresh approach to

the classical problem of epithelial-mesenchymal interactions (see reviews by Tomkins, 1975; Serrero et al, 1979;
Slavkin et al, 1982a). Somewhat surprising, a number of
complex embryonic organ systems appear to be capable of expressing sophisticated developmental programs in serumless
and chemically-defined culture conditions. This paper reports a number of recent observations which describe
morphogenesis and differentiation of complex organ systems
in vitro without serum or hormonal supplementation. In the
absence of serum or hormonal supplementation, dental ectomesenchyme differentiated into odontoblasts which produce
dentine phosphoprotein, ectodermally-derived epithelia differentiated into ameloblasts which produce enamel-specific
proteins, and endodermally-derived lung epithelia differentiated into alveolar type II cells which produce pulmonary surfactant. Mesenchyme-derived regional controls
for epithelial-specific gene expression would appear to reside within a "metabolic cooperativity" resulting from
epithelialmesenchymal interactions associated with embryonic and fetal tooth or lung organogenesis in vitro.

DEVELOPMENT OF SELECTED EMBRYONIC TISSUES USING SERUMLESS,
CHEMICALLY-DEFINED MEDIUM IN ORGAN CULTURE

A useful technique for investigating morphogenesis and
regulatory processes related to cytodifferentiation is
organ culture in vitro (Wessells, 1967). The discovery of
permissive conditions for obtaining both morphogenesis and
differentiation has been dependent upon several critical
experimental decisions: 1) developmental stage (e.g.,
preferably before overt vascularization of the organ rudiment), 2) nutrients in the medium, 3) supplements to the
medium (e.g. serum, embryonic extracts, hormones, growth
factors), 4) physical variables such as substrate (e.g.
biomatrix) used to support the organ explant, 5) concentrations of atmospheric gases, and 6) relative humidity.
Under optimal conditions, determination and differentiation
of specific phenotypes in vitro and the degree of morphogenesis expressed in organ culture should be comparable to
the in vivo developmental processes.

Using a serumless and chemically-defined medium and the
modified Trowell procedure (Trowell, 1954; Yamada et al,
1980), we have cultured a number of different organ systems
in vitro including cap stage tooth organs (see review
Slavkin et al, 1982a) and embryonic lung primordia. In

Table 1. Specific Phenotypes Expressed De Novo in Serum-less, Chemically-Defined Medium Using a Modified Trowell Method of Organ Culture

Selected Organ	Developmental Expression	Reference
Mouse (Mus musculus) (C57BL/6 and Swiss Webster)		
Theiler[a] stage 25 cap stage molars	Dentinogenesis and amelogenesis	b.
Mouse (Mus musculus) (B10.A)		
Theiler stage 20 lung primordia	Alveolar Respiratory Unit Development (e.g. type II cells)	c.

a. Theiler (1972)
b. Yamada et al (1980)
   Slavkin et al (1982b)
c. Jaskoll et al (in press)

each example, our experimental strategy was to test the hypothesis that both differentiation and morphogenesis are determined and maintained in the absence of serum or other exogenous factors. We assumed that the embryonic explants were intrinsically capable of becoming determined and would differentiate and express morphogenesis as the result of reciprocal epithelial-mesenchymal interactions; this suggests a "metabolic cooperativity" between heterotypic tissues as proposed by Tomkins (1975). To test this assumption, careful selection of developmental stage of the embryonic rudiment is imperativeto insure that the cell types were not determined and differentiated before the initiation of the experiment.

CAP STAGE TOOTH ORGAN CULTURE

Molar tooth organs consist of an ectodermally-derived enamel organ epithelia, and a cranial neural crest-derived dental papilla ectomesenchyme. Epithelium immediately adjacent to ectomesenchyme tissue is termed inner enamel epithelia; the juxtaposed ectomesenchyme cells along the perimeter of the dental papilla tissue termed progenitor odontoblasts. As the direct consequence of reciprocal epithelial-mesenchymal interactions, a number of studies have demonstrated dental morphogenesis as well as cytodifferentiation using recombinants of these tissue-types in organ cultures dependent upon serum and embryonic extract supplementation (see reviews by Slavkin, 1979; Slavkin et al, 1984; Kollar, 1983; Kollar, 1972; Koch, 1972). Recently, early mouse cap stage tooth organs have been cultured in serumless and chemically-defined medium and these explants expressed overt morphogenesis and cytodifferentiation (Table 1) (see Yamada et al, 1980; Slavkin et al, 1982a; Slavkin et al, 1982b).

Enamel Proteins. The biochemical phenotype of the mouse ameloblast consists of a family of enamel proteins containing the subfamily of acidic glycoproteins enamelins, and a subfamily of hydrophobic, relatively basic and proline-rich amelogenins (Termine et al, 1980; Slavkin et al, 1982b; Slavkin et al, 1984). The mouse ameloblast appears to express a major enamelin (pI 5.5) and three different amelogenins (pI circa 6.5-7.0)(Snead et al, 1983). Enamelins and amelogenins appear to share common epitopes, and are found to be antigenically cross-reactive using either rabbit anti-mouse amelogenin polyclonal or rabbit anti-human enamelin polyclonal antibodies (see Slavkin et al, 1982b; Zeichner-David et al, 1983; Slavkin et al, 1984). The developmental program for the activation and expression of the enamel proteins during mouse cap stage molar tooth organogenesis in vitro does not depend upon serum or embryonic extract supplementation.

Dentine Phosphoprotein. The biochemical phenotype of the odontoblast is characterized by the non-collagenous acidic dentine phosphoprotein (DPP). In the developing mouse tooth organ, dentine phosphoprotein has a molecular weight of approximately 72 kilodaltons (MacDougall et al, in press). Dot-immunobinding assay, Western transfer techniques and indirect immunofluorescent microscopy procedures have confirmed that odontoblasts differentiate and express DPP in organ culture without serum, embryonic extract or hormone supplementations (MacDougall et al, 1985). These observations suggest that the developmental program for the expression of DPP during odontoblast differentiation is not under hormonal regulation. One curious caveat, however, is that the dentine phosphoprotein is not secreted from odontoblasts in the absence of hormonal supplementation (unpublished observations).

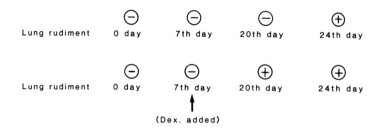

Figure 1. Cultured lung tissue response to dexamethasone.
Lung rudiments have been cultured for up to 24 days in vitro in
serumless and chemically-defined medium and evaluated for the presence
(+) or absence (-) of type II alveolar cells and surfactant proteins.
The addition of dexamethasone (Dex., $10^{-8}M$) to the culture medium
results in the accelerated appearance of type II cells and surfactant
proteins on the 20th day in vitro.

Embryonic Lung Primordia in Organ Culture

The mouse lung develops from paired endodermal epithelial buds embedded in undifferentiated mesenchyme (Hilfer,
1983). Thereafter, epithelial-mesenchymal interactions appear to influence specific epithelial branching patterns
(Spooner and Wessells, 1970; Masters, 1976) and subsequent
epithelial cell differentiation (Smith and Sabry, 1983;
Beer et al, 1984; Jaskoll and Slavkin, 1984). Hormones
(e.g. glucocorticosteroids) appear to stimulate and accelerate lung development (Kotas and Avery, 1971; Kikkawa
et al, 1971; Smith, 1979; Honig et al, 1984). These hormonal effects are probably mediated through the mesenchyme
(Smith, 1979; Beer et al, 1984). Glucocorticosteroids
stimulate fetal lung fibroblasts to release a factor which
enhances alveolar type II cell differentiation and the subsequent synthesis and secretion of pulmonary surfactant
(Smith, 1979). Beer et al (1984) have recently investigated specific [3H] dexamethasone binding in mesenchymal
cells during early stages of mouse lung development. Their
results suggest an hormonal effect on epithelial- mesenchymal interactions during lung morphogenesis.

Recently studies were designed to test the hypothesis
that early embryonic mouse lung primordia become determined
and will differentiate into alveolar type II cells in vitro
in the absence of extrinsic humoral factors. Theiler stage

20 (12 days gestation) mouse lung primordia have been cultured in serumless and chemically-defined medium and these explants expressed overt morphogenesis and cytodifferentiation (Table 1) (Jaskoll et al, in press). Alveolar type II cells are observed after 24 days in vitro (Fig. 1). The addition of dexamethasone (10^{-8}M) on the 7th day in culture results in the appearance of type II cells on the 20th day in vitro (Fig. 1) (Jaskoll et al, in preparation). Surprisingly, the addition of dexamethasone on day zero of culture results in increased cellular necrosis (unpublished data).

Surfactant Proteins. The biochemical phenotype of the alveolar type II cell is characterized by pulmonary surfactant proteins (King, 1979; King and MacBeth, 1979). The major monomeric form of mouse surfactant protein is a non-serum acidic glycoprotein of approximately 35 kilodaltons under reducing conditions; a less abundant form is a 45 kilodalton polypeptide (Jaskoll et al, 1984). Western transfer techniques and indirect immunofluorescence microscopy using rabbit anti-human surfactant proteins polyclonal antibodies have demonstrated the synthesis and secretion of pulmonary surfactant proteins in organ culture in both the presence and absence of hormonal supplementation (Jaskoll et al, in preparation). The developmental program for type II cell cytodifferentiation and the expression of surfactant proteins is not dependent on serum or hormonal supplementation. Hormones appear to regulate the timing and rate of expression during lung morphogenesis.

CONCLUSION

A major problem in developmental biology remains the dissection of intrinsic from extrinsic regulatory processes during embryogenesis. How much regulation is intrinsic to a developing embryonic organ system, and what aspects of organogenesis require extrinsic humoral factors? We have hypothesized that intrinsic epithelial-mesenchymal interactions reflect a unique "metabolic cooperativity" (in the terms of the late Gordon Tomkins) independent from hormonal regulation. We have selected embryonic mouse lung and tooth organogenesis to investigate this problem employing either serum or selected hormone supplementation or cultures using serumless and chemically-defined medium without hormone supplementation. We find that both lung and tooth organogenesis are expressed in terms of morphogenesis as well as cytodifferentiation in serumless and chemically-defined medium without hormone supplementation. Ecto-dermally-derived, ectomesenchyme-derived and endodermal-ly-derived biochemical phenotypes are expressed within the developmental programs of either the tooth or lung organo-gens in vitro. Our preliminary evidence would suggest that hormones effect the timing and rates of expression in the developing lung and tooth organ systems, but intrinsic epithelial-mesenchymal interactions seem to mediate the qualitative changes associated with morphogenesis and cell differentiation.

ACKNOWLEDGEMENTS

We dedicate this paper to Gordon M. Tomkins (1926-1975) who was usually a decade ahead of the intellectual milieu of his time. His critical model for the evolution of bio-logical regulation and the origin of hormone mediated intercellular communication (1975) remains a challenge for all of us. We also wish to thank Mr. Scott Trowbridge for help in preparing this manuscript. These studies were sup-ported in part by research grants DE-02848, DEO-6425, HL-28325 and training grant DE-07006, National Institute of Health.

REFERENCES

Beer DG, Butley MS, Cunha GR, Malkinson AM (1984). Auto-radiographic localization of specific [^{3}H] dexametha-sone binding in fetal lung. Dev Biol 105:351-364.
Dhouailly D, Sengel P (1983). Feather forming properties of the foot integument in avian embryos. In Sawyer RH, Fallon JF (eds) "Epithelial-Mesenchymal Interactions in Development," New York: Praeger Publishers, pp 147-161.
Grobstein C (1967). Mechanisms of organogenetic tissue interaction. Natl Cancer Inst Monogr 26:279-299.
Hilfer SR (1983). Development of terminal buds in the fetal mouse lung. Scan Electron Microsc 3:1387-1401.
Honig LS, Smith BT, Slavkin HC, Donahue HG (1984). Influence of the major histocompatibility complex (H2) on glucocorticoid-stimulated pulmonary surfactant synthesis in two congenic mouse strains. Proc Soc Exp Biol Med 176:419-425.

Jaskoll TF, Don G, Johnson R, Slavkin HC (in preparation). In vitro development of embryonic mouse lung in chemically-defined culture conditions

Jaskoll TF, Johnson R, Don G, Slavkin HC (in press). Embryonic mouse lung morphogenesis in serumless, chemically-defined medium in vitro. In Slavkin HC (ed): "Proceedings of the Tenth Congress of ISDB," New York: Alan R. Liss.

Jaskoll TF, Phelps D, Taeusch HW, Smith BT, Slavkin HC (1984). Localization of pulmonary surfactant protein during mouse lung development. Dev Biol 106:256-261.

Jaskoll TF, Slavkin HC (1984). Ultrastructural and immunofluorescence studies of basal lamina alterations during mouse lung morphogenesis. Differentiation 28:36-48.

Kikkawa Y, Kaibara M, Motoyama EK, Orazalesi MM, Cook CD (1971). Morphologic development of fetal rabbit lung and its acceleration with cortisol. Amer J Pathol 64:423-442.

King RJ (1974). The surfactant system of the lung. Fed Proc 33:2238-2247.

King RJ, MacBeth MC (1979). Physiochemical properties of dipalmitoyl phosphatidylcholine after interaction with an apolipoprotein of pulmonary surfactant. Biochim Biophys Acta 557:86-101.

Koch WE (1972). Tissue interaction during in vitro odontogenesis. In Slavkin HC, Bavetta LA (eds): "Developmental Aspects of Oral Biology," New York: Academic Press, pp 151-164.

Kollar EJ (1972). Histogenetic aspects of dermal-epidermal interactions. In Slavkin HC, Bavetta LA (eds): "Developmental Aspects of Oral Biology," New York: Academic Press, pp 125-149.

Kollar EJ (1983). Epithelial-mesenchymal interactions in the mammalian integumet: Tooth development as a model for instructive induction. In Sawyer RH, Fallon JF (eds): "Epithelial-Mesenchymal Interactions in Development," New York: Praeger Publishers, pp 27-49.

Kotas RV, Avery ME (1971). Accelerated appearance of pulmonary surfactant in the fetal rabbit. J Appl Physiol 30:358-361.

MacDougall M, Zeichner-David M, Bringas P, Slavkin HC (1985). Dentine phosphoprotein expression during in vitro mouse tooth organ culture. In Butler WT (ed): "The Chemistry and Biology of Mineralized Tissues," Birmingham: EBSCO Media, pp 177-181.

MacDougall M, Zeichner-David M, Slavkin HC (in press). Production and characterization of antibodies against murine dentine phosphoprotein. J Biochem.

Masters JRW (1976). Epithelial-mesenchymal interaction during lung development: The effect of mesenchymal mass. Dev Biol 51:98-108.

Saxen L, Karkinen-Jaaskelainen M, Lehtoneu E, Nordling S, Wartiovaara J (1976). Inductive tissue interactions. In Poste G, Nicolson GL (eds): "The Cell Surface in Animal Embryogenesis and Development," New York: North Holland Publishing Co., pp 331-407.

Serrero GR, McClure DB, Sato GH (1979). Growth of mouse 3T3 fibroblasts in serum-free hormone-supplemented media. In Sato GH, Ross R (eds): "Hormones and Cell Culture," Cold Spring, NY: Cold Spring Harbor Laboratory, pp 523-530.

Slavkin HC (1979). The nature and nuture of epithelial-mesenchymal interactions during tooth morphogenesis. J Biol Buccale 6:189-203.

Slavkin HC, Honig LS, Bringas P (1982a). Experimental dissection of avian and murine tissue interactions using organ culture in a serumless medium free from exogenous (nondefined) factors. In Sarnat B, Dixon AD (eds): "Factors and Mechanisms Influencing Bone Growth," New York: Alan R. Liss, pp 217-228.

Slavkin HC, Snead ML, Zeichner-David M, Jaskoll TF, Smith BT (1984). Concepts of epithelial-mesenchymal interactions during development: Tooth and lung organogenesis. J Cell Biochem 26:117-125.

Slavkin HC, Zeichner-David M, MacDougall M, Bringas P, Bessem C, Honig LS (1982b). Antibodies to murine amelogenins: Localization of enamel proteins during tooth organ development in vitro. Differentiation 23:73-82.

Smith BT (1979). Lung maturation in the fetal rat: Acceleration by the injection of fibroblast-pneumocyte factor. Science 204:1094-1095.

Smith BT, Sabry K (1983). Glucocorticoid-thyroid synergism in lung maturation: A mechanism involving epithelial-mesenchymal interactions. Proc Natl Acad Sci USA 80:1951-1954.

Snead ML, Zeichner-David M, Chandra T, Robson KJH, Woo SLC, Slavkin HC (1983). Construction and identification of mouse amelogenin cDNA clones. Proc Natl Acad Sci USA 80:7254-7258.

Spooner BS, Wessells NK (1970). Mammalian lung development: Interactions in primordium formation and branchial morphogenesis. J Exp Zool 175:445-454.

Termine JD, Belcourt AB, Christner PJ, Conn KM, Nylen MU (1980). Properties of dissociatively extracted fetal tooth matrix proteins. I.Principal molecular species in developing bovine enamel. J Biol Chem 255:9760-9768.

Theiler K (1972). "The House Mouse." New York: Springer-Verlag.

Tomkins GM (1975). The metabolic code. Science 189:760-763.

Trowell OA (1954). A modified technique for organ culture in vitro. Exp Cell Res 6:246-258.

Wessels NK (1967). Avian and mammalian organ culture. In Wilt F, Wessels NK (eds): "Methods in Developmental Biology," New York: Thomas Y. Crowell Co., pp 445-456.

Yamada M, Bringas P, Grodin M, MacDougall M, Slavkin HC (1980). Chemically-defined organ culture of embryonic mouse tooth organs: Morphogenesis, dentinogenesis and amelogenesis. J Biol Buccale 8:127-139.

Zeichner-David M, MacDougall M, Slavkin HC (1983). Enamelin gene expression during fetal and neonatal rabbit tooth organogenesis. Differentiation 25:148-155.

Cellular Endocrinology: Hormonal Control of Embryonic and Cellular Differentiation, pages 103-113
© 1986 Alan R. Liss, Inc.

APICAL ECTODERMAL RIDGE MAINTENANCE IN OVO AND IN VITRO

John F. Fallon, Eugenie L. Boutin and
Jill L. Carrington

Department of Anatomy, University of Wisconsin,
Madison, Wisconsin, USA, 53706

OVERVIEW

Vertebrate limb buds are composed of mesoderm and overlying ectoderm. These two tissues participate in what might be described as a dialogue during limb development. Bud shaped structures arise along the body wall in amniote tetrapods. The dorsal and ventral limb bud epithelia are simple cuboidal with overlying simple squamous periderm, while at the apex there is a specialized ridge of epithelium called the apical ectodermal ridge (Saunders, 1948). In reptiles and birds the ridge is a pseudo-stratified columnar epithelium (Fallon and Kelley, 1977).

Saunders (1948) surgically removed the apical ridge from the chick wing bud and demonstrated it is necessary for the determination of skeletal parts. This work also showed that the ridge does not regenerate and that skeletal parts are laid down in a proximal to distal sequence (see also Summerbell, 1974; Rowe and Fallon, 1982). It is clear from these data that the apical ridge is required for the mesodermal component of the limb bud to develop its prospective fate.

Kieny (1960) and Saunders and Reuss (1974) grafted limb level mesoderm, without ectoderm, to non-limb forming flank before the apical ridge had formed. They found that an apical ridge developed in the healed flank ectoderm. This demonstrated that the mesoderm induces the apical ridge in competent ectoderm (see also Carrington and Fallon, 1984a).

Zwilling (1955) designed a technique for combining

limb bud ectoderm and mesoderm from different sources to make a recombinant limb bud. Using trypsin and EDTA to separate the two components it was possible to combine a leg ectodermal jacket with a wing mesodermal core. When this was done a wing developed. In the reverse recombinant a leg developed. This simple, elegant experiment demonstrated that the ridge stimulus to the subjacent mesoderm does not specify the type of appendage which will form. The information for fore- or hindlimb is carried by the mesoderm.

From the foregoing it is clear that the limb bud mesoderm induces the apical ridge which in turn permits the proximal to distal elaboration of limb parts over developmental time.

APICAL RIDGE MAINTENANCE

There is a long history to the possible special relationship of the mesoderm to the maintenance of the morphology and vitality of the apical ridge. Initially Saunders (1949) reported that a thin impermeable mica barrier placed between the mesoderm and apical ridge caused the ridge to flatten. Further, if the ridge was isolated in culture its cells rapidly became necrotic (Searls and Zwilling, 1964; Boutin and Fallon, 1984). Moreover, it would appear that even the brief separation of the limb mesoderm and ectoderm to make a recombinant limb bud caused the ridge to flatten and some of its cells died. However, in such recombinants a healthy ridge was seen 24 hours after recombination (Searls and Zwilling, 1964). Interestingly enough, if somite or flank mesoderm was substituted for limb bud mesoderm in recombinant limbs the ridge flattened, its cells died and no ridge was seen at 24 hours (Searls and Zwilling, 1964).

While there are a variety of possible interpretations of the above results, the simplest one is that the apical ridge requires something from limb mesoderm to maintain its form and to stay alive. Other evidence from the study of chick limb mutants has been adduced to make this same point.

Zwilling used the recombinant limb procedure to advantage in analyzing mutants. Polydactylous limb buds

show more extensive anterior apical ridge thickening than
normal and the limbs develop with extra digits. When
polydactylous limb bud mesoderm was combined with normal
limb ectoderm, the ridge became more extensive anteriorly
and the recombinant developed extra digits (Zwilling and
Hansborough, 1956). In the reverse recombinant the mutant
anterior ridge flattened and no extra digits formed.
Thus, it is a property of the mesoderm which determines
the anterior extent of the apical ridge even after the
ridge is induced. It is possible that this mesodermal
mutant has more extensive maintenance activity than is
normal.

American wingless is a simple Mendelian recessive
gene, carried on an autosomal chromosome, which brings
about no wings and variable leg development in
homozygotes. This is an interesting mutant because limb
buds with apical ridges do arise in all 4 limb sites on
affected embryos. However, the ridges on the wing buds
always regress with resultant forelimb amelia. The leg
bud ridges may regress at varying times, or not at all,
causing ectromelia or normal limbs, respectively. When
recombinant limbs were made using wingless components with
normal limb bud components it was found that neither
wingless ectoderm nor mesoderm gave outgrowths (Zwilling,
1956). Because the apical ridge regressed in wingless and
in the recombinants, Zwilling reasoned wingless lacked the
factor necessary for ridge maintenance and, further, that
the wingless ridge was irreversibly injured by contact
with the wingless mesoderm. This would account for the
mutant ridge's failure to function when combined with
normal mesoderm.

NEW EXPERIMENTAL APPROACHES WITH WINGLESS

Because of its central place in the problem of apical
ridge maintenance we have begun a re-examination of the
wingless mutant to assess the problem of the germ layer
involved (Carrington and Fallon, 1984b) and the
distribution of limb derived muscles (Lanser and Fallon,
in preparation). It was apparent from Zwilling's work
that limb bud recombinant techniques would not permit an
answer to the question of whether limb bud ectoderm or
mesoderm is primarily affected by the mutant gene. We
therefore designed a procedure to combine donor ectoderm

with wing field mesoderm at stage 15 before the limb bud arises (Carrington and Fallon, 1984a). This technique is outlined in Figure 1. Control experiments using quail flank donor ectoderm demonstrated that a ridge was induced in the donor quail ectoderm. Distally complete limbs were produced in the majority (86%) of cases and donor quail ectoderm covered the limb throughout development. When the same procedure was done on wingless embryos a distally complete wing developed in nearly all (90%) of the cases (Figure 1b).

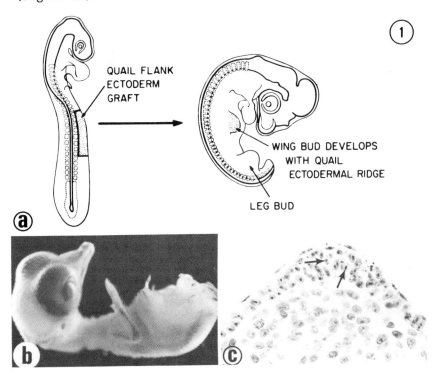

Figure 1. a. Drawing of the pre-limb bud recombinant technique. Stage 15 quail ectoderm grafted to st. 15 prospective chick wing mesoderm. b. Day 11 wingless embryo received a quail flank ectoderm graft at st. 15, a distally complete wing developed. c. Pre-limb bud recombinant sectioned at st. 23. The apical ridge of quail cells is distinguished from chick mesoderm by large heterochromatin clumps in quail nuclei (arrows). The contralateral wingless bud had regressed (X 360).

Under these experimental conditions where the <u>wingless</u>
mesoderm was provided with a normal ectoderm before a bud
formed, a normal ridge was induced in the donor ectoderm
by the mutant mesoderm (Figure 1c). That ridge was also
maintained by the <u>wingless</u> mesoderm and a normal wing
formed. It would appear that <u>wingless</u> is an ectodermal
mutant.

We were faced with the question of why Zwilling could
not get normal wing development by providing <u>wingless</u> limb
bud mesoderm with a normal ectodermal jacket. To begin to
address this we repeated his limb bud recombinant
experiments using normal ectoderm and <u>wingless</u> mesoderm.
Control recombinants gave 70% distally complete
outgrowths. However, <u>wingless</u> limb bud mesoderm plus
normal ectoderm in all cases failed to form wings. In
fact, recognizable wing parts never formed.

These results confirm Zwilling's (1956) data.
However, our data on early recombinants and his (and our
own) data on limb bud recombinants appear to conflict.
There is the possibility that manipulating the <u>wingless</u>
limb bud mesoderm has deleterious effects. Note that the
<u>wingless</u> limb field mesoderm stays in place when the early
recombinant procedure is carried out. To test this we
carried out a double recombinant procedure on normal and
<u>wingless</u> embryos. This is shown in Figure 2.

DOUBLE RECOMBINANT PROCEDURE

When an early recombinant was made at stage 15 on a normal embryo, and the mesoderm of the bud which formed was then used for a limb bud recombinant, normal distally complete limbs formed, Figure 3. When this procedure was done on wingless mesoderm distally complete wings formed. However, when compared to normal mesoderm put through the same procedure these limbs were not as robust and there were fewer distally complete wings.

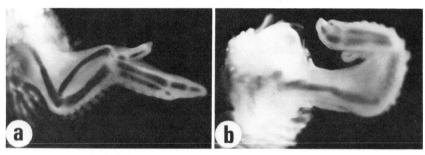

Figure 3. Distally complete limbs resulting from double recombinant procedures using (a) normal mesoderm or (b) wingless mesoderm.

WINGLESS ECTODERM FAILS TO CONFER MAINTENANCE ABILITY ON THE MESODERM

We propose that there is a necessary interaction between the ectoderm and the limb field mesoderm which at a later stage, permits the limb bud mesoderm to maintain the apical ridge. This ectoderm-mesodermal interaction must occur around stage 15. Such an interaction had not been recognized heretofore. It is important to note that if this interaction fails, budding and ridge formation will still occur. However, because the ridge subsequently cannot be maintained the bud is doomed to fail.

We recognize that the wingless gene may also directly affect the mesoderm making it more sensitive to manipulation. It is possible that normal ectoderm may somehow correct the defect. Our experiments do not permit us to distinguish this. Such a dilemma is inherent in all tissue recombinant experiments. Landauer (1944) pointed this out clearly in his critique of these experimental procedures. However, the fact remains that the simplest interpretation of all of the information on the wingless mutant is that the gene affects the ectoderm primarily and the mesoderm secondarily.

HOW IS RIDGE MAINTENANCE ACCOMPLISHED?

With any system as complicated as the developing limb it would be helpful to be able to simplify the system as much as possible. One means of doing this is to place the components in culture. However, as already noted, the apical ridge cells die in isolated culture. Tissue culture studies have demonstrated that the ridge cells will live when cultured in association with limb mesoderm (Globus and Vethameny-Globus, 1976; Solursh et al., 1981) or even when separated by porous filters (Milaire and Mulnard, 1968; Gumpel Pinot, 1981). This raises the possibility that ridge maintenance is accomplished by diffusible factors from the mesoderm. We have just completed a careful fine structure study of the epithelial-mesenchymal interface at the ridge during stages 17-24. It is clear that there was always an intact basal lamina between the two tissues (Fuldner and Fallon, in preparation). This affirms the likelihood of maintenance by diffusible substances.

Interestingly enough there is information that living mesodermal cells may not be required for maintenance. Jorquera et al., (1979) have shown ridge vitality and function can be maintained when cultured in a 33% limb or flank mesodermal extract. This sort of approach is encouraging for it shows the possibility of isolating the maintenance activity and analyzing it. At the same time tissue extracts are extraordinarily complicated to work with.

INSULIN MAINTAINS THE APICAL RIDGE IN CULTURE

We have taken another approach to the problem by testing known growth factors on ridge vitality in culture. The procedure is shown in Figure 4. Among the factors we have tested are insulin, transferrin, selenium, epidermal growth factor and insulin-like growth factor II. Of these, only insulin proved effective in keeping the ridge cells alive in culture. In initial studies (Boutin and Fallon, 1984) we found that 5 ug/ml of insulin

significantly improved survival over controls of stage 20
and 25 ridges cultured for 24 hours. In fact the number
of dying cells was similar to that found at zero time,
while ridge cultures without insulin were massively
necrotic by 12 hours.

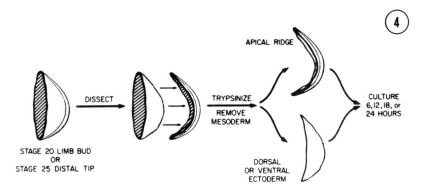

Figure 4. Drawing depicting procedure used to put limb bud
apical ridge into culture.

While 5 ug/ml is standard for tissue culture
supplement, it is much higher than physiological levels.
In fact at this concentration it is known that insulin may
occupy its own receptor and those of the insulin-like
growth factors (IGF's) as well (Rechler et al., 1977). It
is important to establish why insulin has its effect on
ridge cells in culture. We are taking several approaches
to this at the same time. One of these is to lower the
insulin concentration to ranges where one would not expect
to involve IGF receptors. We have been successful in
keeping ridge cells alive for at least 18 hours with an
insulin supplement of 50 ng (8.5 pM)/ml, compare Figure 5a
and 5b. An equally important approach is to demonstrate
insulin binding to ridge cells. These experiments are in
progress. They are difficult at best because of the very
small quantity of material which can be obtained from each
embryo.

Another aspect of the problem is whether ridge
function is retained after 18 to 24 hours in culture.
Because the ridge cells are alive does not mean they have

retained function. These experiments also are in
progress. We have been successful in culturing isolated
ridges in 50 ng/ml of insulin for 12 hours, combining the
ridge with a stage 18 mesoderm and getting distally
complete outgrowths.

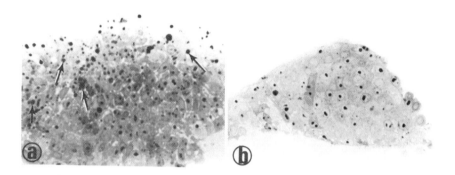

Figure 5. a. Section through a stage 20 apical ridge
grown for 18 hours in culture medium without insulin
supplementation, massive necrosis is evident. Arrows
point to pycnotic nuclei. b. Section through a stage 20
apical ridge grown for 18 hours in culture medium
supplemented with 50 ng/ml insulin, the majority of cells
are healthy.

CONCLUSION

    Many questions and problems remain to be answered on
apical ridge maintenance. It is inferred that limb
mesoderm may be specific in its maintenance ability.
However, the work of Jorquera, alluded to above, indicated
flank mesoderm extracts have some maintenance activity.
Thus, it is possible that the limb mesoderm is high in a
property shared by all mesoderm. In this context it is
interesting that insulin is present in the early chick
embryo (DePablo et al., 1982). It is possible at these
early stages insulin may be acting as a growth factor _in
ovo_ . Considering this we are encouraged to continue our
studies on the premise that _in vitro_ maintenance of the
apical ridge with insulin may have an _in ovo_ correlate.
Another aspect of the problem is to ascertain how a single
gene change can apparently prevent the ectoderm from
conferring the maintenance ability to the mesoderm. As

more is learned about insulin and maintenance we will turn
to the <u>wingless</u> mutant as a possible test system.

ACKNOWLEDGEMENTS

This work was supported by NIH Grant # T32HD07118 and
NSF Grant # PCM8406338. We thank Lucy Taylor for making
the drawings. We express special gratitide to B. Kay
Simandl for her contributions to all aspects of this work
and for typing the manuscript.

REFERENCES

Boutin EL, Fallon JF (1984). An analysis of the fate of
    the chick wing bud apical ectodermal ridge in culture.
    Devel Biol 104:111-116.
Carrington JL, Fallon JF (1984a). The stages of flank
    ectoderm capable of responding to ridge induction in the
    chick embryo. J Embryol Exp Morphol 84:19-34.
Carrington JL, Fallon JF (1984b). Evidence that the
    ectoderm is the affected germ layer in the <u>wingless</u>
    mutant chick embryo. J Exp Zool 232:297-308.
DePablo F, Roth J, Hernandez E, Pruss RM (1982). Insulin
    is present in chicken eggs and early chick embryos.
    Endocrinology 111:1909-1916.
Fallon JF, Kelley RO (1977). The ultrastructural analysis
    of the apical ectodermal ridge during vertebrate limb
    morphogenesis. II. J Embryol Exp Morph 41:223-232.
Globus M, Vethameny-Globus S (1976). An <u>in vitro</u> analogue
    of early chick limb bud outgrowth. Differentiation
    6:91-96.
Gumpel-Pinot M (1981). Ectoderm-mesoderm interactions in
    relation to limb-bud chondrogenesis in the chick
    embryo: Transfilter cultures and ultrastructural
    studies. J Embryol Exp Morphol 65:73-87.
Jorquera B, Molinari E, Goicoechea O, Garrido O (1979).
    Involución <u>in vitro</u> , regeneración y actividad funcional
    de la zona de la cresta apical ectodérmica del esbozo
    del miembro de pollo. Zbl Vet Med C Anat Histol Embryol
    8:262-276.
Kieny M (1960). Rôle inducteur du mésoderme dans la
    différenciation précoce du bourgeon de membre chez
    l'embryon de poulet. J Embrol Exp Morphol 8:457-467.
Landauer W (1944). Transplantation as a tool of

developmental genetics. Am Nat 78:280-284.

Milaire J, Mulnard J (1968). Le rôle de l'épiblaste dans la chondrogénèse du bourgeon de membre chez la souris. J Embryol Exp Morphol 20:215-236.

Rechler MM, Podskalny JM, Nissley SP (1977). Characterization of the binding of multiplication-stimulating activity to a receptor for growth polypeptides in chick embryo fibroblasts. J Biol Chem 252:3898-3910.

Rowe DA, Fallon JF (1982). The proximodistal determination of skeletal parts in the developing chick leg. J Embryol Exp Morphol 68:1-7.

Saunders JW,Jr (1948). The proximo-distal sequence of the origin of parts of the chick wing and the role of the apical ectoderm. J Exp Zool 108:363-404.

Saunders JW,Jr (1949). An analysis of the role of the apical ridge in the development of the limb bud in the chick. Anat Rec 105:567-568.

Saunders JW,Jr, Reuss C (1974). Induction and axial properties of prospective wing bud mesoderm in the chick embryo. Devel Biol 38:41-50.

Searls RL, Zwilling E (1964). Regeneration of the apical ectodermal ridge of the chick limb bud. Devel Biol 9:35-55.

Solursh M, Singley CT, Reuter RS (1981). The influence of epithelia on cartilage and loose connective tissue formation by limb mesenchyme cultures. Devel Biol 86:471-482.

Summerbell D (1974). A quantitative analysis of the effect of excision of the AER from the chick limb bud. J Embryol Exp Morphol 32:651-660.

Zwilling E (1955). Ectoderm-mesoderm relationship in the development of the chick embryo limb bud. J Exp Zool 128:423-442.

Zwilling E (1956). Interaction between limb bud ectoderm and mesoderm. IV. J Exp Zool 132:241-254.

Zwilling E, Hansborough LA (1956). Interaction between limb bud ectoderm and mesoderm in the chick embryo. III. J Exp Zool 132:219-240.

Cellular Endocrinology: Hormonal Control of Embryonic
and Cellular Differentiation, pages 115–126
© 1986 Alan R. Liss, Inc.

EVIDENCE FOR THE TRANSMISSION OF DORSOVENTRAL
INFORMATION TO THE ECTODERM DURING THE EARLIEST
STAGES OF LIMB DEVELOPMENT

Jane S. Geduspan and Jeffrey A. MacCabe

Department of Zoology, University of Tennessee
Knoxville, TN 37996

INTRODUCTION

The early development of the avian limb is characterized
by a series of interactions between the mesodermal and ectodermal
components.   For example, the prospective and early limb
mesoderm induces the formation of the apical ectodermal ridge
(Kieny, 1960; Saunders & Reuss, 1973).   The ectodermal ridge is
then responsible for inducing proximodistal limb outgrowth
(Saunders, 1948; Summberbell, 1974; Rowe and Fallon, 1982).
Development of the anteroposterior axis seems to be under the
sole control of the mesoderm (Zwilling, 1956). In spite of several
published reports on the subject, there are gaps in our knowledge
of the relative roles of the mesoderm and ectoderm in the control
of the dorsoventral (d-v) axis.   After developing the technique
for the separation and recombination of embryonic tissues
(Zwilling, 1955), the late Edgar Zwilling reported that ectoderm
placed onto mesoderm with its dorsoventral axis reversed did not
alter limb development, ie. the composite stage 19-20 (Hamburger
& Hamilton, 1951) limb developed d-v polarity corresponding to
that of the mesoderm (Zwilling, 1956).   Some years later John
Saunders' laboratory reported similar results with younger stages
(12-17) using a different technique for combining the two tissues.
(Reuss and Saunders, 1965; Saunders and Reuss 1974).   Subsequently
MacCabe et al (1973, 1974) and Pautou and Kieny (1973) found an
ectodermal role in the development of dorsoventral differentials.
When the dorsoventral axis of the ectoderm was reversed on
mesoderm from stage 19 to 24, certain leg structures develop
reversed d-v polarity. This ectodermal dorsoventral influence was
confined to the distal regions of the limb and was diagnosed

primarily by the distribution epidermal derivatives. Nevertheless the effect seemed to extend to skeletal elements since the curvature of the toes and flexion of the joints of the foot corresponded to the reversed epidermal structures. Three important questions remain in our understanding of the role of limb ectoderm in the development of dorsoventral polarity. First, does the ectodermal effect extend to muscle and cartilage morphogenesis? Secondly, when does the ectoderm acquire dorsoventral information and finally, does it acquire this from the mesoderm? The experiments reported here answer these questions.

MATERIALS AND METHODS

The chick embryos used in these experiments came from fertile white leghorn eggs acquired from the Animal Science Department of the University of Tennessee, Knoxville. The eggs were stored at 13ºC for up to one week and incubated at 38.5º for two or three days. Windows were cut into the shell and the eggs returned to the incubator until the desired stage of development was reached. Wing buds or prospective wing regions of the somatopleure were excised with tungsten needles and held in cold (2-5ºC) phosphate buffered saline (PBS) until needed. Ectoderms were isolated after a 1.5-3.0 hr. incubation in 1% trypsin (Difco 1:250) in calcium-magnesium-free (CMF) PBS. Mesoderms were isolated after a 20-30 minute incubation (37.5ºC) in 1% EDTA in CMF-PBS. Stage 14-16 mesoderms included adjacent somites, since they provide prospective muscle cells to the wing at these stages (Christ et al., 1983). Ectoderms from left wings were placed onto right wing mesoderms with their dorsoventral axes reoriented by 180º, ie. the dorsoventral polarity of the ectoderm was reversed relative to the mesoderm. The recombined limbs were then transplanted to the flank of stage 19-22 host embryos and returned to the incubator for further development. Controls included normal limbs and limbs recombined with normal axial relationships. The hosts were allowed to develop for an additional 7-9 days, then sacrificed and fixed in Bouin's fixative. The dorsoventral character of the limbs was first described based on feather follicle distribution. Three or four limbs of each stage were then processed for histological examination of muscle, tendon and skeletal morphology. These limbs were embedded in paraffin, serial sectioned at 7μm thickness, stained in Milligan's trichrome stain and compared to controls for evidence of dorsoventral changes.

RESULTS

In the first series of recombinations both the mesoderm and ectoderm of each composite limb were from embryos at the same stage of development. The fully developed recombinant limbs were examined for d-v reversal (in relation to the mesoderm) as diagnosed by the distribution of feather follicles and muscle and cartilage patterns revealed in serial sections (Table I). Reversal

Table I

Results of Reorienting the Dorsoventral Axis of Wing Ectoderm on Mesoderm

stage ectoderm reoriented	no. wings	no. limbs with feather pattern reversal in:			reversed muscle & cartilage
		(upper arm) stylopod	(forearm) zeugopod	(hand) autopod	
14	11	0	1	3a.	0/4b.
15	12	0	6	12	2/4
16	21	2	20	21	3/3
17	16	12	16	16	4/4
18	27	12	27	27	-
19	40	1	40	40	4/4
20	16	0	16	16	-
21	22	0	22	22	4/4

a. This is also the total number of reversed limbs. In no case did a forearm or upper arm reverse without more distal reversal.
b. No. with reversal/no. serial sectioned.

of the feather pattern usually took the form of a bidorsal follicle distribution, particularly a double row of flight feathers. Muscle and cartilage reversals, on the other hand, tended to be more complete and consisted of dorsal muscles in a ventral location and ventral muscles in a dorsal location (Fig. 1) (Table 2). The

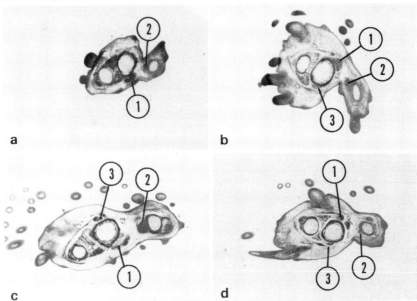

Figure 1. Sections through digits II, III and IV in wings developed after ectoderm dorsoventral reorientation. (a) A wing that developed after ectoderm reorientation at stage 14. It has a normal d-v muscle pattern (compare to control (c), dorsal up, ventral down in all figures). Ectoderm reorientation at stage 16 (b) and stage 18 (d) results in a largely reversed muscle pattern. For example, compare the normal position of the abductor medius (1) in a and c with the position in b and d. The adductor indicis (2) has a ventral origin (at more proximal levels) in a and c and a dorsal origin in b and d. The extensor medius brevis (3) is dorsal to the third metacarpal in the control (c) and (a) (visible only in more proximal sections) but ventral to it in (b) and (d).

shapes of the muscles in cross section were frequently abnormal, so diagnosis was based primarily on origin and insertion sites. Frequently one or more muscles were missing in the experimental limbs. Dorsoventral muscle reversal often affected only distal wing structures. Dorsoventral reversal of skeletal elements could be seen in asymmetric cartilage elements as a mirror image of the normal cross-sectional shape (Fig. 2). The most proximodistally complete reversals occurred at stage 17 and 18, less complete ones occurring both before and after these stages. No muscle and cartilage reversals and few follicle reversals

Table 2

The Extent of Dorsoventral Muscle Reversal in Wing Autopod
Developing with Reoriented Ectoderm

stage ectoderm reoriented		average no. muscles that are:		
		normal	reversed	missing
14	dorsal muscles	4	0	0
	ventral muscles	6	0	0
15	dorsal muscles	2	2	0
	ventral muscles	3	3	0
16	dorsal muscles	1	3	0
	ventral muscles	0	4	2
17	dorsal muscles	0	3	1
	ventral muscles	0	5	1
19	dorsal muscles	1	2	1
	ventral muscles	1	4	1
21	dorsal muscles	1	1	2
	ventral muscles	0	4	2

occurred in limbs recombined prior to stage 15. Limbs recombined
from stage 16-21 all developed some form of d-v reversal. None
of the recombinants developed reversals at the level of the
shoulder or proximal humerus. Thus all of the d-v reversals
induced by ectoderm reorientation were incomplete ones.

Stage 15 seems to be transitionary. Ectoderm reorientation
at this stage resulted in d-v reversal in half the cases. No muscle
and cartilage reversals occur when recombinations are done prior
to this stage and after this stage all recombinants resulted in
some d-v reversal. This seems to suggest a transfer of
dorsoventral information from mesoderm to ectoderm occurs at
stages 14-16.

Another series of recombinations was done using ectoderm
and mesoderm on each side of this transitionary stage (Table 3).
Stage 16 ectoderm reversed dorsoventrally on stage 14 mesoderm
has no effect on subsequent limb development. The reciprocal

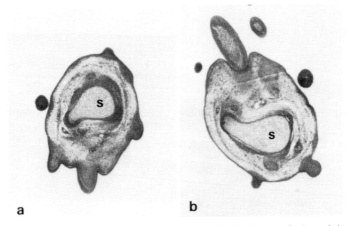

a   b

Figure 2. Section through the proximal phalanx of the third digit in a wing with the ectoderm reoriented at stage 18(a). The shape of this skeletal element (s) is reversed relative to the control wing (b).

Table 3

Results of Reorienting the Dorsoventral Axis Wing Ectoderm on Mesoderm of Different Stages

meso stage	ecto stage	no. limbs	no. with reversed follicle pattern	no. with reversed muscle & cartilage
16	14	6	5	0/4
14	16	7	0	0/3

combination, stage 14 ectoderm reversed on stage 16 mesoderm has only a minimal effect on d-v polarity. Some evidence of follicle pattern reversal was observed but there was no muscle or cartilage reversal. Thus while stage 16 ectoderm can impose polarity on a stage 16 mesoderm (Table 1) it cannot (or at least is less able to) on a stage 14 mesoderm. One possible explanation for this is that the younger mesoderm is unable to respond to the ectodermal message. However because it reaches a stage capable of response soon after recombination, the mesoderms' inability to respond seems an unlikely explanation. Alternatively, stage 14 mesoderm may reprogram stage 16 ectoderm so that its d-v information matches that of the mesoderm, causing the limb to develop d-v polarity in complete conformity to the mesoderm. To test this suggestion, stage 16 ectoderm was reversed on stage 14 mesoderm and allowed to develop for 16 hours. The ectoderm was then removed and placed in normal d-v orientation on stage 19 mesoderm. The resulting wings developed bidorsal d-v axis in both follicle pattern and muscle and cartilage pattern (Table 4)

Table 4

Results of Reorienting Stage 16 Ectoderm for only 16 Hours

meso stage	no. limbs	no. with follicle reversal	no. with muscle & cartilage reversal
14	6	6	3/3
16	6	0	0/3

(Fig. 3a, b). Apparently during the 16 hours the ectoderm was reversed, it obtained new d-v information which it was then capable of imposing on the development of the stage 19 mesoderm. Reversing the ectoderm on a stage 16 mesoderm for 16 hours, then placing it in normal orientation on a stage 19 mesoderm gave limbs with no d-v reversal (Fig. 3c). This suggests the flow of d-v information from mesoderm to ectoderm does not occur after stage 16.

In another series of experiments, wings recombined at stage 20 were examined at various intervals after the host embryos were returned to the incubator to find the earliest morphological indication of d-v reversal. Dorsal and ventral limb bud contours are distinctive, the dorsal side being rather rounded and the ventral somewhat flattened. The recombinant limbs were examined and subjectively evaluated for reversal of these contours (Table 5). The reversal of dorsoventral contours seems to be completed by 15-16 hours after ectoderm reversal. In 15 control limbs which included limbs simply transplanted to hosts and recombinant limbs with normal ectoderm alignment, no shape changes could be detected (Fig. 4).

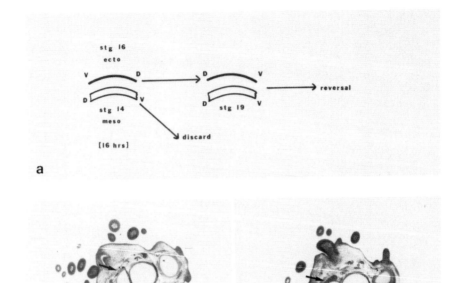

Figure 3. Diagramatic representation of the experiment reversing the ectoderm for only 16 hours (a). This results in a bidorsal pattern when stage 14 mesoderm is used (b). Note the ulnimetacarpalis dorsalis muscle (arrows) is found in both dorsal and ventral locations. When stage 16 mesoderm is used in place of the stage 14, it occupies its normal dorsal location (c).

DISCUSSION

We have shown that the ectoderm can not only affect dorsoventral differences in epidermal structures, (Kieny, 1973; MacCabe et al, 1973, 1974), but also muscle and cartilage patterns - tissues that develop wholly from the mesoderm. This ectodermal effect on mesodermal patterns of differentiation is preceded by

Table 5

Timing of the Dorsoventral Shape Reversal Occurring After Ectoderm Reorientation

hours after reorientation	no. limbs	no. with reversed d-v shape	no. with normal d-v shape
6	5	0	5
8	8	2	6
10	6	4	2
12	12	6	6
13	7	3	4
14	5	3	2
15	4	4	0
16	8	7	1
25	1	1	0
40	1	1	0
72	1	1	0

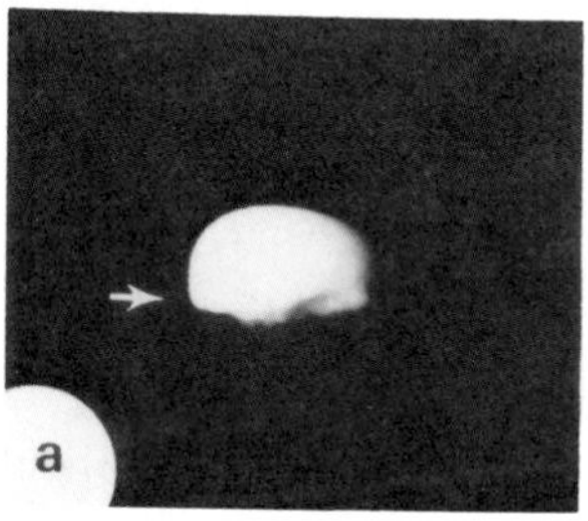

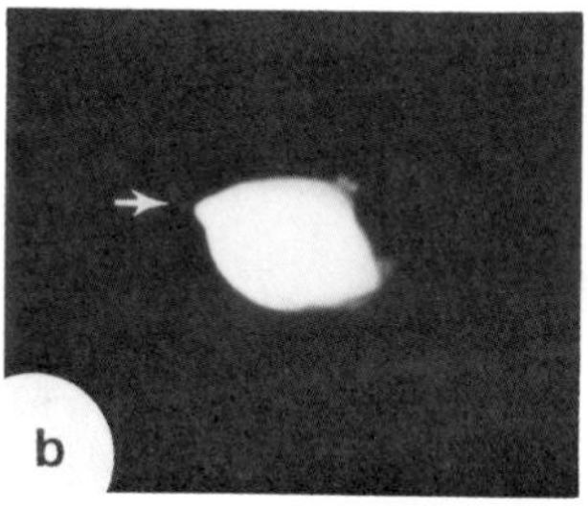

Figure 4. Dorsoventral profile of wing buds 16 hours after recombination with the ectoderm in normal (a) and reversed (b) d-v orientation (arrows indicate the position of the apical ectodermal ridge). The shape of the wing with reoriented ectoderm is reversed (the dorsal side of the mesoderm is up in both pictures).

a dorsoventral change in the shape of the limb bud which reflects the altered d-v polarity. The mechanisms by which the ectoderm influences mesodermal pattern are unknown. However, in view of the rapid effect of ectoderm reversal on mesoderm shape, Harris' "cell-traction" model is an attractive one. (Oster, Murray and Harris, 1983). It not only depends heavily on the overall shape of the tissue, but also on extracellular macromolecules upon which cells exert traction. The distribution of several extracellular macromolecules, as well as mesodermal differentiation, have been shown to be influenced by nearby ectoderm (Stark and Searls, 1973; Kosher, et al, 1979, 1981, 1982; Solursh, et al., 1981; Solursh, 1983; Swalla and Solursh, 1984).

The limb ectoderm can effect patterns of mesodermal differentiation only after stage 14. At stage 14 ectodermal reversal has no effect on dorsoventral development, so the wing develops in accordance with the mesodermal d-v polarity. Since we did not find a consistent ectodermal effect on the d-v axis until stage 16, we conclude that the ectoderm is programmed with d-v information during stages 14-16. Experiments combining stage 14 ectoderm with mesoderm known capable of responding to ectodermal d-v information (stg. 16), confirms the lack of such information in this early ectoderm. These recombinants failed to show any effect of ectoderm reversal. It came as somewhat of a surprise, however, to find the reciprocal combination, stage 16 ectoderm with stage 14 mesoderm, also failed to show a significant effect of ectoderm reversal. Because of this result we conclude that stage 14-16 mesoderm can not only program stage 14 ectoderm with d-v information, but may also program (or perhaps re-program) older ectoderm. This was confirmed by reversing stage 16 ectoderm on stage 14 mesoderm for only 16 hours, then placing it on stage 19 mesoderm in normal d-v orientation. These recombinants were distinctly bidorsal, demonstrating the ectoderm had acquired d-v information during its 16 hours in reversed orientation, and was then capable of imposing this on limb mesoderm. Ectoderm reoriented on stage 16 mesoderm receives no d-v information. Apparently the mesodermal ability to program ectoderm with d-v information, which can then be imposed on the mesoderm, is confined to the earliest stages of limb development. This transfer of information may not be unique to the limb, since stage 19 back ectoderm combined with limb mesoderm gives rise to a bidorsal limb (Errick and Saunders, 1976).

While our results show the ectoderm capable of influencing d-v polarity after stage 14, Saunders and Reuss (1974) report no ectodermal effect as late as stage 17. In Saunders' experiments however, mesoderm was transplanted to a host embryo and the host's ectoderm proliferated over it to accomplish the recombination. We have performed similar experiments with stage 15 and 16 wing mesoderm and obtain the same results, namely, the mesoderm controls polarity under these conditions. Possibly proliferating ectoderm loses d-v information, only to be reprogrammed by the limb mesoderm over which it migrates.

Our results indicate the mesoderm is initially responsible for the control of the limbs' dorsoventral polarity. However at stages 14-16 dorsoventral information is transmitted to the ectoderm. Once this occurs the ectoderm can influence the d-v develoment of the mesoderm. Reversing the d-v polarity of the ectoderm on the mesoderm reveals this influence, by causing a partial reversal of the polarity of mesodermal structrures. The significance of this ectodermal d-v information during normal limb development is not clear. Ectoderm without d-v information (stg 14) combined with mesoderm which has lost most of its' ability to transmit d-v information (stg 16), nevertheless give rise to limbs with normal axes. Perhaps embryonic development is best served by a certain amount of informational redundancy, or there may be more subtle roles for the ectoderm not yet detected.

REFERENCES

Christ B, Jacob HJ, Wachtler F (1983). On the origin, distribution and determination of Avian limb mesenchymal cells. In, "Limb Development and Regeneration B, Kelly RO, Goetinck PF, MacCabe JA, eds. Alan R. Liss Inc., New York. pp. 281-291.

Errick JE, Saunders JW Jr. (1976). Limb outgrowth in the chick embryo induced by dissociated and reaggregated cells of the apical ectodermal ridge. Develop Biol 50: 26-34.

Hamburger V, Hamilton HL (1951). A series of normal stages in the develoment of the chick embryo. J Morphol 88:49-92.

Kieny M (1960). Role inducteur du mesoderme Jans la differenciation proecuce du bourgeon de membre chez l'embryon de poulet. J Embryol Exp Morphol 8:457-467.

Kosher RA, Savage MP, Chan S-C (1979). In vitro studies on the morphogenesis and differentiation of the mesoderm subjacent to the apical ectodermal ridge of the embryonic chick limb-bud. J Embryol Exp Morph 50:75-97.

Kosher RA, Savage MP, Walker KH (1981). A gradation of hyaluronate accumulation along the proximodistal axis of the embryonic chick limb bud. J Embryol Exp Morph 63:85-98.

Kosher RA, Walker KH, Ledger PW (1982). Temporal and spatial distribution of fibronectin during development of the embryonic chick limb bud. Cell Differentiation 11:217-228.

MacCabe JA, Errick JE, Saunders JW JR. (1974). Ectodermal control of the dorsoventral axis in the leg bud of the chick embryo. Develop. Biol. 39:69-82.

MacCabe JA, Saunders JW Jr., Pickett M (1973). The control of the anteroposterior and dorsoventral axes in embryonic chick limbs constructed of dissociated and reaggregated limb-bud mesoderm. Develop Biol 31:323-335.

Oster GF, Murray JD, Harris AK (1983). Mechanical aspects of mesenchymal morphogenesis. J Embryol Exp Morph 78:83-125.

Pautou M-P, Kieny M (1973). Interaction ectomesodermique dans l'etablissement de al polarite' dorsoventrale du pied de l'embryon de poulet. CR Acad Sci Ser D 227:1225-1228.

Reuss, C. Saunders JW Jr. (1965). Inductive and axial properties of prospective limb mesoderm in the early chick embryo. Amer Zool 5:214.

Rowe DA, Fallon JF (1982). The proximodistal determination of skeletal parts in the developing chick leg. J Embryol Exp Morph 68:1-7.

Saunders JW Jr. (1948). The proximodistal sequence of origin of the parts of the chick wing and the role of the ectoderm. J Exptl Zool 108:363-404.

Saunders JW Jr., Reuss C (1974). Inductive and axial properties of prospective wing-bud mesoderm in the chick embryo. Develop Biol 38:41-50.

Solursh M (1983). Cell interaction during in vitro limb chondrogenesis. In Limb Development and Regeneration B, Kelley RO, Goetinck PF, MacCabe, JA, eds., Alan R. Liss Inc., New York. pp. 139-148.

Solursh M, Singley CT, Reiter RS (1981). The influence of epithelia on cartilage and loose connective tissue formation by limb mesenchyme cultures. Develop Biol 86:471-482.

Stark RJ, Searls RL (1974). The establishment of the cartilage pattern in the embryonic chick wing, and evidence for a role of the dorsal and ventral ectoderm in normal wing development. Develop Biol 38:51-63.

Swalla BJ, Solursh M (1984). Inhibition of limb chondrogenesis by fibronectin. Differentiation 26:42-48.

Summerbell D (1974). A quantitative analysis of the effect of excision of the AER from the chick limb-bud. J Embryol Exp Morph 32:651-660.

Zwilling E (1955). Ectoderm - mesoderm relationship in the development of the chick embryo limb bud. J Exp Zool 128:423-441.

Zwilling E (1956). Interaction between limb bud ectoderm and mesoderm in the chick embryo I Axis establishment. J Exp Zool 132:157-171.

Cellular Endocrinology: Hormonal Control of Embryonic
and Cellular Differentiation, pages 127–139
© 1986 Alan R. Liss, Inc.

INTERACTIONS OF MIGRATING NEURAL CREST CELLS WITH FIBRONECTIN

Jean-Loup Duband*, Sylvie Rocher*, Kenneth M.
Yamada+ and Jean Paul Thiery*
*Institut d'Embryologie du CNRS et du Collège de
France, 49 bis avenue de la Belle Gabrielle,
94130 Nogent sur Marne, France, and +Laboratory
of Molecular Biology, National Cancer Institute,
Bethesda, Maryland 20205

During embryogenesis, the behavior of cells depends largely on their degree of interaction with the extracellular matrix. Although each cell type exhibits a specificity in its shape and function, only a limited repertoire of molecules are responsible for the adhesive properties of the cells. These include collagens, fibronectin, vitronectin, laminin, hyaluronic acid, proteoglycans, and a few other molecules present in highly specialized tissues (e.g. chondronectin, chondrocalcin, and osteonectin in cartilages and bones). The glycoprotein fibronectin has been studied intensively because of its striking biological effects on cells and because of its possible medical importance. The purpose of the present report is to illustrate the role of this glycoprotein during embryogenesis, and particularly during avian neural crest cell migration.

STRUCTURE AND FUNCTIONS OF FIBRONECTIN

Fibronectins (FNs) constitute a class of high molecular weight glycoproteins that consist of two similar but not identical polypeptide subunits of 220 kd linked by disulfide bonds (see for reviews Ruoslahti et al., 1981; Hynes and Yamada, 1982; Yamada, 1983). FN is present in large amounts in the plasma (0.3 mg/ml) as a soluble dimer (plasma FN). FN is also found as an insoluble form in 10 nm fibrils around mesenchymal cells and in the basal surface of epithelia (cellular FN). Plasma FN is synthesized in the liver, while cellular FN is produced by a large variety of cell types (reviewed by Hynes and Yamada, 1982).

The primary structure of FN has now been completely established (Petersen et al., 1983; Kornblihtt et al., 1983, 1984, 1985). It reveals highly conserved amino acid sequences both between the two FN forms and among FN from different species. FN polypeptide has three different types of internal repeats (homology types I, II, and III). The differences between FN subunits are due in part to the variability of internal primary sequences. The various FN molecules are generated by transcription of a single gene into a common mRNA precursor which undergoes alternative splicing (Schwarzbauer et al., 1983; Vibe-Pedersen et al., 1984). The splicing concerns two sequences called ED and IIICS. Splicing in the IIICS region generates at least five different motifs and, in the ED region, it results in two peptides (Kornblihtt et al., 1983, 1985; Schwarzbauer et al., 1983). Interestingly, the ED segment is absent in hepatocytes mRNAs which code for plasma FN, while it is present in mRNAs from other cell types (Kornblihtt et al., 1983, 1984).

Several distinct functional domains have been mapped along the molecule using limited proteolytic digestion (Furcht, 1983; Yamada, 1983). They mainly consist of binding sites for a variety of molecules such as collagen, heparin, fibrin, actin, and possibly DNA. Furthermore, a cell binding sequence has been precisely mapped. It consists of a peptide in which the very hydrophilic sequence Arg-Gly-Asp-Ser (RGDS) is absolutely required for the adhesion of cells to FN (Pierschbacher and Ruoslahti, 1984; Yamada and Kennedy, 1984). Interestingly, this sequence is found in several other molecules such as vitronectin, fibrinogen, the receptor for phage λ on E. coli, the Sendai virus coat protein. The wide distribution of this sequence suggests that it may act as a "glue" sequence without any high specificity.

In contrast to plasma FN, cellular FN self-associates to form polymers. However, so far, the sequences responsible for fibrillogenesis have not been yet identified. A possible candidate is the 90 amino-acid peptide coded by the ED sequence (Schwarzbauer et al., 1983; Kornblihtt et al., 1983, 1984). Alternatively, the codistribution of FN and collagens in fibers (Furcht et al., 1980) suggests that collagen could constitute a framework for FN polymerization.

Cellular FN is implied in the adhesion, spreading and migration of cells, and in the organization of the ECM (reviewed in Yamada, 1983). In the blood, plasma FN is involved in wound healing and haemostasis through its binding to fibrin (Ruoslahti and Vaheri, 1975) and in opsonization (Van de Water et al., 1981). In addition, the behavior of a cell (i.e. migratory vs stationary) depends on the synthesis of FN, on the relative concentration of FN in the milieu, and on the mode of interaction of FN with the cell membrane. Exogenous FN, when present as small plaques on the cell surface, greatly enhances cell motility. Conversely, the synthesis by the cells themselves of a dense fibrillar meshwork of FN provokes the cessation of movement and the anchorage of a cell (Couchman et al, 1982).

FIBRONECTIN RECEPTOR

The modest affinity of FN to cell membrane (10^{-6}M; Akiyama and Yamada, 1985) greatly hampered the isolation of FN receptor(s). A number of candidates have been proposed, including heparan sulfate (Laterra et al., 1983) and gangliosides (Kleinman et al., 1979; Spiegel et al., 1985). Recently, two different approaches, one using monoclonal antibodies that interfere with cell attachment (Greve and Gottlieb, 1982; Brown and Juliano, 1985; Chen et al., 1985a; Damsky et al., 1985; Knudsen et al., 1985) and the other based on affinity between the cell-binding sequence of FN and solubilized membrane proteins (Pytela et al., 1985), have lead to the identification of a complex of three glycoproteins of approximately 120, 140 and 160kd involved in the interaction of cells with FN. This complex is located on fibroblasts, myoblasts, and other cell types at the cell-to-substratum contact sites and codistributes with FN fibers (Chen et al., 1985a, b; Damsky et al., 1985). The number of receptor molecules on fibroblasts has been estimated to approximately 3×10^{5} molecules/cell (Akiyama and Yamada, 1985; Akiyama et al., submitted). Finally, this complex has been shown recently to also act as a laminin receptor (Horwitz et al., submitted).

FIBRONECTIN AND AVIAN NEURAL CREST CELL MIGRATION

The neural crest is an embryonic structure lying along the entire dorsal border of the neural tube. After their appearance, crest cells detach from the neural tube and migrate to various sites of the embryo. Their differentiation gives rise to numerous cell types, including neurons and glia of the peripheral nervous system, pigments and, in the head and neck, mesenchyme, muscles, bones, and cartilages (for review, see Le Douarin, 1982). A variety of transplantation experiments (Weston, 1963; Le Douarin and Teillet, 1974; Noden, 1975, 1978; Le Douarin, 1982) have suggested that the routes of migration and the fate of crest cells depend largely on the environment encountered by the cells. The remarkable properties of FN prompted us to examine the distribution and possible role of this molecule during neural crest cell migration.

Fibronectin as a Marker of the Migratory Pathways of Neural Crest Cells

Various markers such as the quail nucleolar marker (reviewed in Le Douarin, 1982), acetylcholinesterase (Cochard and Coltey, 1983), and the monoclonal antibody NC-1 (Vincent and Thiery, 1984) have provided complementary data on the routes of migration of crest cells (for a comparative study, see Le Douarin et al., 1984). However, the structure and topology of the pathways have been mostly elucidated through the use of FN (Duband and Thiery, 1982; Thiery et al., 1982). Even though they are greatly influenced by the morphology of the embryo, the structure of the routes of migration remains constant throughout the embryo. They are cell-free spaces limited by one or two basal laminae of epithelia.

FN is a major component of the pathways of crest migration. The presence of migrating crest cells is always correlated with the presence of FN and, in most cases, cessation of movement is accompanied by the disappearance of FN among the cells (Duband and Thiery, 1982; Thiery et al., 1982; Duband et al., 1985). However, FN is not the only molecule found in crest pathways; collagen types I and III (Duband et al., in preparation), hyaluronic acid (Derby, 1978, Pratt et al., 1975), and vitronectin (Newgreen, personal communication) are also abundant. On the other hand, there are areas in the embryo which exhibit high quantities of FN, but are not invaded by crest cells. The presence of FN in acellular spaces is thus necessary but not sufficient for crest migration. For example, crest cells do not invade the notochordal area and the space between the ectoderm and the dermatome, areas particularly rich in chondroitin sulfate (Derby, 1978; Thiery et al., 1982); this component has been shown not favor cell displacement (Newgreen et al., 1982; Tucker and Erickson, 1984).

So far, it has been impossible to detect any spatial and temporal variations in the composition of the ECM present in crest pathways (Duband and Thiery, 1982; Thiery et al., 1982). It thus seems improbable that a gradient of adhesiveness (haptotactism) or a chemotactic mechanism, as suggested by Greenberg et al. (1981), is responsible for the orientation of migration of crest cells. The three-dimensional structure of the ECM does not appear to influence the direction of crest migration by a mechanism of contact guidance (Weston and Butler, 1966; Erickson et al., 1980). With the possible exception of the amphibian embryo (Löfberg et al., 1980), the meshwork does not seem to exhibit any particular orientation (Tosney, 1978).

The morphology of the embryo is responsible for the structure of the pathways of migration. Various tissues may constitute obstacles or guides to crest migration. In the head, the presence of local thickening of the neural tube (optic vesicle) or of the ectoderm (ectodermal placodes) prevent ventral migration of crest cells (Noden, 1975; Duband and Thiery, 1982; Cochard and Coltey, 1983). In the trunk, the migration of crest cells is mainly guided by metamerized structures, the somites (Thiery et al., 1982; Duband et al., 1985; Duband et al., in preparation). Depending on their location with respect to the somite, crest cells move between two consecutive somites or between the somite and neural tube. Those using the first pathway rapidly reach the aorta where they will provide the sympathetic ganglia. Crest cells facing the somites accumulate only in the anterior part of each segment or migrate more ventrally along the basement membrane of the myotome; they will give rise to the spinal ganglia and to the Schwann cells along the motor nerve

(Weston, 1963; Thiery et al., 1984; Duband et al., in preparation).

Role of Fibronectin in Neural Crest Adhesion and Migration

The effect of FN on the crest cell adhesion and migration has been examined and compared with that of other extracellular matrix molecules (Greenberg et al., 1981; Newgreen et al., 1982; Rovasio et al., 1983; Tucker and Erickson, 1984). FN alone, associated with collagen in two- and three-dimensional lattice, or deposited by fibroblasts greatly promotes the spreading and the movement of crest cells (Greenberg et al., 1981; Newgreen et al., 1982; Rovasio et al., 1983; Tucker and Erickson, 1984). In vitro, crest cells do not attach to pure collagen deposited on two-dimensional substrate (Newgreen et al., 1982; Rovasio et al., 1983), but they are able to move in three-dimensional collagen gels, with the restriction that collagen must be native and at a low concentration. However, the speed of movement is low as compared to that in the presence of FN (Tucker and Erickson, 1984). Likewise, hyaluronate in two- and three-dimensional gels is a very poor substrate of migration (Newgreen et al., 1982; Tucker and Erickson, 1984), but due to its hydration properties, it expands spaces (Pratt et al., 1975; Pintar, 1978) and indirectly enhances the speed of migration (Tucker and Erickson, 1984). From this point of view, it is interesting to note that crest cells synthesize hyaluronate at the onset of their migration (Greenberg and Pratt, 1977; Pintar, 1978). In vitro, chondroitin sulfate is not a good substrate for movement (Newgreen et al., 1982; Tucker and Erickson, 1984); it is almost absent from crest pathways (Derby, 1978; Brauer et al., 1985) and its presence has been correlated with the arrest of crest cells (Derby, 1978). Finally, laminin is also a poor substrate for crest migration but rather induces crest cell aggregation (Rovasio et al., 1983).

The crucial role of FN in crest cell displacement has been approached in an in vitro system and in perturbation experiments. When crest cells are confronted with alternative stripes of FN and coated serum proteins, they migrate exclusively on the FN ones. When stripes of laminin were used instead, few crest cells could move on laminin and tended to form aggregates (Rovasio et al.,

1983). Monovalent antibodies directed against the cell binding site of FN reversibly block the migration of crest cells both in vitro and in vivo (Rovasio et al., 1983; Thiery, 1985). When a decapeptide containing the RGDS sequence is used to compete with the cell binding site of FN, crest cells do not move in vitro; in vivo, they are not seen on the sides of the neural tube, but rather form a bulk in the neural tube lumen (Boucaut et al., 1984). Finally, antibodies to the 140kd FN-receptor complex inhibit the adhesion and migration of motile neural crest cells in vitro (Duband et al., submitted). All together, these studies strongly suggest that a direct interaction with FN is necessary for active crest cell migration.

Behavior of Neural Crest Cells

The final distribution of crest cells at the end of their migration does not result solely from the structure of the pathways and from the properties of FN. Crest cells or pigment cells, when grafted in normal crest migratory pathways, distribute in the normal sites of arrest in contrast to fibroblasts from somite, limb bud and lateral plate which remain intact at the site of the graft. Interestingly, other motile cells such as tumor cells exhibit the same behavior as crest cells (Erikson et al., 1980). These data strongly suggest that crest cells exhibit a specific migratory behavior.

In contrast to stationary somitic and notochordal fibroblasts, migratory crest cells do not show any polarized shape but rather have many cell processes. Crest cells display very little organized microfilament fibers (Tucker et al., 1985; Duband et al., submitted), low numbers of focal contacts and limited amounts of localized vinculin, and α-actinin (Duband et al., submitted). In addition, crest cells do not synthesize FN (Newgreen and Thiery, 1980; Sieber-Blum et al., 1981), and exert a weak tractional force on their substratum (Tucker et al., 1985). This behavior has been suggested to be necessary for a good displacement on a FN substrate (Couchman and Rees, 1979; Couchman et al., 1982; Koliga et al., 1982). Finally, the 140kd FN-receptor complex is present on crest cells both in vivo and in vitro; however, in contrast to mesenchymal cells where it is enriched in the cell-to-substratum contact sites, the receptor complex is diffusely organized on motile crest cells, thus allowing a labile adhesion of the cell to the substratum and an ability of the cell to rapidly establish new contacts with the substratum (Duband et al., submitted).

On FN, isolated crest cells move very actively but their effective distance is very small in contrast to crest cells among a cell population which move in a precise direction (Newgreen et al., 1979; Rovasio et al., 1983, Erickson and Olivier, 1984). The unidirectional translocation of crest cells could thus result from a population pressure in limited pathways of migration and from contact inhibition of movement (Newgreen et al., 1982; Rovasio et al., 1983; Erickson, 1985).

CONCLUDING REMARKS

The neural crest is a striking example of cell migration; during embryogenesis, only a limited number of cells are capable of such an autonomous displacement. It seems that, in order to acquire motile properties, a cell population must benefit from a conjunction of favorable conditions such as a substratum suitable for movement, transient and defined pathways of migration, specific cytoskeleton organization, and particular interactions of the cell membrane with the substratum. However, this does not exclude the possibility that other cell types use different ways to migrate, for example chemotactism, haptotactism, and contact guidance (see Thiery, 1984, for a review).

AKNOWLEDGMENTS

The authors are particularly grateful to their colleages involved in the original work described in the present paper. Research by the authors is supported by grants from INSERM (CRL 83-4017), CNRS (ATP 950 906), MRT (84-C1312), the Ligue Nationale Française contre le Cancer, the Fondation pour la Recherche Médicale, the Association pour la Recherche contre le Cancer (ARC 6455), and the U.S. Public Health Service.

REFERENCES

Akiyama SK, Yamada KM (1985). The interaction of plasma fibronectin with fibroblastic cells in suspension. J Biol Chem 260: 4492-4500.

Boucaut JC, Darribère T, Poole TJ, Aoyama H, Yamada KM, Thiery JP (1984). Biological active synthetic peptides as probes of embryonic development: A competitive peptide inhibitor of fibronectin function inhibits gastrulation in amphibian embryos and neural crest cell migration in avian embryos. J Cell Biol 99: 1822-1830.

Brauer PR, Bolender DL, Markwald RR (1985). The distribution and spatial organization of the extracellular matrix encountered by mesencephalic neural crest cells. Anat Rec 211: 57-68.

Brown PJ, Juliano RL (1985). Selective inhibition of fibronectin-mediated cell adhesion by monoclonal antibodies to a cell-surface glycoprotein Science 228: 1448-1450.

Chen WT, Hasegawa E, Hasegawa T, Weinstock C, Yamada KM (1985a). Development of cell surface linkage complexes in cultured fibroblasts. J Cell Biol 100: 1103-1114.

Chen WT, Greve JM, Gottlieb DI, Singer SJ (1985b). Immunocytological localization of 140 kd cell adhesion molecules in cultured chicken fibroblasts, and in chicken smooth muscle and intestinal epithelial tissues. J Histochem Cytochem 33: 576-586.

Cochard P, Coltey P (1983). Cholinergic traits in the neural crest: Acetylcholinesterase in crest cells of the chick embryo. Dev Biol 98: 221-238.

Couchman JR, Rees DA (1979). The behaviour of fibroblasts migrating from chick heart explants: Changes in adhesion, locomotion and growth, and in the distribution of actomyosin and fibronectin. J Cell Sci 39: 149-165.

Couchman JR, Rees DA, Green MR, Smith CG (1982). Fibronectin has a dual role in locomotion and anchorage of primary chick fibroblasts and can promote entry into the division cycle. J Cell Biol 93: 402-410.

Damsky CH, Knudsen KA, Bradley D, Buck CA, Horwitz AF (1985). Distribution of the cell substratum attachment (CSAT) antigen on myogenic and fibroblastic cells in culture. J Cell Biol 100: 1528-1539.

Derby MA (1978). Analysis of glycosaminoglycans within the extracellular environments encountered by migrating neural crest cells. Dev Biol 66: 321-336.

Duband JL, Thiery JP (1982). Distribution of fibronectin in the early phase of avian cephalic neural crest cell migration. Dev Biol 93: 308-323.

Duband JL, Tucker GC, Poole TJ, Vincent M, Aoyama H, Thiery JP (1984). How do the migratory and adhesive properties of the neural crest govern ganglia formation in the avian peripheral nervous system? J Cell Biochem 27: 189-203.

Erickson CA (1985). Control of neural crest cell dispersion in the trunk of the avian embryo. Dev Biol in press.

Erickson CA, Olivier KR (1983). Negative chemotaxis does not control quail neural crest cell dispersion. Dev Biol 96: 542-551.

Erickson CA, Tosney KW, Weston JA (1980). Analysis of migratory behavior of neural crest and fibroblastic cells in embryonic tissues. Dev Biol 77: 142-156.

Furcht LT (1983). Structure and function of the adhesive glycoprotein fibronectin. Modern Cell Biology 1: 53-117.

Furcht LT, Smith D, Wendelschafer-Crabb G, Woodbridge PA, and Foidart JP (1980). Fibronectin presence in native collagen fibrils of human fibroblasts: Immunoperoxidase and immunoferritin localization. J Histochem Cytochem 28: 1319-1333.

Greenberg JH, Pratt RM (1977). Glycosaminoglycan and glycoprotein synthesis by cranial neural crest cells in vitro. Cell Diff 6: 119-132.

Greenberg JH, Seppä A, Seppä H, Hewitt TA (1981). Role of collagen and fibronectin in neural crest cell adhesion and migration. Dev Biol 87: 259-266.

Greve JM, Gottlieb DI (1982). Monoclonal antibodies which alter the morphology of cultured chick myogenic cells. J Cell Biochem 18: 221-229.

Hynes RO, Yamada KM (1982). Fibronectins: Multifunctional modular glycoproteins. J Cell Biol 95: 369-377.

Kleinman HK, Martin GR, Fishman PH (1979). Ganglioside inhibition of fibronectin mediated cell adhesion to collagen. Proc natl Acad Sci USA 76: 3367-3371.

Knudsen KA, Horwitz AF, Buck CA (1985). A monoclonal antibody idientifies a glycoprotein complex involved in cell-substratum adhesion. Exp Cell Res 157: 218-226.

Koliga J, Shure MF, Chen W-T, Young ND (1982). Rapid cellular translocation is related to close contact formed between various cultured cells and their substratum. J Cell Sci 44: 23-34.

Kornblihtt AR, Vibe-Pedersen K, Baralle FE (1983). Isolation and characterization of cDNA clones for human and bovine fibronectins. Proc natl Acad Sci USA 80: 3218-3223.

Kornblihtt AP, Umezawa K, Vibe-Pedersen K, Baralle FE (1985). Primary structure of human fibronectin: Differential splicing may generate at least 10 polypeptides from a single gene. EMBO J 4: 1755-1759.

Kornblihtt AR, Vibe-Pedersen K, Baralle FE (1984). Human fibronectin: Cell specific alternative mRNA splicing generates polypeptide chains differing in the number of internal repeats. Nucl Acid Res 12: 5853-5868.

Le Douarin NM (1982). The Neural Crest. Cambridge University press.

Le Douarin NM, Cochard M, Vincent M, Duband JL, Tucker GC, Teillet MA, Thiery JP (1984). Nuclear, cytoplasmic and membrane markers to follow neural crest cell migration: A comparative study. In Trelstad RL (ed): "The role of extracellular matrix in development". New York: Alan R. Liss, pp 373-398.

Le Douarin NM, Teillet MA (1974). Experimental analysis of the migration and differentiation of neuroblasts of the autonomic nervous system and of neuroectodermal mesenchymal derivatives, using a biological cell marking technique. Dev Biol 41: 162-184.

Löfberg J, Ahlfors K, Fällstrom C (1980). Neural crest cell migration in relation to extracellular matrix organization in the embryonic axolotl trunk. Dev Biol 75: 148-167.

Newgreen D, Thiery JP (1980). Fibronectin in early avian embryos: Synthesis and distribution along the migration pathways of neural crest cells. Cell Tiss Res 211: 269-291.

Newgreen DF, Gibbins IL, Sauter J, Wallenfels B, Wütz R (1982). Ultrastructural and tissue-culture studies on the role of fibronectin, collagen and glycosaminoglycans in the migration of neural crest cells in the fowl embryo. Cell Tiss Res 221: 521-549.

Newgreen DF, Ritterman M, Peters EA (1979). Morphology and behaviour of neural crest cells of chick embryo in vitro. Cell Tiss Res 203: 115-140.

Noden DM (1975). An analysis of the migratory behavior of avian cephalic neural crest cells. Dev Biol 42: 106-130.

Noden DM (1978). The control of avian cephalic crest cell

cytodifferentiation. Dev Biol 67: 296-329.
Petersen TE, Thogersen HC, Skortengaard K, Vibe-Pedersen K, Sahl P, Sottrup-Jensen L, Magnusson S (1983). Partial primary structure of bovine plasma fibronectin: Three types of internal homology. Proc Natl Acad Sci USA 80: 137-141.
Pierschbacher MD, Ruoslahti E (1984). Cell attachment activity of fibronectin can be duplicated by small synthetic fragments of the molecule. Nature 309: 30-33.
Pintar JE (1978). Distribution and synthesis of glycosaminoglycans during quail neural crest morphogenesis. Dev Biol 67: 444-464.
Pratt RM, Larsen MA, Johnston MC (1975). Migration of cranial neural crest cells in a cell-free hyaluronate-rich matrix. Dev Biol 44: 298-305.
Pytela R, Pierschbacher MD, Ruoslahti E (1985). Identification and isolation of a 140dk cell surface glycoprotein with properties expected of a fibronectin receptor. Cell 40: 191-198.
Rovasio RA, Delouvée A, Yamada KM, Timpl R, Thiery JP (1983). Neural crest cell migration: Requirement for exogenous fibronectin and high cell density. J Cell Biol 96: 462-473.
Ruoslahti E, Engwall E, Hayman EG (1981). Fibronectin: Current concepts of its structure and functions. Coll Rel Res 1: 95-128.
Ruoslahti E, Vaheri A (1975). Interaction of soluble fibroblast antigen with fibrinogen and fibrin. Identity with cold insoluble globulin of human plasma. J Exp Med 141: 497-501.
Schwarzbauer JE, Tamkun JW, Lemischka IR, Hynes RO (1983). Three different fibronectin mRNAs arise by alternative splicing within the coding region. Cell 35: 421-431.
Sieber-Blum M, Sieber F, Yamada KM (1981). Cellular fibronectin promotes adrenergic differentiation of quail neural crest cells in vitro. Exp Cell Res 133: 285-295.
Spiegel S, Yamada KM, Hom BE, Moss J, Fishman PH (1985). Fluorescent gangliosides as probes for the retention and organization of fibronectin by ganglioside-deficient mouse cells. J Cell Biol 100: 721-726.
Thiery JP (1984). Mechanisms of cell migration in the vertebrate embryo. Cell Diff 15: 1-15.
Thiery JP (1985). Roles of fibronectin in embryogenesis. In Mosher DF (ed): "Fibronectin". New York: Academic Press, in press.
Thiery JP, Delouvée A, Grumet M, Edelman G (1985). Initial

appearance and regional distribution of the neuron-glia cell adhesion molecule (Ng-CAM) in the chick embryo. J Cell Biol 100: 442-456.

Thiery JP, Duband JL, Delouvée A (1982). Pathways and mechanism of avian trunk neural crest cell migration and localization. Dev Biol 93: 324-343.

Tosney KW (1978). The early migration of neural crest cells in the trunk region of the avian embryo. An electron microscopic study. Dev Biol 62: 317-333.

Tucker RP, Erickson CA (1984). Morphology and behavior of quail neural crest cells in artificial three dimensional extracellular matrices. Dev Biol 104: 390-405.

Tucker RP, Edwards BF, Erickson CA (1985). Tension in the culture dish: Microfilament organization and migratory behavior of quail neural crest cells. Cell Motility 5: 225-237.

Van de Water L, Schroeder S, Creshaw EB, Hynes RO, (1981). Phagocytosis of gelatin-latex particles by a murine macrophage line is dependent on fibronectin and heparin. J Cell Biol 90: 32-39.

Vibe-Pedersen K, Kornblihtt AR, Baralle FE (1984). Expression of a human α-globin/fibronectin gene hybrid generates two mRNAs by alternative splicing. EMBO J 3: 2511-2516.

Vincent M, Thiery JP (1984). A cell surface marker for neural crest and placodal cells: Further evolution in peripheral and central nervous system. Dev Biol 103: 468-481.

Weston JA (1963). A radioautographic analysis of the migration and localization of trunk crest cells in the chick. Dev Biol 6: 279-310.

Weston JA, Butler SL (1966). Temporal factors affecting localization of neural crest cells in the chicken embryo. Dev Biol 14: 246-266.

Yamada KM (1983). "Cell Interactions and Development: Molecular Mechanisms". New york: John Wiley and Sons, pp 287.

Yamada KM, Kennedy DW (1984). Dualistic nature of adhesive protein function: Fibronectin and its biologically active peptide fragments can auto inhibit fibronectin function. J Cell Biol 99: 29-36.

Cellular Endocrinology: Hormonal Control of Embryonic
and Cellular Differentiation, pages 141–146
© 1986 Alan R. Liss, Inc.

HORMONAL/INTERCELLULAR CONTROL OF LUNG MATURATION

Barry T. Smith, Joanna Floros, and Martin Post

Department of Pediatrics, Harvard Medical
School, Boston, MA 02115 U.S.A.

The growth and maturation of the fetal lung are critical to postnatal survival. As the fetus nears term, the
fetal alveolar epithelial type II cell acquires the ability
to synthesize and secrete the pulmonary surfactant which is
required for normal postnatal air breathing. The regulation
of acquisition of this function has provided information
which may be applicable to the development of other fetal
organs, particularly other foregut derivatives.

The development of the foregut has long fascinated
developmental biologists (His, 1874) since its deceptively
simple and undifferentiated epithelial lining layer, the
endoderm, gives rise to a number of highly differentiated
and widely divergent epithelia (Rudnick, 1933). These
include endocrine glands (thyroid and parathyroids), exocrine glands (the salivary glands and exocrine pancreas),
the respiratory system, the liver, and the varying specialized epithelia of the upper digestive tube (posterior pharynx, esophagus, stomach, and small intestine). The processes
by which differentiation of primitive endodermal cells along
one or other of these pathways is promoted are termed direc-
tive induction (Saxen, 1977). The focus of this paper is,
however, upon permissive induction (Saxen, 1977): that is,
processes by which cells already committed to a given differentiated state are stimulated to fully express their differentiated potential. In many of the foregut derivatives
under consideration, such permissive induction occurs late

in fetal life, in anticipation of independent existence and need for the various foregut functions. The processes involved are a blend of earlier regulatory tissue interactions (primarily mesenchymal-epithelial interactions) and a more classically mature mode of regulation, hormonal regulation, in this case primarily by glucocorticoids.

That glucocorticoids directly affect the fetal lung with respect to surfactant synthesis has been established by demonstrating stimulation of this process in fetal lung organ cultures (Adamson and Bowden, 1975; Ekelund et al., 1975; Gross et al., 1978), organotypic cultures (Sanders et al., 1981), or mixed monolayer cultures of fetal lung cells (Smith et al., 1974). All of these systems are characterized by varying degrees of cellular heterogeneity and contain at least two cell types: epithelial alveolar type II cells (which synthesize pulmonary surfactant) and fetal lung fibroblasts. Surprisingly, when techniques were developed to isolate pure cultures of fetal lung alveolar type II cells (Tanswell and Smith, 1980; Post et al., 1984d; Milo et al., 1984), no glucocorticoid stimulation of surfactant synthesis was demonstrable (Smith, 1978; Tanswell and Smith, 1980; Post et al., 1984d). This implied to us that the presence of the fetal lung fibroblast was necessary for the alveolar type II cell to demonstrate increased surfactant synthesis in response to glucocorticoids. Indeed, subsequent studies show that the fibroblast plays a central role in the response.

Glucocorticoids act on the fetal lung fibroblast to induce synthesis of a small protein, fibroblast-pneumonocyte factor (FPF), which in turn stimulates pulmonary surfactant synthesis by the alveolar type II cell (Smith, 1978). The production of FPF is organ specific (Smith, 1978, 1981a) but not species specific (Smith, 1981a), and only occurs developmentally during the time that the ability to synthesize surfactant is being acquired by the type II cell (Smith, 1981b).

This glucocorticoid-induced synthesis of FPF by the fetal lung fibroblast has been shown to be blocked by actinomycin D and cycloheximide (Floros et al., 1985), indicating the need for RNA and protein synthesis. This is in keeping with previous observations that these inhibitors prevent glucocorticoid-induced surfactant lipid synthesis in fetal lung organ cultures (Gross et al., 1983).

Cell-free translation products from size-fractionated mRNA from glucocorticoid-treated fetal lung fibroblasts demonstrate FPF biological activity (Floros et al., 1985). The active fraction is approximately 500 nucleotide bases in size, in rough agreement with previous estimates of the molecular weight of FPF (Smith, 1979, 1981a). These results indicate that glucocorticoid regulation of FPF production is pretranslational.

Exogenous FPF stimulates fetal lung maturation in vivo (Smith, 1979) and monoclonal antibodies against FPF delay lung maturation in vivo (Post et al., 1984c), indicating the physiologic relevance of this system. With fetal type II cells, FPF stimulates saturated phosphatidylcholine synthesis from radiolabelled precursors (Post et al., 1984d; Post and Smith, 1984a) and specifically affects surfactant-associated lipids in vitro (Post and Smith, 1984a) and in vivo (Smith, 1979).

In both adult (Post et al., 1984b) and fetal (Post et al., 1984a) alveolar epithelial type II cells the enzyme cholinephosphate cytidylyltransferase (CP-CYT) is rate limiting in the synthesis of phosphatidylcholine. It is now apparent that FPF acts on the fetal type II cell to stimulate CP-CYT activity (Post and Smith, 1984b).

When used clinically for the acceleration of fetal lung maturation (Collaborative Group on Antenatal Steroid Therapy, 1981), glucocorticoids must be given at least 24 hours prior to delivery to be effective. In mixed fetal lung cell cultures, a similar time course was observed (Torday et al., 1975). We now know that the pretranslational regulation of FPF production is relatively slow (Floros et al., 1985) while the effect of FPF on type II cell CP-CYT activity is maximal within 60 minutes (Post and Smith, 1984b). Thus future availability of large amounts of this protein could improve prenatal acceleration of fetal lung maturation, since the time factor is a major limitation in the current use of glucocorticoids.

As noted above, it is reasonable to predict that this endocrine/paracrine mechanism might occur in other developing tissues, especially the foregut derivatives. Indeed, Dow et al. (1983) have provided evidence for this in the liver. They described fibroblast-hepatocyte factor which is very similar to FPF, but which is antigenically different (Dow et al., 1983) and cannot mimic the action of FPF on pulmonary cells, just as FPF is ineffective with hepatic cells (Post, Dow and Smith, unpublished observations). Following the terminology of Sirbasku (Sirbasku and Benson, 1979), these two molecules which we have operationally termed as fibroblast-pneumonocyte factor and fibroblast-hepatocyte factor may represent a related family of glucomedins. If so, determination of their structure and genetic regulation will be of considerable interest in view of the widely divergent evolutionary timetables of the various foregut derivatives.

REFERENCES

Adamson IYR, Bowden D (1975). Reaction of cultured adult and fetal lung to prednisolone and thyroxine. Arch Pathol 99:80-85.
Collaborative Group on Antenatal Steroid Therapy (1981). Effect of antenatal dexamethasone on the prevention of RDS. Amer J Obstet Gynecol 141:276-287.
Dow KE, Sabry K, Smith BT (1983) Evidence for epithelial-mesenchymal interactions mediating glucocorticoid effects in developing chick liver: Fibroblast-hepatocyte factor. Cell Tiss Res 231:83-91.
Ekelund L, Arvidson G, Astedt B (1975). Cortisol-induced accumulation of phospholipids in organ culture of human fetal lung. Scand J Clin Lab Invest 35:419-423.
Floros J, Post M, Smith BT (1985). Glucocorticoids affect the synthesis of pulmonary fibroblast-pneumonocyte factor at a pretranslational level. J Biol Chem 260:2265-2267.
Gross I, Ballard PL, Ballard RA, Jones CT, Wilson CM (1983). Corticosteroid stimulation of phosphatidylcholine synthesis in cultured fetal rabbit lung: Evidence for de novo protein synthesis mediated by glucocorticoid receptors. Endocrinology 112:829-837.
Gross I, Walker-Smith GJ, Maniscalco WM, Czajka MR, Wilson CM, Rooney SA (1978). An organ culture model for study of biochemical development of fetal rat lung. J Appl Physiol 45:355-362.
His W ( ). Unsere koperform und das physiologische problem ihrer. Entstehung Vogel, Leipzig.
Milo GE, Ackerman GA, Sanders RL (1984). Growth characteristics, morphology, and phospholipid composition of human type II pulmonary alveolar cells grown in a collagen-free microenvironment. In Vitro 20:899-911.

Post M, Batenburg JJ, Smith BT, VanGolde LMG (1984a). Pool-sizes of precursors for phosphatidylcholine formation in adult rat lung type II cells. Biochim Biophys Acta 795: 552-557.

Post M, Batenburg JJ, VanGolde LMG, Smith BT (1984b). The rate-limiting reaction in phosphatidylcholine synthesis by alveolar type II cells isolated from fetal rat lung. Biochim Biophys Acta 795:558-563.

Post M, Floros J, Smith BT (1984c). Inhibition of lung maturation by monoclonal antibodies against fibroblast-pneumonocyte factor. Nature 308:284-286.

Post M, Torday JS, Smith BT (1984d). Alveolar type II cells isolated from fetal rat lung organotypic cultures synthesize and secrete surfactant-associated phospholipids and respond to fibroblast-pneumonocyte factor. Exper Lung Res 7:53-65.

Post M, Smith BT (1984a). Effect of fibroblast-pneumonocyte factor on the synthesis of surfactant phospholipids in type II cells from fetal rat lung. Biochim Biophys Acta 793:297-299.

Post M, Smith BT (1984b). Fibroblast-pneumonocyte factor purified with the aid of monoclonal antibodies stimulates cholinephosphate cytidylyltransferase activity in fetal type II cells. Pediatr Res 18:401A.

Rudnick D (1933). Ann N Y Acad Sci 16:109.

Sanders RL, Engle MJ, Douglas WHJ (1981). Effect of dexamethasone upon surfactant phosphatidylcholine and phosphatidylglycerol synthesis in organotypic cultures. Biochim Biophys Acta 664:380-388.

Saxen L (1977). In Lash JW, Burger MM (eds): "Cell and Tissue Interactions," Raven Press, pp 1-10.

Sirbasku DA, Benson RH (1979). Estrogen-inducible growth factors that may act as mediators (estromedins) of estrogen-promoted tumor cell growth. Cold Spring Conferences on Cell Proliferation 6:477-497.

Smith BT (1978). Fibroblast-pneumonocyte factor. In Stern L, (ed): "Neonatal Intensive Care, Volume 2, New York: Masson, pp 25-32.

Smith BT (1979). Lung maturation in the fetal rat: Acceleration by the injection of fibroblast-pneumonocyte factor. Science 204:1094-1095.

Smith BT (1981a). Lack of species-specificity in production of fibroblast-pneumonocyte factor by perinatal lung fibroblasts. In Minkowski A (ed): "Physiological and Biochemical Basis for Perinatal Medicine," Karger:Basel, pp 54-58.

Smith BT (1981b). Differentiation of the pneumonocyte:
Optimization of production of fibroblast-pneumonocyte
factor by rat fetal lung fibroblasts. In Ritzen M, et al
(eds): "The Biology of Normal Human Growth," New York:
Raven Press, pp 157-162.

Smith BT, Torday JS, Giroud CJP (1974). Evidence for different gestation-dependent effects of cortisol on cultured
fetal lung cells. J Clin Invest 53:1518-1526.

Tanswell AK, Smith BT (1980). Clonal isolation of human
fetal alveolar type II cells. Birth Defects Original
Article Series 16:249-259.

Torday JS, Smith BT, Giroud CJP (1975). The rabbit fetal
lung as a glucocorticoid target tissue. Endocrinology
96:1462-1467.

Cellular Endocrinology: Hormonal Control of Embryonic
and Cellular Differentiation, pages 147–156
© 1986 Alan R. Liss, Inc.

GROWTH FACTORS AND THE EMBRYONIC KIDNEY

Werner Risau and Peter Ekblom

Max-Planck-Institut für Entwicklungsbiologie and
Friedrich-Miescher-Laboratorium der Max-Planck-
Gesellschaft, Spemannstrasse 35-39, D-7400
Tübingen Federal Republic of Germany

During embryonic development the number of cells
increases dramatically and this growth is much more rapid
than in most other biological processes. Malignant cells do
not usually grow with a similar speed. It is likely that
soluble growth factors are involved in most growth
dependent processes. It is therefore important to determine
the nature, specificity and activity of growth factors
during embryonic development. This can be achieved by
studying growth factor requirements for embryonic cells in
model systems which mimick normal development.

THE KIDNEY MODEL SYSTEM

In most embryonic organs, several cell types are found
already at onset of organogenesis. These cell types may
have different growth factor requirements. The cellular
heterogeneity thus often complicates growth factor studies.
This is the case also in the the developing kidney, the
model system presented here. In spite of this, the
developing kidney is well suited to study the role of
growth factors in development. The availability of an in
vitro model makes it possible to study the development of
some cell lineages in isolation.

During onset of kidney differentiation, three cell
lineages can be detected, the nephrogenic mesenchyme, the
ureter epithelium, and the endothelium. The mesenchyme
stimulates the growth of the epithelium, and the

epithelium, in turn, induces the mesenchyme to differentiate into an epithelium. Because some mesenchymal cells actually convert into epithelium, the adult kidney contains two ontogenetically different epithelia. All the four major cell types, the mesenchyme, the endothelium, and the two interconnected epithelial sheets seem to respond to different growth factors.

A major advantage of the kidney model system is that the differentiation of one cell lineage, the nephrogenic mesenchyme, can be studied separately without the presence of the other cell lineages. In vivo, the ureter bud acts as an inducer for differentiation of the mesenchyme, but it can be microsurgically separated, and the mesenchyme can be induced to differentiate in vitro by heterologous inducers. For example, the embryonic spinal cord is a very potent inducer of the mesenchyme (Grobstein 1956; Saxen et al., 1968). The conversion of the mesenchyme to epithelium and the concomitant proliferation of the induced cells can thus be studied separately from the epithelial cells of the ureter bud. Furthermore, no endothelial cells are present in these experiments (Ekblom et al., 1985). Similar model systems are not available for the other cell lineages, but other types of experiments can be used to determine their growth factor requirements.

Kidney development is naturally not dependent only on growth factors, but other aspects have been thoroughly reviewed previously (Saxen et al., 1968; Ekblom et al., 1985).

TRANSFERRIN IS A MITOGEN FOR THE EPITHELIAL CELLS
DERIVED FROM THE NEPHROGENIC MESENCHYME

The in vitro culture system was used to identify the nature of the serum mitogens required for proliferation of the induced mesenchyme. Thymidine-incorporation studies of in vitro induced kidney mesenchymes show that there is a burst of DNA-synthesis at about 24 hours of in vitro culture (Fig.1). No differentiation and proliferation occurs in the absence of serum nor in the absence of inducer tissue even in the presence of serum. This suggests that the inducer tissue itself is mitogenic, and that serum growth factors also are required. The serum factor has been identified as transferrin (Ekblom et al.,1983). However, it cannot replace the effect of the inducer tissue. During the conversion of the mesenchyme to an epithelium, there is thus an induction-dependent proliferation and a subsequent transferrin-dependent proliferation.

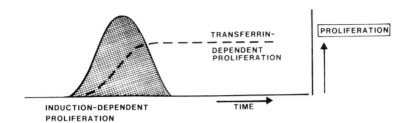

Figure 1. Proliferation during in vitro induction of the mesenchyme. The cells are stimulated by the induction and then by transferrin (see Ekblom et al., 1983).

A synthetic iron chelator can replace transferrin as a stimulator of proliferation. (Landschulz et al.1984). This shows that iron itself is sufficient to stimulate proliferation, and transferrin itself is merely required as an iron carrier. Thus, it seems unlikely that other mitogens could have the same effect as iron-transferrin in this system. Epidermal growth factor (EGF) and multiplication stimulating activity (MSA) have been tested, but they cannot replace transferrin as stimulators of the induced mesenchyme.

Transferrin is present in the serum of 11 day old mouse embryos. The major sources of serum transferrin in the embryo are the liver and the yolk sac, and the kidney does not seem to produce it. Transferrin is therefore present in vivo during onset of kidney differentiation, but it has to be transported through the circulation to the kidney. The continued growth of the epithelial cells thus requires the presence of blood vessels (Ekblom et al.,1985).

EGF MAY STIMULATE THE NEPHROGENIC MESENCHYME

Although EGF does not seem to be important for the the induced mesenchyme, it could have other functions. It is now known that EGF can serve as a mitogen for a multitude of cell types, and its actions are not restricted to epithelial cells (Schlessinger et al., 1983). In several embryonic tissues, EGF is mitogenic and often the mesenchmal cells are major targets (Yoneda and Pratt, 1981). For example, application of EGF during in vitro tooth development leads to a drastic increase of certain mesenchymal cell types, and this has profound effects on development (Partanen et al., 1985).

Studies in other embryonic tissue therefore raise the possibility that the nephrogenic mesenchyme like many other mesenchymes could respond to EGF. Our preliminary studies with isolated, uninduced mesenchymes are in line with this proposal. The mesenchyme can apparently respond to EGF as long as it is not induced but once it is induced to differentiate, it loses this capacity and instead responds to transferrin (unpublished observations). Our data therefore suggest that the cell interactions which are required for differentiation alter the response to serum mitogens. It will therefore be of importance to measure the amount of transferrin receptors and EGF receptors during induction of the nephrogenic mesenchyme. Our data raise the possibility that induction decreases the amount of EGF receptors and increases the amount of transferrin receptors.

ANGIOGENESIS FACTORS AND THE DEVELOPING KIDNEY

Induced mesenchymes from embryonic kidneys strongly stimulate the ingrowth of blood vessels when transplanted on the chorioallantoic membrane (CAM). When embryonic kidneys are transplanted on the quail CAM, the distinct morphology of the quail nucleus (LeDouarin, 1973) can be used to study the cellular origin of the endothelium. Such studies demonstrate that quail endothelial cells invade the mouse kidney, and the endothelium is therefore not derived from the nephrogenic mesenchyme (Sariola et al., 1983). It is noteworthy that the uninduced mesenchyme will not be vascularized on the CAM. Taken together, all data suggest that the differentiation of the mesenchyme into epithelium leads to a secretion of angiogenesis factors (Sariola, 1985).

Until recently very little was known about the mechanisms of angiogenesis and the nature of angiogenesis factors, although it is well known that angiogenesis plays a major role in various growth processes (Folkman, 1985).

Most of the previously identified angiogenesis factors have been isolated from adult tissues. Most of them seem to be growth factors for endothelial cells. No angiogenesis factors have so far been isolated from embryonic tissues. This is not surprising, because the factors from adult tissues are usually isolated from kilogram amounts of tissue. This amount is of course not available from embryonic kidneys. Since this organ, however, induces such a strong vascular effect on the CAM, it is conceivable that embryonic tissues contain a large amount of angiogenesis factors.They may in this respect be comparable with tumors.

Our preliminary evidence suggests that the embryonic kidney produces a growth factor for endothelial cells. It seems to bind to heparin, and its molecular weight is very similar to that of other heparin-binding growth factors (Shing et al., 1984). The recent advances in the purification of endothelial mitogens by heparin-Sepharose affinity chromatography (Klagsbrun and Shing, 1985; Gospodarowicz et al., 1985), should allow us to characterize and purify the growth factor from the embryonic kidney. It is possible that the secretion of this factor is differentiation-dependent.

OTHER GROWTH FACTORS

There are still other growth factors which may participate in the regulation of growth in the embryonic kidney. High levels of mRNA for insulin-like-growth factor II (IGF-II, also called MSA) have been found fetal tissues, including the the embryonic kidney (Scott et al., 1985). Other insulin-like growth factors may also be produced by the embryonic kidney (D`Ercole et al., 1980). The level of IGF-II is low in adult tissues suggesting that this growth factor has a function in embryogenesis (Moses et al., 1980). Interestingly, the level of IGF-II mRNA remains high in childhood kidney tumors. It is possible that the production of IGFs influences the growth of the tumor, although this has not yet been directly demonstrated (Reeve et al., 1985). Similarly, we do not yet know whether

the production of IGFs by the embryonic kidney influences
kidney growth during embryogenesis. These studies clearly
suggest, however, that that there is an endogenous
production of growth factors by the embryonic kidney. Our
present knowledge on the growth factors that could be
involved in kidney development is summarized in Table 1.

TABLE 1. Growth factors and the embryonic kidney

MITOGEN	SOURCE	TARGET
A. Endogenous		
- Angiogenesis factor	Kidney	Endothelium
- IGF-II	Kidney	Unknown
B. Exogenous		
- Transferrin	Liver Yolk sac	Induced mesenchyme
- EGF	Salivary gland Other tissues?	Uninduced mesenchyme

As Table 1. shows, the developing kidney can respond
to certain exogenous mitogens, but there is also an
endogenous growth factor production. The best characterized
event is the iron delivery by transferrin to the induced
mesenchyme, and the role of the other growth factors in
kidney development is not yet well known. It is tempting to
speculate, however, that the listed growth factors are
involved in kidney development and our present working
hypotheses on the impact of these growth factors is
therefore briefly summarized.

IMPACT OF GROWTH FACTORS ON KIDNEY DEVELOPMENT

Transferrin is clearly required as an iron carrier for the proliferation of those epithelial cells that are derived from the nephrogenic mesenchyme. Since transferrin is not produced by the kidney, it must be transported by the bloodstream from the embryonic liver and the yolk sac. Blood vessels are therefore required rather early to support the continuous growth of the epithelium. Blood vessel ingrowth, in turn, seems to be regulated by a production of an embryonic-kidney-derived angiogenesis factor (EKdAF), possibly secreted by the differentiating epithelium. The mode of action of the kidney angiogenesis factor would thus be paracrine as outlined in our scheme in Fig 2.

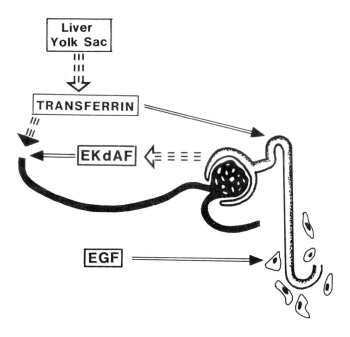

Figure 2. Scheme of postulated growth factor production, delivery, and target specificity of growth factors during kidney development.

The physiological role of EGF in the system is not known. It is apparently mitogenic for the uninduced mesenchymal cells. A continued increase in the number of these stem cells is a prerequisite for the formation of new nephric units during development.the adult kidney contains millions of nephric units, and each unit is derived from mesenchymal cells as a result of an induction. EGF-like polypeptides could be the mitogens responsible for the increase in the mesenchymal cell mass.

Our scheme does not include IGFs, although it seems very likely that they are produced by the embryonic kidney. Data on the biological role of these in kidney growth is at present too scanty. IGF-II is apparently not mitogenic for induced mesenchymal cells (Ekblom et al., 1985), but there may naturally be other target cells in the embryonic kidney.

Only a few years ago, almost nothing was known about growth factor requirements for the developing kidney. The development of chemically defined media for kidney organogenesis according to previously established procedures for cell lines (Barnes and Sato, 1980) has rapidly changed the situation, and several other approaches are now being used to study the growth factor requirements. Perhaps these approaches also will increase our knowledge of the first proliferative event, the one seen in direct response to induction of the nephrogenic mesenchyme. This induction-dependent proliferation still remains the least well understood event, although various aspects of this phenomenon have been studied for about 30 years.

REFERENCES

Barnes D, Sato G (1980). Serum-free culture: A unifying approach. Cell 22:649-655.
D'Ercole AJ, Applewhite GT, Underwood LE (1980). Evidence that somatomedin is synthesized by multiple tissues in the fetus. Dev Biol 75:315-328.
Ekblom P, Thesleff I (1985). Control of kidney differentiation by soluble factors secreted by the embryonic liver and the yolk sac. Dev Biol 110:29-38.

Ekblom P, Thesleff I, Saxen L, Miettinen A, Timpl R (1983). Transferrin as a fetal growth factor. Acquisition of responsiveness related to embryonic induction. Proc Natl Acad Sci USA 80:2651-2655.

Ekblom P, Thesleff I, Sariola H (1985). The extracellular matrix in tissue morphogenesis and angiogenesis. In Edelman G, Thiery JP (eds): "The cell in contact," New York: J. Wiley & Sons, pp 365-392.

Folkman J (1985). Tumor angiogenesis. Adv Cancer Res 43:175-203.

Gospodarowicz D, Chen J, Lui G, Baird A, Böhlent P (1984). Isolation of brain fibroblast growth factor by heparin-Sepharose affinity chromatography. Identity with pituitary fibroblast growth factor. Proc Natl Acad Sci USA 81:6963-6967.

Grobstein C (1956). Trans-filter induction of tubules in mouse metanephrogenic mesenchyme. Exp Cell Res 10:424-440.

Klagsbrun M, Shing Y (1985) Heparin affinity of anionic and cationic capillary endothelial cell growth factors. Proc Natl Acad Sci USA 82:805- 809.

Landschulz W, Thesleff I, Ekblom P (1984). A lipophilic iron chelator can replace transferrin as a stimulator of proliferation and differentiation. J Cell Biol 98:596-601.

LeDouarin N (1973). A biological labeling technique and its use in experimental embryology. Dev Biol 30:217-222.

Moses AC, Nissley SP, Short PA, Rechler MW, White RM, Knight AB, Higa OZ (1980). Increased levels of of multiplication-stimulating-activity, an insulin-like growth factor, in fetal serum. Proc Natl Acad Sci USA 77:3649-3653.

Partanen AM, Ekblom P, Thesleff I (1985). Epidermal growth factor inhibits morphogenesis and cell differentiation in cultured mouse embryonic teeth. Dev Biol 11:84-94.

Reeve AE, Eccles M, Wilkins R, Bell G, Millow L (1985). Expression of insulin-like growth factor transcripts in Wilms tumour. Nature 317:258-260.

Sariola H (1985). Interspecies chimeras: an experimental approach for studies on embryonic angiogenesis. Med Biol 63:43-65.

Sariola H, Ekblom P, Lehtonen E, Saxen L (1983).Differenti-
    ation and vascularization of   the metanephric mesenchyme
    grafted on the chorionallantoic membrane.   Dev Biol
    96:427-435.
Saxen L, Koskimies O, Lahti A, Miettinen H, Rapola J,
    Wartiovaara J (1968). Differentiation of   kidney
    mesenchyme in an experimental model   system. Adv Morphog
    7:251-293.
Schlessinger J, Schreiber A, Levi I, Lax I, Liberman I,
    Yarden Y (1983). Regulation of cell   proliferation by
    epidermal growth factor. Crit   Rev Biochem 14:93-112.
Scott J, Cowell J, Robertson ME, Priestley LM, Wadey R,
    Hopkins B, Pritchard J, Bell GI,Rall LB, Graham CF,
    Knott TJ (1985). Insulin-like growth factor-II gene
    expression in Wilms tumour and embryonic tissues. Nature
    317:260-262.
Shing Y, Folkman J, Sullivan R, Butterfield C, Murray J,
    Klagsbrun M (1985). Heparin affinity: purification of a
    tumor-derived capillary endothelial cell growth factor.
    Science 223:1296-1298.
Yoneda T, Pratt RM (1981). Mesenchymal cells from   the
    human embryonic palate are highly responsive   to
    epidermal growth factor. Science 213:563-565.

Section 3. MODEL SYSTEMS TO STUDY HORMONAL CONTROL OF DIFFERENTIATION MULTIPOTENT CELLS

Cellular Endocrinology: Hormonal Control of Embryonic
and Cellular Differentiation, pages 159-174
© 1986 Alan R. Liss, Inc.

EXTRAEMBRYONIC TISSUES AS SOURCES AND SINKS OF HUMORAL
FACTORS IN DEVELOPMENT: TERATOCARCINOMA MODEL SYSTEMS

Eileen D. Adamson

La Jolla Cancer Research Foundation, La Jolla,
California 92037

INTRODUCTION

The hypothesis presented in this paper is that among
the broadly recognized but poorly understood functions of
the extraembryonic tissues is the responsibility for
providing the first humoral factors that stimulate or
regulate the development of the mouse embryo. In addition, extraembryonic tissues express receptors for humoral
factors and may provide a means, together with non-specific micropinocytosis, for removing excess factors from the
embryonic environment. This paper describes some of the
factors that may be involved in providing the correct
embryonic/fetal environment. Very little is known about
the regulation of the production of these factors by
extraembryonic tissues, but one aspect of their metabolism
is provoking. Why should tissues that have no future
beyond the gestational period express growth factor
receptors? What role do such tissues play after endocy-
tosing growth factors and serum factors? Is it reasonable
to conclude that they may either crudely (micropinocytosis) or finely (by receptor internalization) control the
removal as well as the production (synthesis and secretion) of growth-stimulating factors for the developing
fetus? To illustrate this thesis, I will examine the
synthesis and expression of transferrin and its receptors
and briefly touch upon epidermal growth factor (EGF)-like
factors and their receptors in the developing mouse fetus
and in murine teratocarcinoma cells. Finally, some
relationships between growth factors, receptors, and
oncogenes in extraembryonic tissues will be discussed.

EXPRESSION OF GROWTH FACTORS AND RECEPTORS BY EXTRA-EMBRYONIC TISSUES

The term placenta is a complex multi-factory of stimulatory factors and their receptors. Among the peptide secretory products detected are transforming growth factor type β (TGFβ; Stromberg et al., 1982), insulin-like growth factors (IGFs; D'Ercole and Underwood, 1981), nerve growth factor (NGF; Goldstein et al., 1978), insulin (Liu et al., 1985), platelet-derived growth factor (PDGF; Goustin et al., 1985), chorionic gonadotropin (CG in human placenta; Thiede and Choate, 1963), and placental lactogen (Hertz, 1977). The visceral yolk sac (VYS) synthesizes alphafetoprotein (AFP), α1-anti-trypsin, apolipoprotein A1, albumin, and transferrin (see below) which are all normal serum proteins also synthesized later by the fetal liver (reviewed by Adamson, 1986). Extra-embryonic mesoderm tissues, amnion, and allantois synthesize an IGF-II-like factor (J. Heath, personal communication). Other secretory products of the placenta include peptide hormone-releasing factors, β-endorphin, steroid hormones, and plasminogen activator.

Specific receptors for a wide range of humoral factors are expressed by extraembryonic tissues. In addition to transferrin and EGF receptors (see below), receptors for IGFs (Massague and Czech, 1982; Bhaumick and Bala, 1985; reviewed by Perdue, 1984), insulin (Bhaumick et al., 1982), PDGF (Goustin et al., 1985; Rizzino and Bowen-Pope, 1985), transcobalamin (Nexø and Hollenberg, 1980), and Fc (Johnson et al., 1980) occur among others. It is clear that humoral factors must constantly be circulated from these extraembryonic sources, and their levels could also be regulated by uptake and endocytosis, although it remains to be shown if there is systematic control of individual growth factor levels such as by feed-back inhibition.

TRANSFERRIN SYNTHESIS

This glycoprotein (80,000 mol. wt.) is a major component of serum (2-4 mg/ml) where it functions as a carrier of iron and other heavy metals. Each molecule of transferrin provides two roughly equivalent and reversible metal binding sites. The provision of iron, however,

probably only partially accounts for the dependence of
growing tissues on transferrin. There is some evidence
that suggests that kidney morphogenesis (Ekblom et al.,
1981,1983), white blood cell development (Tormey et al.,
1972; Broxmeyer et al., 1980; Pelus et al., 1981; Brock,
1981; Anderson et al., 1982; Gentile and Broxmeyer, 1983),
myogenesis (Cohen and Fischbach, 1977; Kuromi et al.,
1981; Podlewski et al., 1978; Markelonis et al., 1982;
Beach et al., 1983, 1985), tooth formation (Partanen et
al., 1984), as well as erythrocyte development, may all
require transferrin. Recently, transferrin has become an
increasingly relevant growth-promoting substance with
possibly general mitogenic activity, since it has some
homology with a transforming gene, B-lym, detected in
chicken and human B lymphomas (Goubin et al., 1983;
Diamond et al., 1983). In addition, a cell surface
glycoprotein (p97) present in most human melanomas is
structurally and functionally related to transferrin
(Brown et al., 1982).

In adults, the main source of transferrin appears to
be the liver, but during mouse development, maternal
transferrin apparently does not cross the placenta (Renfree and McLaren, 1974), and this may account for the very
early synthesis of transferrin by the embryo. Newly-syn-
thesized transferrin is detected by immunoprecipitation of
labelled 80 kDa protein from metabolically-labelled mouse
embryos on the 7th day of gestation (the first day is when
the copulation plug is detected; Adamson, 1982). Immunoperoxidase staining with a specific antibody indicates
that transferrin may be produced earlier than this and
that its major source is the visceral endoderm layer of
the egg cylinder stage. By a combination of metabolic
labelling followed by immunoprecipitation and enzyme-
linked immunosorbent assays, the 13th-day visceral yolk
sac (presumably the endoderm layer predominantly) appears
to be the most important producer of transferrin in the
mouse fetus. By the 15th day of gestation, the fetal
liver is an approximately equal source. After this, the
rapid development of the fetal liver ensures that this
organ becomes the major source (Meek and Adamson, 1985).
No synthesis of transferrin is detected in the placenta,
amnion, or parietal yolk sac, but small amounts are
synthesized by several fetal organs. Minor sources of
transferrin include 15th-day spinal cord, brain, and skin
and 19th-day spinal cord, spleen, lung, and rib cage (Meek

and Adamson, 1985). Transferrin is stored in several
fetal tissues besides the visceral yolk sac and liver:
15th-day limbs contain a high proportion and muscle and
skin tissues mainly account for this. Nervous tissues
including spinal cord, brain, and adult sciatic nerve
contain relatively high stores of transferrin. The rib
cage and vertebrae also contain high levels and this
probably originates in the bone marrow. Other laboratories have examined levels of transferrin mRNA in rat
fetal tissues and, in contrast, find the highest levels in
skeletal and cardiac muscle (Levin et al., 1984), whereas
we could detect only occasional traces of synthesized
protein in fetal mouse muscle. Levin et al. (1984) found
that lung, spleen, kidney, and small intestine all tran-
scribe the transferrin gene with changing expression
during gestation. Mouse fetal brain, spleen, testis, and
small intestine all express the transferrin gene and
produce transcripts at 50-100 times lower amounts than in
the liver (Meehan et al., 1984). Levels of transferrin
mRNA in the 13th day mouse visceral yolk sac are several-
fold higher than in fetal or adult liver, thus confirming
the findings on protein levels. A small amount of transferrin mRNA is detectable in the parietal yolk sac, and
this conflicts with earlier protein results (Meehan et
al., 1984; Adamson, 1982). Since several tissues produce
transferrin during fetal development, it may be speculated
that: a) spinal cord could supplement the supply of
transferrin delivered by a still undeveloped blood circu-
latory system to the nearby kidneys; b) the nerves growing
into developing muscle tissue may be able to deliver the
essential iron-bearing transferrin needed for muscle
maturation; c) hematopoietic cells may provide autocrine
or "symbiotic" growth-stimulating factors, including
transferrin, to adjacent cells in the bone marrow.

The relative lack of tissue specificity in the
production of transferrin by embryonic tissues is also
seen in teratocarcinoma cells. It appears, however, that
embryonal stem cells (ECC) synthesize little or no transferrin, except for F9 cells which are therefore thought to
be partially differentiated (Adamson and Hogan, 1984). We
may extrapolate to suggest that embryonic ectoderm cells
do not synthesize transferrin. Several ECC lines, such as
PC13, P19, and OC15, start to synthesize transferrin after
they differentiate. Other differentiated teratocarcinoma
cell lines, such as 1H5 and PSA5E, but not PYS-2 or

F9ACc19, do synthesize transferrin and allow the conclusion that transferrin is largely the product of visceral endoderm-like cells in these cultures. The production of transferrin by some teratocarcinoma cell lines is enhanced by the addition of retinoic acid to the medium and by culture as aggregates (Figure 1), suggesting that cell-cell interactions play a part in the regulation of the transferrin gene as they do for the AFP gene (Hogan et al., 1981; Adamson and Hogan, 1984).

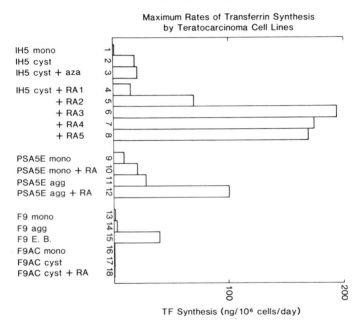

Figure 1. Comparison of the rates of transferrin synthesis by teratocarcinoma cell lines: stimulation of rate by cell geometry and retinoic acid. Transferrin secreted into the medium was assayed by ELISA as described by Meek and Adamson (1985) and expressed as ng transferrin per 10^6 cells per day. 1H5 = primitive endoderm-like epithelial cell line (Kahan and Adamson, 1983); PSA5E = visceral endoderm-like; F9AC = parietal endoderm-like. Mono = monolayers; aza = 5-azacytidine treated; RA = retinoic acid (10^{-6} M); RA1 = 10^{-8} M; RA2 = 10^{-7} M; RA3 = 10^{-6} M; RA4 = 2×10^{-6} M; RA5 = 3×10^{-6} M; agg = aggregates cultured in bacteriological dishes; EB = embryoid body (Grover et al., 1983).

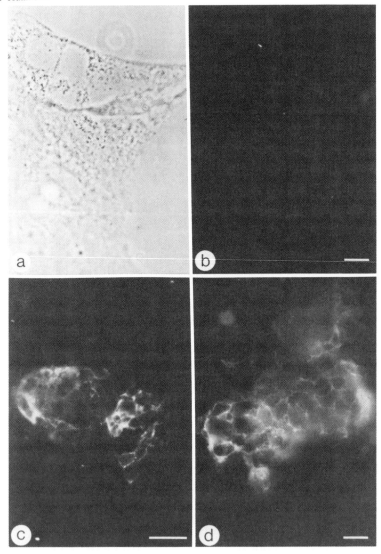

Figure 2. Immunofluorescent reactions for transferrin
receptor on cells of blastocyst outgrowths. a) phase, b)
fluorescent (negative) reaction of trophoblast giant cells
shown in (a) with antibody to transferrin receptors
(Trowbridge et al., 1982), bar = 20 microns; c) endoderm
cells left after inner cell mass detached, bar = 50
microns; d) endoderm and inner cell mass, bar = 20
microns.

TRANSFERRIN UPTAKE BY EXTRAEMBRYONIC TISSUES

With the ubiquitous production of transferrin by
embryonic and fetal cells, a means of removal and regulation may be predicted. This could occur at two levels and
extraembryonic tissues must be the most important func-
tionaries in this respect, especially at early times in
gestation when extraembryonic tissues predominate over
embryonic. First, transferrin together with other peptide
factors could be pinocytosed by the notably proficient
trophoblast and endodermal cells of the early embryo.
Secondly, transferrin (and other) receptors could bind and
internalize ligands and lead to their destruction (EGF) or
recycle (transferrin).

In immunofluorescence reactions, blastocyst outgrowth
on coverslips allowed to react with anti-transferrin
receptor give no staining on trophoblast giant cells, but
a positive reaction is seen on endodermal and inner cell
mass cells (these could not be distinguished) (Figure 2).
This result is not unexpected because, in sections of
mouse placenta, transferrin receptors are largely confined
to the labyrinth region (inner placenta) while the spongiotrophoblast and giant cells are largely negative
(Muller et al., 1983; Figure 3). Sections of 18th day
visceral yolk sac and amnion and 14th day parietal yolk
sac weakly stain with the anti-receptor antibody and show
that very low levels of transferrin receptor are present
on amnion and visceral yolk sac endoderm. In contrast,
immunofluorescence tests and ELISA for transferrin in
extraembryonic membranes at all stages of development show
that very high levels of transferrin are present in spite
of low levels of receptor (Adamson, 1982; Meek and Adamson, 1985). Our interpretation is that transferrin
receptors are present on every rapidly growing cell type
such as embryonic ectoderm, primitive endoderm, and stem
cells of all kinds, including embryonal carcinoma cells
(Karin and Mintz, 1981). They are sparse or absent from
fully differentiated, non-proliferating cell types such as
in adult tissues and trophoblast giant cells. The placenta is a special case since transferrin receptors are
needed together with transferrin to adsorb the iron that
passes through the placental barrier to the fetus.
Extraembryonic tissues such as VYS and PYS probably
provide a similar transport function both before and after
the formation of the placenta. They cannot do so via

transferrin receptors but because of the high rate of
production of transferrin (VYS) and by adsorption by
endocytosis (VYS, PYS). The large size of the extraembryonic tissues then makes them important sources and stores
or sinks of transferrin and other growth factors.

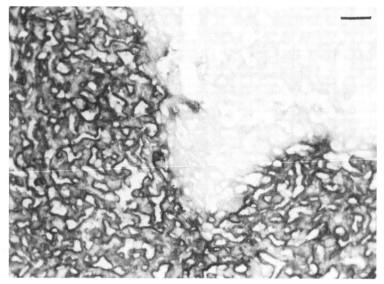

Figure 3. Immunoperoxidase reactions for transferrin
receptor on sections of mouse placenta. Dark staining in
the labyrinth portion denotes a positive reaction. The
spongiotrophoblast, giant cells, and decidua of the outer
portion of the placenta show little specific staining.
Bar = 50 microns.

EGF RECEPTORS ON EXTRAEMBRYONIC TISSUES

Although most fetal tissues express some degree of
^{125}I-EGF binding activity, which increases with gestational age, 6.5-day trophoblast cells in blastocyst
outgrowths express the earliest demonstrable binding
activity (Adamson and Meek, 1984). The highest density of
EGF receptors per mg protein is seen on late-stage amnion,
but all extraembryonic tissues except the parietal endoderm are capable of binding EGF. Embryonic rat and mouse
extracts immunoprecipitated with a rabbit antibody to
human EGF receptor incorporate γ-^{32}P-labelled phosphate
groups from ATP into a 170 kDa band on polyacrylamide

gels, thus demonstrating that 11th day-mouse embryos express EGF receptors that can autophosphorylate (Hortsch et al., 1983). In apparent conflict with EGF binding data, VYS appears to be incapable of phosphorylating the 170 kDa protein. Other results suggest either that phosphorylation activity appears later than EGF binding activity in embryonic EGF receptors or that the immunoprecipitation and phosphorylation assay is less sensitive than binding activity.

Embryonal carcinoma cells (except for F9) do not express EGF receptors, although their differentiated cell products may do so (Rees et al, 1979; Adamson and Hogan, 1984; Mummery et al., 1985). Parietal endoderm cell types do not, while visceral endoderm, fibroblasts, and epithelial cells can express EGF receptors. This is in accord with the hypothesis that primitive ectodermal stem cells are not subject to mitogenic regulation by EGF-like peptides but their differentiated products may be responsive.

Clearly, extraembryonic tissues express EGF receptors, but whether the active peptide is EGF or an EGF-like molecule like transforming growth factor is not yet known. EGF-like substances have been detected in mouse (Nexø et al., 1980) and rat (Proper et al., 1982) embryos and in normal rat tissues (Lee et al., 1985). Both EGF and TGF occur as larger precursor polypeptides that are membrane bound, and many tissues appear to produce small amounts (Rall et al., 1985). The largest stores of EGF, however, occur in male mouse submandibulary salivary glands although the precise significance of this is unknown and cannot affect fetal development since the stores are only built up after birth.

DISCUSSION

The necessity for some vital function provided by extraembryonic membranes is evident since cultures of mouse and rat fetuses and embryos in vitro only develop when the membranes are left in place (New, 1978). The kind of support provided, however, is not clear but nutritive stimulatory factors must play a role. These include transferrin, albumin, α1-anti-trypsin, apolipoproteins, TGFβ, PDGF, and IGF-II. Receptors for some of these factors have been detected on extraembryonic tissues, namely EGF, transferrin, and PDGF receptors. The first two of these receptors have been shown to have homologies to oncogenes, namely c-erb-B and B-lym, respectively. A third oncogene known to be expressed at very high levels in extraembryonic tissues (Muller et al., 1983a), c-fms, has been identified as the receptor for hematopoietic cell stimulating factor, CSF-1 (Sherr et al., 1985).

There is a clear but ill-defined relationship between growth factor action and several oncogenes. For instance, when PDGF or serum is added to quiescent fibroblasts, c-fos oncogene is rapidly transcribed (within a few minutes) followed by c-myc (Greenberg and Ziff, 1984; Kruijer et al., 1984; Muller et al., 1984). Activation of the latter cellular oncogene is associated with cell proliferation in many cell types including the early human placenta where c-sis (homologous to PDGF) is also expressed during the first trimester. In the case of the placenta, an autocrine effect is suggested by the simultaneous presence of c-sis transcripts, PDGF-like activity, and PDGF receptors (Goustin et al., 1985). It is more difficult to explain why c-fos transcription (Muller et al., 1982,1983b,1983c; Adamson et al., 1983) and translation (Adamson et al., 1985) should be so high in amnion, VYS, and placenta. Levels of expression increase with age of gestation which is consistent with other findings that increasing differentiation accompanies increasing c-fos expression. However, as we have seen above, c-fos activation is also related to growth factor response. Although early trophoblast has invasive properties, mid- to late-gestation placenta, amnion, and VYS are not tumorigenic in nude mice (Adamson et al., 1985). The c-fos expressed therefore is incapable of transforming these cells, even though it is known that c-fos can act as a transforming gene (Miller et al., 1984). It may be concluded that because of the high levels of growth factors and serum proteins that abound in the amniotic fluid and fetal serum, extraembryonic membranes adsorb and regulate levels of such factors. In doing so, these tissues could become permanently stimulated thus expressing c-fos at ever increasing levels. Extraembryonic tissues, however, have devices that prevent their transformation. This could be by rapid breakdown or by processing c-fos to higher apparent molecular weight forms (p55 c-fos is succeeded by p60, p62, p68, and p72) that are not able to transform.

In summary, extraembryonic tissues are acting as growth factor sources and sinks for the regulation of the important processes of embryonic cell proliferation and differentiation. Some of these growth factors and receptors are related to oncogenes. Some oncogenes such as c-fos may only be activated incidentally after growth factors produced by these and other tissues have initiated a growth factor response. This satisfactorily explains why c-fos oncogene should be highly active in tissues that are not destined to survive beyond the gestational period. The basis for c-fms expression in placenta may relate to its ability to adsorb CSF-1 specifically, though the source of this growth factor remains to be studied.

ACKNOWLEDGEMENTS

I thank I. S. Trowbridge for antibody to transferrin receptor. Support by NIH grants 18782 and 28427 is gratefully acknowledged. This paper is dedicated to the memory of Geoffrey V. Goldin.

REFERENCES

Adamson ED (1982) The location and synthesis of transferrin in mouse embryos and teratocarcinoma cells. Dev Biol 91:227-234.

Adamson ED (1986) Cell lineage-specific gene expression in development. In Rossant J, Pedersen R (eds): "Experimental Approaches to Mammalian Embryonic Development," New York: Cambridge University Press (in press).

Adamson ED, Hogan BLM (1984) Expression of EGF receptor and transferrin by F9 and PC13 teratocarcinoma cells. Differentiation 27:152-157.

Adamson ED, Meek J (1984) The ontogeny of epidermal growth factor receptors during mouse development. Dev Biol 103:62-71.

Adamson ED, Meek J, Edwards SA (1985) Product of the cellular oncogene, c-fos, observed in mouse and human tissues using an antibody to a synthetic peptide. EMBO J 4:941-947.

Adamson ED, Muller R, Verma I (1983) Expression of c-onc genes c-fos and c-fms in developing mouse tissues. Cell Biol Int Rep 7:557-558.

Anderson WL, Chase CG, Tomasi TB (1982) Transferrin support of stimulated lymphocytes. In Vitro 18:766-774.

Beach RL, Popiela H, Festoff BW (1983) The identification of neurotrophic factor as transferrin. FEBS Lett 156:151-156.

Beach RL, Popiela H, Festoff RW (1985) Specificity of chicken and mammalian transferrin in myogenesis. Cell Differ 16:93-100.

Bhaumick B, Armstrong GD, Hollenberg RD, Bala RM (1982) Characterization of the human placenta receptor for basic somatomedin. Can J Biochem 60:923-932.

Bhaumick B, Bala RM (1985) Ontogeny and characterization of basic somatomedin receptors in rat placenta. Endocrinology 116:492-498.

Brock JH (1981) The effect of iron and transferrin on the response of serum-free cultures of mouse lymphocytes to Concanavalin A and lipopolysaccharide. Immunology 43:387-398.

Brown P, Hewick RM, Hellstrom L, Hellstrom KE, Doolittle RF, Dreyer WJ (1982) Human melanoma-associated antigen p97 is structurally and functionally related to transferrin. Nature 296:171-173.

Broxmeyer HE, de Sousa M, Smithyman A, Hamilton RP, Kurland JI, Bognacki J (1980) Specificity and modulation of the action of lactoferrin, a negative feedback regulator of myelopoiesis. Blood 55:324-333.

Cohen SA, Fischbach GD (1977) Clusters of acetylcholine receptors located at identified nerve-muscle synapses in vitro. Dev Biol 59:24-38.

D'Ercole AJ, Underwood LE (1981) Growth factors in fetal growth and development. In Novy MJ, Resko JA (eds): "Fetal Endocrinology," New York: Academic Press, pp 155-182.

Diamond A, Cooper GM, Ritz J, Lane MA (1983) Identification and molecular cloning of the human Blym transforming gene activated in Burkitt's lymphomas. Nature 305:112-116.

Ekblom P, Thesleff I, Miettinen A, Saxen L (1981) Organogenesis in a defined medium supplemented with transferrin. Cell Differ 10:281-288.

Ekblom P, Thesleff I, Saxen L, Miettinen A, Timpl R (1983) Transferrin as a fetal growth factor: Acquisition of responsiveness related to embryonic induction. Proc Natl Acad Sci USA 80:2651-2655.

Gentile P, Broxmeyer HE (1983) Suppression of mouse myelopoiesis by administration of human lactoferrin in vivo and the comparative action of human transferrin. Blood 61:982-993.

Goldstein LD, Reynolds CP, Perez-Ford JR (1978) Isolation of human NGF from placental tissue. Neurochem Res 3:175-181.

Goubin G, Goldman DS, Luce J, Neiman PE, Cooper GM (1983) Molecular cloning and nucleotide sequence of a trans-forming gene detected by transfection of chicken B-cell lymphoma DNA. Nature 302:114-119.

Goustin AS, Betsholtz C, Pfeifer-Ohlsson S, Persson H, Rydnert J, Bywater M, Holmgren G, Heldin C-H, Westermark B, Ohlsson R (1985) Coexpression of the sis and myc proto-oncogenes in developing human placenta suggests autocrine control of trophoblast growth. Cell 41: 301-312.

Greenberg ME, Ziff EB (1984) Stimulation of 3T3 cells induces transcription of the c-fos proto-oncogene. Nature 311:433-437.

Grover A, Oshima RG, Adamson ED (1983) Epithelial layer formation in differentiating aggregates of F9 embryonal carcinoma cells. J Cell Biol 96:1690-1696.

Hertz R (1977) "The Trophoblast in Choriocarcinoma and Related Gestational Trophoblastic Tumors in Women." New York: Raven Press, pp 1-12.

Hogan BLM, Taylor A, Adamson ED (1981) Cell interactions modulate embryonal carcinoma cell differentiation into parietal or visceral endoderm. Nature 291:235-237.

Hortsch M, Schlessinger J, Gootwine E, Webb CG (1983) Appearance of functional EGF receptor kinase during rodent embryogenesis. EMBO J 2:1937-1941.

Johnson PM, Brown PJ, Faulk WP (1980) Immunobiological aspects of the human placenta. In Finn CA (ed): "Oxford Reviews of Reproductive Biology," Vol 2, U.K.: Oxford University Press, pp 1-40.

Kahan B, Adamson ED (1983) A teratocarcinoma-derived bipotential cell line with primitive endoderm proper-ties. Cold Spring Harb Conf Cell Prolif 10:131-141.

Karin M, Mintz B (1981) Receptor mediated endocytosis of transferrin in developmentally totipotent mouse terato-carcinoma stem cells. J Biol Chem 256:3245-3252.

Kruijer W, Cooper JA, Hunter T, Verma IM (1984) PDGF induces rapid but transient expression of the c-fos gene. Nature 312:711-716.

Kuromi H, Gonoi T, Hasegawa S (1981) Neurotrophic substance develops tetrodotoxin-sensitive action potential and increases curare-sensitivity of acetylcholine responses in cultured rat myotubes. Devel Brain Res 1:369-379.

Lee DC, Rose TM, Webb NR, Todaro GJ (1985) Cloning and sequence analysis of a cDNA for rat transforming growth factor-α. Nature 313:489-492.

Levin MJ, Tuil D, Uzan G, Dreyfus J-C, Kahn A (1984) Expression of the transferrin gene during development of non-hepatic tissues: high level of transferrin mRNA in fetal muscle and adult brain. Biochem Biophys Res Commun 122:212-217.

Liu K-S, Wang C-Y, Mills N, Gyves M, Ilan J (1985) Insulin-related genes expressed in human placenta from normal and diabetic pregnancies. Proc Natl Acad Sci USA 82:3868-3870.

Markelonis GJ, Bradshaw RA, Oh TH, Johnson JL, Bates OJ (1982) Sciatin is a transferrin-like polypeptide. J Neurochem 39:315-320.

Massague J, Czech MP (1982) The subunit structure of 2 distinct receptors for insulin-like growth factors I and II and their relationship to the insulin receptor. J Biol Chem 257:5038-5045.

Meehan RR, Barlow DP, Hill RE, Hogan BLM, Hastie ND (1984) Pattern of serum protein gene expression in mouse visceral yolk sac and foetal liver. EMBO J 3:1881-1885.

Meek J, Adamson ED (1985) Transferrin in fetal and adult mouse tissues: synthesis, storage, and secretion. J Embryol Exp Morph 86:205-218.

Miller AD, Curran T, Verma IM (1984) c-Fos protein can induce cellular transformation: a novel mechanism of activation of a cellular oncogene. Cell 36:51-60.

Muller R, Slamon DJ, Tremblay JM, Cline MJ, Verma IM (1982) Differential expression of cellular oncogenes during pre- and postnatal development of the mouse. Nature 299:640-644.

Muller R, Slamon DJ, Adamson ED, Tremblay JM, Muller D, Cline MJ, Verma IM (1983a) Transcription of cellular oncogenes c-ras^{Ki} and c-fms during mouse development. Mol Cell Biol 3:1062-1069.

Muller R, Verma IM, Adamson ED (1983b) Expression of c-onc genes: c-fos transcripts accumulate to high levels during development of mouse placenta, yolk sac, and amnion. EMBO J 2:679-684.

Muller R, Tremblay JM, Adamson ED, Verma IM (1983c) Tissue and cell type-specific expression of two human c-onc genes. Nature 304:454-456.

Muller R, Bravo R, Burckhardt J, Curran T (1984) Induction of c-fos gene and protein by growth factors precedes activation of c-myc. Nature 312:716-720.

Mummery CL, Feijen A, VanderSaag PT, vandenBrink CE, deLaat SW (1985) Clonal variants of differentiated P19 embryonal carcinoma cells exhibit epidermal growth factor receptor kinase activity. Dev Biol 109:402-410.

New DA (1978) Conditions for the culture of whole embryos. Biol Rev 53:81-122.

Nexø E, Hollenberg MD (1980) Characterization of the particulate and soluble acceptor for transcobalamin II from human placenta and rabbit liver. Biochim Biophys Acta 628:190-200.

Nexø E, Hollenberg MD, Figueroa A, Pratt RM (1980) Detection of epidermal growth factor - urogastrone: and its receptor during mouse fetal development. Proc Natl Acad Sci USA 77:2782-2785.

Partanen A-M, Thesleff I, Ekblom P (1984) Transferrin is required for early tooth morphogenesis. Differentiation 27:59-66.

Pelus LM, Broxmeyer HE, de Sousa M, Moore MAS (1981) Heterogeneity among resident murine peritoneal macrophages: separation and functional characterization of monocytoid cells producing granulocyte-macrophage colony stimulating factor (GM-CSF) and responding to regulation by lactoferrin. J Immunol 126:1016-1021.

Perdue JF (1984) Chemistry, structure, and function of insulin-like growth factors and their receptors: a review. Can J Biochem Cell Biol 62:1237-1245.

Podlewski TR, Axelrod D, Ravdin P, Greenberg L, Johnson MM, Salpeter MM (1978) Nerve extract induces increase and redistribution of acetylcholine receptors on cloned muscle cells. Proc Natl Acad Sci USA 75:2035-2039.

Proper JA, Bjornson CL, Mosco HL (1982) Mouse embryos contain polypeptide growth factor(s) capable of inducing a reversible neoplastic phenotype in nontransformed cells in culture. J Cell Physiol 110:169-174.

Rall LB, Scott J, Bell GI, Crawford RJ, Penschow JD, Niall HD, Coughlan JP (1985) Mouse prepro-epidermal growth factor synthesis by the kidney and other tissues. Nature 313:227-231.

Rees AR, Adamson ED, Graham CF (1979) Epidermal growth factor receptors increase during the differentiation of embryonal carcinoma cells. Nature 281:309-311.

Renfree MB, McLaren A (1974) Foetal origin of transferrin in mouse amniotic fluid. Nature 252:150-161.

Rizzino A, Bowen-Pope DF (1985) Production of PDGF-like growth factors by embryonal carcinoma cells and binding of PDGF to their endoderm-like differentiated cells. Dev Biol 110:15-22.

Sherr CJ, Rettenmier CW, Sacca R, Roussel MF, Look AT, Stanley ER (1985) The c-fms proto-oncogene product is related to the receptor for the mononuclear phagocyte growth factor, CSF-1. Cell 41:665-676.

Stromberg K, Pigott DA, Ranchalis JE (1982) Human term placenta contains transforming growth factors. Biochem Biophys Res Commun 106:354-361.

Thiede H, Choate JW (1963) Chorionic gonadotropin localization in the human placenta by immunofluorescent staining. II. Demonstration of HCG in the trophoblast and amnion epithelium of immature and mature placentas. Obstet Gynecol 22:433-445.

Tormey DC, Imrie RC, Mueller GC (1972) Identification of transferrin as a lymphocyte growth promoter in human serum Exp Cell Res 74:163-169.

Trowbridge IS, Lesley J, Schulte R (1982) Murine cell surface transferrin receptor: studies with an anti-receptor monoclonal antibody. J Cell Physiol 112: 403-410.

Cellular Endocrinology: Hormonal Control of Embryonic
and Cellular Differentiation, pages 175–179
© 1986 Alan R. Liss, Inc.

THE MECHANISM OF CHEMICALLY-INDUCED DIFFERENTIATION
OF A MOUSE EMBRYONAL CARCINOMA CELL LINE

Micheal W. McBurney, Jose Campione-Piccardo,
Steven C. Smith and John C. Bell

Departments of Medicine and Biology, University
of Ottawa, 451 Smyth Road, Ottawa, Canada,
K1H 8M5

Murine embryonal carcinoma (EC) cells can
differentiate into a diverse spectrum of cell types both
in vivo and in vitro. Our interest is to investigate
the developmental processes which occur in
differentiating EC cultures to learn (a) what are the
signals which induce the EC cell to initiate
differentiation and (b) how does any one differentiating
cell choose between the various developmental lineages
available to it.

The P19 line of EC cells (McBurney and Rogers,
1982) has a euploid male karyotype and grows readily in
culture in the absence of feeders. Aggregates of P19
cells exposed to drugs such as retinoic acid (RA) or
dimethyl sulfoxide (DMSO) are induced to differentiate.
The cell types which develop depend on the drug concentration (Edwards and McBurney, 1983; Edwards et al,
1983). At the lowest effective doses of either drug,
rhythmically contracting cardiac muscle appears
(McBurney et al, 1982); at higher doses, skeletal muscle
develops; and at still higher doses, neurons and glial
cells are formed (Jones-Villeneuve et al, 1982; 1983).
All of the differentiated cell types appear to be
embryonic and they develop in a sequence similar to that
in the embryo. The fact that both RA and DMSO have the
same dose-related effects on the P19 cultures, suggests
that both drugs affect the same developmental
decision-making system in the cells. Since quantitative
changes in drug dose result in qualitative changes in
the cell types developing, models are suggested in which

the intracellular system responsible for lineage choice consists in part of a ligand interacting with a variety of receptors with various affinities for that ligand. The lineages which develop could be determined by the extent of receptor titration. If models of this type were correct, one of the effects of RA and DMSO might be the induction of the intracellular ligand.

When P19 cells are aggregated with mutant cells no longer responsive to RA, the P19 cells respond to the drug as efficiently in the mixed aggregates as in aggregates consisting only of P19 cells. The response to RA is, therefore, cell autonomous and suggests that RA-induced differentiation of P19 cells is a result of interaction of the drug with an intracellular target (Campione-Piccardo et al, 1985). It seems likely that RA induces differentiation by binding to the cells' cytoplasmic receptor protein (cRABP) because analogues of RA induce P19 cell differentiation with the same rank order of effectiveness as they bind to the cRABP (Jones-Villeneuve et al, 1983).

The target of DMSO action is much less clear. When aggregates of P19 cells are mixed with mutant cells no longer responsive to DMSO, the P19 cells within the mixed aggregate do not differentiate in DMSO (Campione-Piccardo et al, 1985). Thus, the neighbourhood of EC cells prevents DMSO-induced differentiation of cells which are responsive if aggregated by themselves. DMSO did not induce the differentiation of P19 cells grown as monolayers on plastic surfaces (McBurney et al, 1982) and did not induce differentiation of aggregates containing only small numbers of P19 cells. Indeed, DMSO induced development of muscle occurs only if aggregates contain more than 50 cells. The evidence is circumstantial, but the above results suggest that cells differentiate in a cooperative fashion in the presence of DMSO and further suggests that the DMSO may be acting by interacting with an extracellular molecule.

In DMSO-treated aggregates, cells around the outside of the aggregate are the first to become overtly differentiated. By 3 to 4 days, each aggregate is surrounded by a single layer of cells which contain intermediate filaments which stain with an antibody (TROMA-1, Kemler et al, 1981) reactive with a cytokeratin. These cells do not have receptors for dolichos bifluorus agglutinin (DBA), a marker for derivatives of the extra embryonic endoderm (Noguchi et al, 1982). Thus, this rapidly forming epithelial cell type appears to be distinct from the endoderm-like cells (TROMA-1[+], DBA[+]) which spontaneously develop around aggregates of P19 and a variety of other multipotent EC cell lines (Martin and Evans, 1975).

Muscle cells appear in DMSO-treated aggregates at 5-6 days. These muscle cells rarely appear on the surface of an aggregate or in the aggregate center. Rather, the majority of muscle cells develop 1-3 cell diameters beneath the aggregate surface. The facts that the muscle appears 1-2 days after the epithelial layer comes to surround each aggregate and that muscle develops in close proximity to this epithelium suggests that the epithelial cell may play an instructive role in the differentiation of <u>cells</u> into the myogenic lineage.

Because our indirect evidence suggested that DMSO might interact with an extracellular molecule, we examined the possibility that epithelial cells might release, into culture medium, factors which induce differentiation of P19 cells. Medium conditioned by F9-derived endoderm cells does appear to contain an activity which induces differentiation of P19 cells growing on solid substrates. The differentiated P19 cells become TROMA-1[+] DBA[-] and thus resemble the epithelial layer formed around DMSO-treated aggregates. Our preliminary indications are that the active material is insensitive to trypsin, heat stable (30 mins./at $100^{0}C$) and small (less than 10 kd). The activity in this conditioned medium appears to be enhanced in the presence of DMSO. We are attempting further characterization of this activity to determine whether it is a natural morphogenetically important factor.

It seems clear from work on the mouse embryo that many developmental signals originate from outside the cell. A responsive cell which receives a signal reacts by changing both qualitatively and quantitatively nuclear gene transcription. The signal must, therefore, be transduced through the plasma membrane and the cytoplasm. A possibility suggested by the inverse correlation between proliferation and differentiation is

that the protein products of proto-oncogenes might be
components of the intracellular system used to transduce
developmental signals. Were this true, one might expect
that the flow of differentiation information could be
disrupted by the presence of an altered proto-oncogene
product. Since oncogenes incodes such products, we
transfected into P19 cells DNA from a cloned plasmid
containing the human Ha-ras^{EJ}-1 oncogene (Shih and
Weinberg, 1982). The product of this gene is a 21 kd
protein (p21^{EJ}) identical to the proto-oncogene
product (p21) except for the substitution of valine for
glycine at amino acid 12. The Ha-ras^{EJ}-1 gene
malignantly transforms immortal mouse cell lines.

Some of the transfected P19 cells carried and
expressed the oncogene. These P19(ras$^+$) cells
expressed the Ha-ras^{EJ}-1 oncogene mRNA and protein at
levels at least 10 times higher than the endogenous
Ha-ras-1 proto-oncogene. Nevertheless, the P19(ras$^+$)
cells differentiated when aggregated in the presence of
RA and differentiated into normal neurons and glial.
Since the presence of the p21^{EJ} failed to affect the
differentiation of EC cells, it seems unlikely that p21
is a component of the intracellular system the cell uses
to transduce developmental signals from outside the cell
into the nucleus.

REFERENCES

Campione-Piccardo J, Sun JJ, Craig J, McBurney MW (1985)
    Cell-cell interaction can influence drug-induced
    differentiation of murine embryonal carcinoma cells.
    Dev Biol 109:25-31.
Edwards MKS, Harris JF, McBurney MW (1983). Induced
    muscle differentiation in an embryonal carcinoma cell
    line. Mol Cell Biol 3:2280-2286.
Edwards MKS, McBurney MW (1983). The concentration of
    retinoic acid determines the differentiated cell types
    formed by a teratocarcinoma cell line. Dev Biol
    98:187-191.
Jones-Villeneuve EMV, McBurney MW, Rogers KA, Kalnins VI
    (1982). Retinoic acid induces embryonal carcinoma
    cells to differentiate into neurons and glial cell.
    J Cell Biol 94:253-262.

Jones-Villeneuve EMV, Rudnicki MA, Harris JF, McBurney MW (983). Retinoic acid-induced neural differentiation of embryonal carcinoma cells. Mol Cell Biol 3:2271-2279.

Kemler R, Brulet P, Schnebelin M-T, Gaillard J, Jacob F (1981). Reactivity of monoclonal antibodies against intermediate filament proteins during embryonic development. J Embryol Exp Morphol 64:45-60.

Martin GR, Evans MJ (1975). Differentiation of clonal lines of teratocarcinoma cells: formation of embryoid bodies in vitro. Proc Natl Acad Sci (USA) 72:1441-1445.

McBurney MW, Jones-Villeneuve EMV, Edwards MKS, Anderson PJ (1982). Control of muscle and neuronal differentiation in a cultured embryonal carcinoma cell line. Nat 299:165-167.

McBurney MW, Rogers BJ (1982). Isolation of male embryonal carcinoma cells and their chromosome replication patterns. Dev Biol 89:503-508.

Noguchi M, Noguchi T, Watanabe M, Muramatsu T (1982). Localization of receptors for dolichos biflorus agglutinin in early post implantation embryos in mice. J Embryol Exp Morph 72:39-52.

Shih C, Weinberg RA (1982). Isolation of a transforming sequence from a human bladder carcinoma cell line. Cell 29:161-169.

Cellular Endocrinology: Hormonal Control of Embryonic
and Cellular Differentiation, pages 181–189
© 1986 Alan R. Liss, Inc.

The Regulation of Collagen Type IV(α1) and Other Genes
During the Retinoic Acid Induced Differentiation of Wild
Type and Mutant Mouse Teratocarcinoma Stem Cells

Lorraine J. Gudas and Sho-Ya Wang

Department of Pharmacology, Harvard Medical
School, and Dana-Farber Cancer Institute, 44
Binney St., Boston, MA   02115

INTRODUCTION

Mouse teratocarcinomas contain malignant stem cells
which resemble early embryonic cells, and thus, these stem
cells can be used as a model system for studying early
mammalian development. One teratocarcinoma stem cell line,
F9, differentiates in monolayer cultures into a homogeneous
population of primitive endoderm cells in response to
retinoic acid (RA), and into a population of more
differentiated parietal endoderm cells in response to RA and
dibutyryl cyclicAMP (Strickland et al., 1980). This
differentiation response of F9 cells is irreversible, fairly
synchronized, and reasonably rapid (within 24-48 hours)
(Strickland and Mahdavi, 1978). Although dibutyryl
cyclicAMP, or other compounds which elevate intracellular
cyclicAMP, can enhance the differentiation of these
teratocarcinoma cells in response to retinoic acid,
dibutyryl cyclicAMP alone does not cause differentiation of
the cells (Strickland et al., 1980).

In addition to teratocarcinoma stem cells, vitamin A
and its derivatives (retinoids) can influence
differentiation in several types of cultured cells,
including human promyelocytic leukemia cells (Breitman et
al., 1980), melanoma cells (Lotan and Lotan, 1980), and
human neuroblastoma cells (Haussler et al., 1983).
Retinoids have also been shown to influence the developing
chick limb bud (Tickle et al., 1982), and regenerating
amphibian limbs (Maden, 1982).

The mechanism(s) by which retinoids regulate differentiation and in some cases, loss of tumorigenicity, are unclear at the present time. We are studying the differentiation of mouse teratocarcinoma stem cells in response to retinoic acid in order to determine how retinoic acid acts in this system. In this article, we describe the isolation and characterization of specific gene sequences that are regulated in F9 cells by low concentrations of retinoic acid. In future experiments, we will be able to use these molecular probes to determine which sequences are required for retinoic acid to regulate the expression of these genes.

METHODS

The procedures used for these studies have been previously described (Wang and Gudas, 1983; Wang and Gudas, 1984; Wang et al., 1985).

RESULTS

PolyA$^+$ RNA was prepared from differentiated F9 cells (treated with 5×10^{-7}M retinoic acid and 500µM dibutyryl cyclicAMP for 72 hours), and double stranded cDNA was synthesized (Wang et al., 1985). Poly(dC) tailed cDNA of sizes from 500-2000 base pairs was hybridized to pST1 digested poly(dG)-tailed pBR322 and used to transform E. coli 600. About 100-200 tetracycline resistant colonies were obtained per nanogram of input cDNA, and 85% of these were sensitive to ampicillin. Colony hybridization was then performed by using ^{32}P-labelled cDNAs from either F9 stem cell poly A$^+$ RNA, or RNA from F9 cells treated with RA and dibutyryl cyclicAMP. Of approximately 1000 bacterial colonies which were screened, about 12 colonies showed increased hybridization with the ^{32}P-cDNA probe synthesized from the RA and dibutyryl cyclicAMP treated F9 cell RNA (Fig. 1). We then identified one of these colonies which exhibited increased hybridization with the probe from the differentiated cell RNA as collagen type IV(α1) (Wang and Gudas, 1983; Wang et al., 1985).

a   b

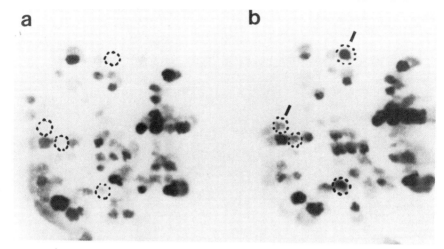

Figure 1. Differential screening of the cDNA library made
from differentiated F9 cell RNA. The two panels are
autoradiograms of replica plated colonies that have been
lysed and hybridized to P³²-labelled cDNA from either F9
stem (Panel A) or retinoic acid and dibutyryl cyclicAMP
treated F9 cells (Panel B), as described in Wang and Gudas
(1983). The circles denote the locations of clones which
contain retinoic acid inducible gene sequences.

     The collagen type IV(α1) gene is expressed only to a
very small extent in F9 undifferentiated stem cells (Fig.
2). Between 24 to 48 hours after retinoic acid addition,
collagen type IV(α1) gene expression is observed, with a
maximal expression occurring at 48 to 72 hours after
retinoic acid addition (Wang et al., 1985). The degree of
expression of collagen type IV(α1), and another parietal
endoderm specific gene, F117, is also dependent on the
concentration of retinoic acid in the medium, and on the
presence of dibutyryl cyclicAMP in the medium. Collagen
type IV(α1) specific mRNA expression reaches a maximum level
in the presence of 5×10^{-8}M retinoic acid, whereas in the
presence of both retinoic acid and dibutyryl cyclicAMP, the
maximum level of collagen type IV(α1) expression occurs at 2
$\times 10^{-7}$M retinoic acid (Fig. 2). Dibutyryl cyclicAMP
greatly enhances the expression of the differentiation
specific gene F117 (Fig. 2). The maximal level of
expression of F117 in the presence of retinoic acid and

dibutyryl cyclicAMP occurs at approximately 2 x 10^{-7}M
retinoic acid.

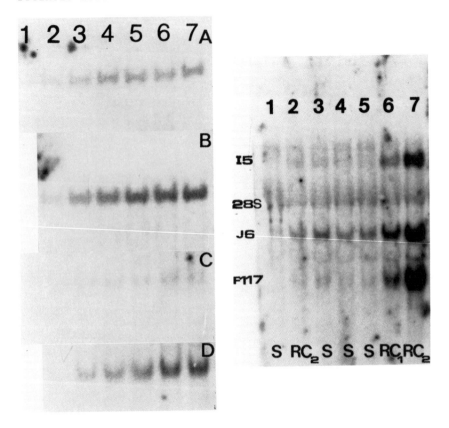

Figure 2. Dose response of I5 and F117 to various
concentrations of retinoic acid. F9 teratocarcinoma cells
were exposed to various concentrations of RA, with (Panels
B,D) or without (Panel A,C) 500μM dibutyryl cyclicAMP, and
500μM theophylline, for 48 hours. Total cellular RNA was
isolated, and 5μg of each RNA sample was fractionated on a
1% agarase/formaldehyde gel, transferred to nitrocellulose
filters, and hybridized to P^{32}-labelled pcI5 (A,B) or
P^{32}-labelled F117 probe (C,D). Lanes: (1) F9 stem
cells; (2) 1 x 10^{-9}M RA; (3) 1 x 10^{-8}M RA; (4) 5 x
10^{-8}M RA; (5) 2 x 10^{-7}M RA; (6) 5 x 10^{-7}M RA; (7) 2
x 10^{-6}M RA.

Figure 3. Analysis of retinoic acid inducible mRNAs from wild type and mutant cell lines. F9 teratocarcinoma stem cells were treated with 5 x 10^{-7}M retinoic acid, 500µM dibutyryl cyclicAMP, and 500µM theophylline for either 24 or 48 hours. Total cell RNA was extracted, and 5µg of each preparation was fractionated, transferred to nitrocellulose filters, and hybridized to P^{32}-labelled plasmids I5, J6, and F117. RNA was isolated from: (1) RA 3-10 mutant stem cells; (2) RA 3-10 mutant cells which had been treated for 48 hours with retinoic acid and dibutyryl cyclicAMP; (3,4,5) F9 wild type stem cells; (6) F9 wild type cells treated for 24 hours, or (7), 48 hrs. with retinoic acid and dibutyryl cyclicAMP.

The expression of collagen type IV(α1) mRNA is not only dependent on the retinoic acid concentration, and on the time RA addition. Expression of the collagen type IV(α1) gene also depends on the presence of a functional binding protein or receptor for retinoic acid. We have previously isolated a mutant, RA 3-10, which lacks a functional cellular retinoic acid binding protein (Wang and Gudas, 1984). When the expression of collagen type IV(α1) mRNA was studied in wild type F9 cells versus RA 3-10 mutant cells grown in the presence of RA and dibutyryl cyclicAMP, we found that no collagen type IV(α1) specific mRNA was expressed in the RA 3-10 mutant (Fig. 3). There was also no increase in other differentiation specific gene expression in the RA 3-10 mutant after RA addition (Fig. 3, see J6 and F117). Thus, in the teratocarcinoma differentiation system, the expression of a number of differentiation specific mRNAs, including collagen type IV(α1), is dependent on the presence of a functional retinoic acid binding protein.

In order to determine whether the regulation of these differentiation specific genes is a primary effect of retinoic acid, we also measured the sensitivity of the induction of mRNA specific for several RA inducible genes, including collagen IV(α1), to inhibitors of protein synthesis. RNA was isolated from F9 cells that had been treated for 20 hours with RA (with or without dibutyryl cyclicAMP), in the presence or absence of either of the protein synthesis inhibitors cycloheximide or puromycin.

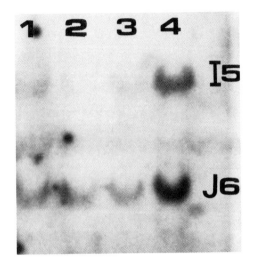

Figure 4. The effect of cycloheximide on mRNA
accumulation. F9 cells were treated for 20 hours with 5 x
10^{-7}M RA, 500μM dibutyryl cyclicAMP, and 500μM
theophylline in the presence or absence of 1μg/ml
cycloheximide. Total cell RNA was extracted, and 5μg of
each total RNA preparation was fractionated on a 1%
agarose/formaldehyde gel, transferred to a nitrocellulose
filter, and hybridized to the P^{32}-labelled nick translated
recombinant plasmids pcI5 and pcJ6. The lanes contain RNA
from: (1) control F9 stem cells; (2) cycloheximide
treated stem cells; (3) RA, dibutyryl cyclicAMP,
theophylline, and cycloheximide treated cells; (4) RA,
dibutyryl cyclicAMP, and theophylline treated F9 cells.

We then hybridized the ^{32}P-labelled recombinant plasmid
pcI5 (collagen type IV(α1)) to RNA from the treated cells.
Both cycloheximide (Fig. 4) and puromycin (data not shown)
inhibit the RA induction of mRNA specific for the collagen
type IV(α1) gene, and for another differentiation specific
gene, J6 (Fig. 4). Thus, this result is evidence that the
induction of the collagen type IV(α1) gene is not a primary
effect of retinoic acid. Appropriate controls were
performed in order to demonstrate that the cycloheximide
treatment for 20 hours was not toxic to the cells. For
example, we demonstrated that metallothionein I specific RNA

could be induced by zinc or cadmium in F9 stem cells even after a 20 hour treatment with cycloheximide (data not shown).

DISCUSSION

We have isolated a number of retinoic acid inducible gene sequences, including the gene for collagen type IV(α1). Maximal induction of these sequences occurs between 48 and 72 hours after RA addition (Wang et al., 1985). RA treatment alone causes the induction of these mRNAs, but to a lower maximal level than the induction seen in the presence of both RA and dibutyryl cyclicAMP (Fig. 2).

In some respects, the action of retinoic acid may be similar to that of steroid hormones (for review, Lotan, 1980). Steroid hormones cause a primary response by directly inducing transcription of a few specific genes, and the products of these genes may then activate other genes (for review, Yamamoto and Alberts, 1976). If the action of RA is similar to that of steroid hormones, then the slow induction response and the sensitivity of the induction to protein synthesis inhibitors such as cycloheximide (Fig. 4) suggest that these RA inducible genes, including collagen type IV(α1), may be indirectly regulated by retinoic acid.

We have also demonstrated that these RA-inducible genes exhibit differing responses at the RNA level to changes in the concentration of RA (Fig. 2). The response of these genes to increasing RA concentrations is gradual and increases proportionally as the concentration of RA increases.

The activity of retinoic acid is also similar to that of steroid hormones with respect to its dependence on a functional receptor or binding protein. We have demonstrated this by utilizing a mutant which lacks a functional retinoic acid binding protein. Using this mutant, we have shown that collagen type IV(α1) specific mRNA is not expressed following RA addition (Fig. 3). This result is similar to the result of Yamamoto et al. (1974), who demonstrated that mutations in the glucocorticoid receptor could prevent the response of S49 cells to glucocorticoid hormone.

In contrast to the response of most genes to steroid hormones, the increase in the expression of most of these RA-inducible genes appears to be stable upon removal of exogenous RA (Wang et al., 1985). In addition, we have not been able to clearly demonstrate the presence of the cellular retinoic acid binding protein:retinoic acid complex in nuclei from F9 cells that have been treated with RA (McGovern and Gudas, unpublished).

By analyzing the expression of specific genes in this model differentiation system, we have already learned much about the regulation of specific genes by retinoic acid. Our next goal is to determine which gene sequences interact, either directly or indirectly, with RA and its binding protein to achieve the resultant increases in differentiation specific messages. In order to do this, we are currently in the process of isolating genomic clones for a number of these differentiation specific genes. We are also attempting to isolate full length cDNA clones for several of the differentiation specific genes, including collagen type IV(α1) (Brinker et al., 1985).

REFERENCES

Breitman TR, Selonick S, Collins SJ (1980). Induction of differentiation of the human promyelocytic leukemia cell line (HL-60) by retinoic acid. Proc. Natl. Acad. Sci.USA 71:2936-2940.

Brinker JM, Gudas LJ, Loidl H, Wang S-Y, Rosenbloom J, Kefalides NA, Myers JC (1985). Restricted homology between human α1 type IV and other procollagen chains. Proc. Natl. Acad. Sci. USA 82:3649-3653.

Haussler M, Sidell N, Kelly M, Donaldson C, Altman A, Mangelsdorf D (1983). Specific high-affinity binding and biologic action of retinoic acid in human neuroblastoma cell lines. Proc. Natl. Acad. Sci. USA 80:5525-5529.

Lotan R (1980). Effects of vitamin A and its analogs (retinoids) on normal and neoplastic cells. Biochim. Biophys. Acta 605:33-91.

Lotan R, Lotan D (1980). Stimulation of melanogenesis in a human melanoma cell line by retinoids. Cancer Res. 40:3345-3350.

Maden M (1982). Vitamin A and pattern formation in the regenerating limb. Nature 295:672-675.

Strickland S, Mahdavi V (1978). The induction of differentiation in teratocarcinoma stem cells by retinoic acid. Cell 15:393-403.

Strickland S, Smith KK, Marotti KR (1980). Hormonal induction of differentiation in teratocarcinoma stem cells: Generation of parietal endoderm by retinoic acid and dibutyryl cAMP. Cell 21:347-355.

Tickle C, Alberts B, Wolpert L, Lee J (1982). Local application of retinoic acid to the limb bud mimics the action of the polarizing region. Nature (London) 296:564-566.

Wang S-Y, Gudas LJ (1983). Isolation of cDNA clones specific for collagen IV and laminin from mouse teratocarcinoma cells. Proc. Natl. Acad. Sci. USA 80:5880-5884.

Wang S-Y, Gudas LJ (1984). Selection and characterization of F9 teratocarcinoma stem cell mutants with altered responses to retinoic acid. J. Biol. Chem. 259:5899-5906.

Wang S-Y, LaRosa GJ, Gudas LJ (1985). Molecular cloning of gene sequences transcriptionally regulated by retinoic acid and dibutyryl cyclic AMP in cultured mouse teratocarcinoma cells. Dev. Biol. 107:75-86.

Yamamoto KR, Alberts BM (1976). Steroid receptors: Elements for modulation of eukaryotic transcription. Annu. Rev. Biochem. 45:721-746.

Yamamoto KR, Stampfer MR, Tomkins GM (1974). Receptors from glucocorticoid-sensitive lymphoma cells and two classes of insensitive clones: Physical and DNA-binding properties. Proc. Natl. Acad. Sci. USA 71:3901-3905.

Cellular Endocrinology: Hormonal Control of Embryonic
and Cellular Differentiation, pages 191–204
© 1986 Alan R. Liss, Inc.

ENDOCRINE AND AUTOCRINE CONTROL OF GROWTH AND DIFFERENTIA-
TION OF TERATOMA-DERIVED CELL LINES

Ginette Serrero

W. Alton Jones Cell Science Center, Inc.
10 Old Barn Road, Lake Placid   NY   12946

For the past few years, our laboratory has been interested in studying the hormonal control of adipose differentiation using C3H mouse teratoma-derived cell lines as in
vitro model system. As these cells can proliferate and
undergo differentiation in defined medium, they represent a
suitable system with which to identify the hormones and
growth factors influencing either positively or negatively
the processes of growth and differentiation. For this
purpose, we have characterized two cell lines: the adipogenic cell line 1246 (Darmon et al., 1981; Serrero and
Sato,   1982;   Serrero   and   Khoo,   1982),   and   an
insulin-independent variant cell line, 1246-3A isolated
from 1246 cells which has lost the ability to differentiate
(Serrero, 1985). The study of these cell lines has allowed
us to demonstrate the existence of an autocrine control of
growth   and   differentiation   in   addition   to   the
identification of the endocrine factors influencing both
processes.

HORMONAL CONTROL OF 1246 CELL DIFFERENTIATION

a)   1246 Cell Line Proliferates and Differentiates in
      Defined Medium

      1246 is a triglyceride-accumulating cell line that has
been clonally isolated from the C3H mouse myogenic cell
line C17-S1-D-T984. Although, 1246 cells will primarily
undergo adipose differentiation, when cells are plated at

high cell density or treated with 5-azacytidine at low cell density, they can be induced to form patches of myotubes (Darmon et al., 1981). Since the 1246 cells which had accumulated triglycerides presented the same biochemical and biological characteristics of mature adipocytes (Serrero and Khoo, 1982), it was considered as a suitable system to study adipose differentiation in vitro. Our approach to identify the hormones and growth factors controlling adipose proliferation and differentiation has been to establish a defined medium in which 1246 cells could grow and to determine in which conditions they would differentiate. The defined medium allowing the best growth of undifferentiated 1246 cells consisted of DME-F12 medium supplemented with insulin, transferrin, fibroblast growth factor (FGF) and fibronectin (Serrero and Sato, 1982). This medium called 4F medium supported a growth rate similar to the one measured for cells maintained in DME-F12 medium containing 10% FBS. When the confluent 1246 cells cultivated in 4F medium were treated with dexamethasone (2 x 10^{-7} M) and isobutylmethylxanthine (2 x 10^{-4} M), they underwent adipose differentiation. In these conditions, the 1246 cells developed activities controlling lipid metabolism and acquired characteristics of mature adipocytes such as morphological changes, increase in enzymatic activities controlling lipogenesis and lipolysis including the hormone sensitive lipase which is a specific marker of adipocytes, de novo synthesis of fatty acids and triglycerides, development of response to lipolytic hormones and cytoplasmic accumulation of triglycerides (Serrero and Khoo, 1982; Serrero and Sato, 1982). These experiments indicated that 1246 cells could undergo differentiation in the absence of fetal bovine serum in the culture medium whereas other adipogenic cell lines such as $3T3-L_1$, 3T3-F442A and Ob17 could grow in defined medium but required the presence of FBS in the culture medium in order to differentiate (Serrero et al., 1979; Gaillard et al., 1984). Based on these results, the 1246 cell line is an adequate system to examine: 1) the effect of individual components of the 4F medium on proliferation and differentiation; 2) the effect of hormones and growth factors added to the 4F medium on adipose differentiation; 3) the possibility that 1246 cells produce their own adipogenic factor thus by-passing the need for an exogenous factor provided by fetal bovine serum.

b)   Insulin is Stringently Required to Support 1246 Cell
     Proliferation and Differentiation

The effect of individual component of the 4F medium on
1246 cell growth and differentiation, was examined by
inoculating 1246 cells either in 4F medium (positive control) or in 4F medium from which either insulin, transferrin, FGF or fibronectin had been omitted. Proliferation
and differentiation were followed by measuring cell number
and glycerol-3-phosphate dehydrogenase specific activity,
respectively (Table 1).

TABLE 1. Effect of the Omission of Individual Component on
Growth and Differentiation

Condition	Cell growth % of control	G3PDH mU/mg protein
4F	100	100
4F-fibronectin	60	80
4F-insulin	20	0
4F-FGF	20	100
4F-transferrin	80	20

Culture conditions have been described elsewhere (Serrero
and Sato, 1982).

As shown in Table 1, insulin was the only hormone
whose omission impaired both growth and differentiation.
In the absence of insulin, 1246 cells did not grow but
remained viable and their differentiation did not take
place. Omission of transferrin also impaired differentiation, but in contrast to what was observed with insulin,
differentiation of 1246 cells maintained in the absence of
transferrin was only delayed (data not shown). Growth of
1246 cells was stimulated by insulin concentrations as low
as 1 ng/ml with an ED50 of 10 ng/ml whereas differentiation
was stimulated by insulin concentrations of 10 ng/ml with
an ED50 of 30-100 ng/ml (Serrero, 1984). Binding experiments performed on 1246 cells before and after differentiation indicated that 1246 cells possessed two categories of
insulin receptors for insulin (Kd 10^{-10} M; 6,000 sites/cell
and Kd 10^{-8} M; 10^5 sites/cell) and that insulin receptor
number increased during the differentiation process
(Gazzano and Serrero, submitted to publication).

c)   Effect of Growth Hormone on 1246 Cell Differentiation

Growth hormone is known to control adipose tissue development in vivo (Murakawa and Vrana, 1968) and to stimulate the adipose conversion of pre-adipocyte cell lines in vitro (Morikawa et al. 1982; Nixon and Green, 1983, 1984). As insulin appeared as a regulator of 1246 cell differentiation, the effect of growth hormone on 1246 differentiation was examined in the presence and in the absence of insulin.

TABLE 2.   Effect of Insulin and Growth Hormone on 1246 Adipose Differentiation

Condition	G3PDH mU/mg protein
3F 4F	120
3F (4F-insulin)	0
4F + GH 10 ng/ml	610
3F + GH 10 ng/ml	0

1246 Cells were inoculated at a density of 30,000 cells/35 mm dish either in 4F medium (DME-F12 supplemented with insulin, transferrin, FGF and fibronectin) or 3F medium (4F medium deprived of insulin) in the presence or absence of 10 ng/ml of human growth hormone. Cells were treated with DEX-MIX for 48 hours and harvested at day 15 to measure G3PDH specific activity.

As shown in Table 2, growth hormone at an optimal concentration of 10 ng/ml stimulated by 5-fold, G3PDH specific activity of 1246 cells cultivated in 4F medium. However, when insulin was removed from the defined medium, differentiation did not take place even in the presence of growth hormone, indicating the growth hormone was inactive in the absence of insulin.

Experiments are underway to examine if this corresponds to changes in receptor numbers or affinity for growth hormone.

d)   1246 Conditioned Medium Replaces Fetal Calf Serum to
Stimulate Adipose Differentiation of 3T3-L$_1$ Cells

As indicated above, 1246 cells can proliferate and
differentiate in defined medium whereas 3T3-L$_1$ cells can
proliferate in defined medium but require the presence of
fetal bovine serum to undergo adipose differentiation.
This may be explained by the fact that 1246 cells can
synthesize and secrete an adipogenic factor in the culture
medium, therefore by-passing the need for an exogenous
serum adipogenic factor to control the onset of adipose
differentiation. In order to test this hypothesis, 3T3-L$_1$
cells were cultivated in defined medium (see legend of
Table 3) alone or in the presence of either 2% FBS or
conditioned medium collected from differentiated 1246
cells, added at the time when 3T3-L$_1$ cells reached
confluency. As indicated in Table 3, 3T3-L$_1$ cells
maintained in defined medium failed to differentiate
(absence of G3PDH activity). However, when 2% FBS were
added at confluency to 3T3-L$_1$ cells cultivated in defined
medium, differentiation took place as measured by the increase of G3PDH specific activity. Interestingly, the
cells cultivated in defined medium in the presence of 20%
1246-CM instead of serum could also differentiate into
adipocytes. However, the level of G3PDH activity was
2-fold lower than the one found in cells cultivated with 2%
FBS.

TABLE 3. Glycerophosphate Dehydrogenase (GPDH) Specific
Activity in 3T3-L$_1$ Cells Maintained in Various Conditions

Culture condition	GPDH mU/mg protein
1. 4F	ND
2. 4F+GH+T3	90
3. 4F+GH+T3+1246CM	480
4. 4F+GH+T3+2%FBS	910

3T3-L$_1$ cells were maintained in DME-F12 medium containing
insulin 10 μg/ml, transferrin 10 μg/ml, FGF 10 ng/ml and
HDL (50 μg/ml). At confluency various factors were added
to the cells which have been treated for 48 hours with
DEX-MIX: 1) 4F medium alone; 2) 4F medium containing
growth hormone 50 ng/ml (GH) and T3 10^{-11} M; 3) same as in
(2) but, supplemented with 20% of 1246 conditioned medium
1246-CM; 4) same as in (2) but, supplemented with 2% fetal
bovine serum. Cells were harvested on day 21 and glycero-

phosphate dehydrogenase specific activity determined in each condition. 1246 CM had been collected from 1246 cells undergoing differentiation in serum-free medium. ND = Not Detectable.

Preliminary biochemical characterization of the activity present in the 1246-CM has indicated that it was destroyed by incubation of the 1246-CM fraction with immobilized pronase, was heat-sensitive and had an apparent molecular weight of 10,000 daltons. Experiments are underway to characterize the adipogenic stimulating activity produced by the 1246 cell line and to compare its nature to already known hormones and growth factors and to adipogenic activity characterized from serum (Grimaldi et al., 1982).

FACTORS PRODUCED BY THE INSULIN-INDEPENDENT CELL LINE 1246-3A INFLUENCING 1246 CELL GROWTH AND DIFFERENTIATION

As mentioned earlier, if insulin is removed from the 4F medium, 1246 cells do not grow but remain viable and their differentiation is blocked. Based on this observation, insulin-independent variant cells able to proliferate in the absence of insulin were isolated from 1246 cells maintained in defined medium deprived of insulin (in conditions in which they would not proliferate). These cells were isolated and subsequently cloned in 3F medium (4F medium deprived of insulin). One of the clones, called 1246-3A was characterized (Serrero, 1985). Unlike the parent cell line 1246, the insulin-independent variant cell line 1246-3A has the following properties: it can proliferate in the absence of insulin; it has lost the ability to undergo adipose differentiation even in the most optimal conditions (in the presence of fetal calf serum); it develops into tumors when injected into syngeneic hosts C3H mice at a density of 10^6 cells per animal; it produces in its culture medium factors able to replace insulin to stimulate the growth of the parent cell line 1246 but not its differentiation (Serrero, 1985). Based on this observation, two possibilities could account for the fact that 1246-3A CM could replace insulin only to stimulate 1246 cell growth: 1) the factor produced by 1246-3A cells was different from insulin and insulin-like growth factors (IGF) which are known to replace insulin to stimulate both 1246 cell proliferation and differentiation; 2) 1246-3A cells produced a factor similar to insulin or IGF and secreted also an inhibitor of adipose differentiation which would block the effect of insulin or related factors on the differentiation process. In order to investigate these various possibilities, the factors contained in the 1246-3A CM were characterized using several bioassays described as follows: cell proliferation assay to measure the ability of 3A-produced factor to stimulate the growth of 1246 cells in the absence of insulin; radioimmunoassays for insulin and IGF-s to determine if 1246-3A cells secreted insulin or IGF-related molecules; radioreceptor assays for insulin and IGF to determine if 1246-3A CM contained factors able to competitively displace radiolabeled insulin and IGF from 1246 cell surface receptors; differentiation assays using 1246 cells cultivated in defined medium either with or without insulin, to determine the presence of negative or positive regulators of differentiation in 1246-3A CM. Based on these various assays, it has been possible to demonstrate the existence of two types of activities in the 1246-3A conditioned medium: a factor called insulin-related factor, IRF, which is immunologically and biochemically similar to pancreatic insulin, and an inhibitor of adipose differentiation. Characterization of these activities has been carried out using factor and hormone-free 1246-3A conditioned medium (1246-3A CM).

a)   Characterization of the Insulin-Related Factor, IRF, Produced by 1246-3A Cells

When 1246-3A CM was chromatographed on a Sephadex G50 column equilibrated with 1 M acetic acid, the growth promoting activity was eluted in two peaks, one in the void volume, the other one with an apparent molecular weight of 6 kDa (Yamada and Serrero, 1986). It was demonstrated that only the 6 kDa fraction presented immunological and biochemical similarities with pancreatic insulin as measured by radioimmuno- and radioreceptor assays. However, none of the fractions from 1246-3A CM eluted from the Sephadex G50 column contained immunoreactive IGF-I and IGF-II. Biochemical characterization of the 6 kDa fraction indicated that the growth promoting activity was destroyed by incubation with immobilized pronase, by treatment at 100°C for 5 minutes and by incubation with 0.1 M 2-mercaptoethanol. Dialysis of the fraction against 0.1 M acetic acid did not affect the growth stimulatory activity (Yamada and Serrero, 1986). Because of its similarities with insulin, the growth factor contained in the 6 KDa fraction was called, insulin-related factor (IRF). IRF was purified to homogeneity from 1246-3A CM using a three step purification procedure including ion exchange chromatography on Amberlite CG50 resin equilibrated with 20 mM ammonium acetate, pH 6.0 and elution with 0.1 and 0.7 M ammonium hydroxyde; immunoaffinity chromatography on Affi-Gel 10 coupled to an anti-insulin monoclonal antibody and high pressure liquid chromatography on an octadecyl support and elution with 35% acetonitrile containing 0.1% trifluoroacetic acid (Yamada and Serrero, submitted to publication). Throughout the purification procedure, growth promoting activity and radioimmunoassayable insulin comigrated. After the HPLC step, both activities coeluted in a single homogenous peak which gave rise to a single band with the same mobility as pancreatic insulin when analyzed by SDS-PAGE both in dissociating and in non-dissociating conditions. The degree of final purification of IRF was 3,210-fold with a recovery of 16% (Yamada and Serrero, submitted to publication). HPLC-IRF was equipotent to insulin to stimulate 1246 cell growth, to displace ^{125}I-insulin specifically bound to 1246 cell surface receptors (Yamada and Serrero, submitted to publication), to stimulate adipose differentiation of 1246 cells and 3T3-L$_1$ cells (Serrero, submitted to publication) and to stimulate the phosphorylation of partially purified immunoprecipitated insulin receptors from 1246 and 1246-3A cells (Gazzano and Serrero, manuscript in preparation). Experiments are currently underway to determine IRF amino-acid sequence and compare it to mouse pancreatic insulin I and II.

b)   IRF Acts as an Autocrine Growth Factor

Preliminary results (Yamada and Serrero, 1986) had shown that 1246-3A cells bound 43% less ^{125}I-insulin than 1246 cells; however, specific insulin binding to 1246-3A cells was restored to the level found in 1246 cells by acid pre-wash of 1246-3A cells, which is known to dissociate excess growth factor bound to their cell surface receptors. Binding of ^{125}I-IRF was performed on intact 1246 and 1246-3A cells with or without acid pre-wash and in the absence or in the presence of anti-insulin or anti-IGF monoclonal antibody added at a concentration of 3×10^{-7} M. Specific IRF binding was lower on 1246-3A cells than on 1246 cells. Acid pre-wash and incubation with the anti-insulin monoclonal antibody restored IRF binding on 1246-3A cells to a value similar to the one found for IRF binding to 1246 cells. In contrast, incubation of 1246-3A cells with anti-IGF monoclonal antibody failed to increase IRF binding to 1246-3A cells (Yamada and Serrero, submitted to publication). These results indicate that cell surface receptors on 1246-3A cells are being partially occupied by IRF secreted in their culture medium. In addition, we have demonstrated that an incubation of 1246-3A cells in 3F medium with anti-insulin monoclonal antibody blocked not only the binding of secreted IRF but also inhibited the growth of the producer cells 1246-3A by 50% (Yamada and Serrero, submitted to publication). These data are in agreement with the autocrine hypothesis (Sporn and Todaro, 1980), and indicate that ectopic IRF acts as an autocrine growth factor for the insulin-independent cell line 1246-3A.

c)   1246-3A Cells Produce a Differentiation Inhibitor in Their Conditioned Medium

As mentioned in the preceding paragraph, pure IRF was able to replace insulin to stimulate not only the growth of the parent cell line 1246 but also its differentiation at concentrations similar to insulin. In contrast, crude conditioned medium was able to replace insulin only to stimulate the growth but not the differentiation of 1246 cells maintained in 3F medium. One could assume that either IRF was present in the 1246-3A CM at concentrations too low to stimulate the differentiation of 1246 cells or the 1246-3A CM contained a factor that would inhibit differentiation of 1246 cells even in the presence of IRF or insulin. To examine this later hypothesis, fractions derived from the chromatography of 1246-3A CM on amberlite CG50 resin were added to 1246 cells cultivated in 4F medium. Differentiation was determined by measuring G3PDH specific activity.

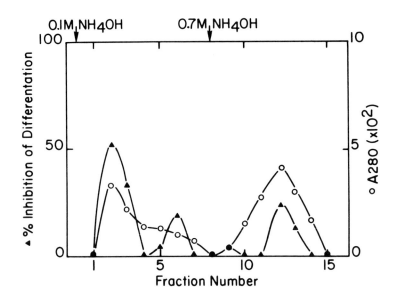

Figure 1. Ion exchange chromatography of 1246-3A CM on amberlite CG50.

As indicated in Figure 1, two peaks of differentiation inhibiting activity were eluted, with 0.1 M ammonium hydroxide, another one with 0.7 M ammonium hydroxide. The peak eluted with 0.7 M ammonium hydroxide eluted at a higher pH (pH 11) than IRF (eluted at pH 9). Thus, chromatography of 1246-3A CM on amberlite CG50 allowed us to separate IRF and the differentiation inhibitory factors in one step. The partially purified fractions from 1246 CM were unable to block adipose differentiation of 1246 cells. To determine if the inhibiting factor produced by 1246-3A cells acted directly by inhibiting the differentiation process or by blocking insulin action, we investigated if the active fractions eluted from CG50 column could block adipose differentiation of 3T3-L$_1$ cells maintained in medium supplemented with 10% FBS, for their differentiation was under the control of serum and growth hormone (Morikawa et al., 1982). It was found that 3T3-L$_1$ differentiation was blocked by the CG50 fractions. The determination of the chemical nature of differentiation inhibitor is currently under investigation. Meanwhile, we examined if known growth factors could act as differentiation inhibitors for both 1246 cells and 3T3-L₁ cells. We have found that EGF and transforming growth factors α and β blocked 1246 cell differentiation when added in the 4F medium (Serrero, submitted to publication). The effect of TGF-β on 1246 differentiation is in agreement with the recent report of Ignotz and Massague (1985), who have shown that TGF-β blocked adipose differentiation of 3T3-L₁ cells cultivated in the presence of 10% FBS. However, interestingly, the effect of EGF and TGF-α on the adipose differentiation of 3T3-L₁ cultivated in the presence of 10% FBS was quite different from that observed on 1246 cells. In contrast to what was observed with 1246 cells, EGF and TGF-α failed to inhibit adipose differentiation of 3T3-L₁ cells even when added at concentrations that induced complete inhibition of 1246 cell differentiation (Table 4).

TABLE 4. Effect of EGF and TGF-β on the Adipose Differentiation of 1246 and 3T3-L₁ Cells

Conditions	G3PDH specific activity % of control	
	1246	3T3-L₁
Control	100	100
+ EGF (10 ng/ml)	5	200
+ TGF-β (0.3 ng/ml)	10	20

1246 cells cultivated in 4F medium as described previously served as positive control (Serrero, 1985). For 3T3-L₁ cells, positive control was represented by 3T3-L₁ cells cultivated in the presence of 10% FBS. The concentrations of EGF and TGF-β represent optimal concentrations as determined by dose-response experiments. TGF-α had the same effect as EGF (data not shown) on 1246 and 3T3-L₁ differentiation. Values are expressed in percentage of the G3PDH specific activity measured in the control plates taken as 100%.

In fact, EGF stimulated the increase of G3PDH specific activity in 3T3-L₁ cells undergoing differentiation.

Experiments are underway to examine these differences in response to the growth factors between these two cell lines. The determination of relationship with the differentiation inhibitors in the 1246-3A CM and TGF-α or -β, awaits further experimentations.

CONCLUSION

The model system presented in this paper consists of two cell lines: the 1246 cell line which is able to proliferate and undergo adipose differentiation in defined medium and the insulin-independent variant cell line 1246-3A which can proliferate in the absence of insulin, has lost the ability to differentiate and has acquired tumorigenic properties in vivo. In our study, we have demonstrated that the teratoma-derived cell lines synthesize three types of factors which influence pre-adipocyte growth and differentiation: adipogenic factor produced by the adipogenic cell line 1246; insulin-related factor, IRF synthesized and secreted by the insulin-independent variant cell line 1246-3A; differentiation inhibiting activity produced by the 1246-3A cells. There is strong evidence to suggest that among the factors produced by 1246 and 1246-3A cells, at least IRF acts as an autocrine growth factor for the 1246-3A cells. It would be interesting to investigate if the adipogenic factor and the adipogenic inhibitor also act as autocrine regulators of differentiation for the cells that produce them. It has been postulated that cell-produced growth factors and altered responsiveness to different hormones at various stages during development could play an important role in mediating early growth and differentiation (Sporn and Todaro, 1980). Based on these observations and on our results, one could postulate a role for extra-pancreatic insulin as a growth and differentiation factor in the embryo at a pre-pancreatic stage and a role for paracrine and autocrine regulators of differentiation during tissue development, in particular during adipose tissue development. Such autocrine or paracrine control via positive and negative regulators could affect the maintenance of a balance between undifferentiated and differentiated cellular pools in the adipose tissue. We are currently investigating these hypothesis.

This work was supported by grants from the National Science Foundation DCB-834050582, from the National Institute of Health 1-PO1 CA 37589 and from the Juvenile Diabetes Foundation file #185221.

REFERENCES

Darmon M, Serrero G, Rizzino A, Sato, G (1981) Isolation of myoblastic, fibroadipogenic and fibroblastic clonal cell lines form a common precursor and study of their requirements for growth and differentiation. Exp Cell Res 132:313-327.

Gaillard D, Negrel R, Serrero G, Cermolacce C, Ailhaud G (1984) Growth of preadipocyte cell lines and cell strains from rodents in serum free, hormone-supplemented medium. In Vitro 20:79-88.

Grimaldi P, Djian P, Negrel, R, Ailhaud, G (1982) Differentiation of Ob17 preadipocytes to adipocytes: Requirement of adipose conversion factor(s) for fat cell cluster formation. EMBO J 6:687-692.

Ignotz RA, Massague J (1985) Type β transforming growth factor controls the adipogenic differentiation of 3T3 fibroblasts. Proc Natl Acad Sci USA 82:8530-8534.

Morikawa M, Nixon T, Green H (1982) Growth hormone and the adipose conversion of 3T3 cells. Cell 31:783-789.

Murakawa S, Raben MS (1968) Effect of growth hormone and placental lactogen on DNA synthesis in rat costal cartilage and adipose tissue. Endocrinology 87:645-650.

Nixon T, Green H (1983) Properties of growth hormone receptors in relation to the adipose conversion of 3T3 cells. J Cell Physiol 115:291-296.

Nixon T, Green H (1984) Contribution of growth hormone to the adipogenic activity of serum. Endocrinology 114:527-532.

Serrero G (1984) Growth and differentiation of preadipocytes cell lines in serum-free medium in mammalian cell cultures. In Mather, JP (ed): "The use of serum-free hormone-supplemented media," New York and London: Plenum Press, pp 53-75.

Serrero G (1985) Tumorigenicity associated with loss of differentiation and of response to insulin in the adipogenic cell line 1246. In Vitro Cell and Dev Biology 21:537-540.

Serrero G, Khoo JC (1982) An in vitro model to study adipose differentiation in serum-free medium. Anal Biochem 120:351-359.

Serrero G, Sato G (1982). Growth and differentiation of a teratoma-derived fibroadipogenic cell line in serum-free medium, In Sato, GH, Pardee, AB, Sirbasku, DA (eds): "Growth of Cells in Hormonally Defined Media," Vol 9, Cold Spring Harbor Conferences on Cell Proliferation, Cold Spring Harbor Laboratory, New York, pp. 943-955.

Serrero G, McClure D, Sato, G (1979) Growth of mouse 3T3 fibroblasts in serum-free hormone-supplemented media, In Sato, GH, Ross, R (eds): "Hormones and Cell Culture", Vol 6, Cold Spring Harbor Conference on Cell Proliferation, Cold Spring Harbor Laboratory, New York, pp 523-530.

Sporn MB, Todaro GJ (1980). Autocrine secretion and malignant transformation of cells. New Engl J Med 303:878-880.

Yamada Y, Serrero G (1986) Characterization of an insulin-related factor secreted by a teratoma-cell line. Biochem Biophys Res Commun 135:533-540.

Cellular Endocrinology: Hormonal Control of Embryonic
and Cellular Differentiation, pages 205-213
© 1986 Alan R. Liss, Inc.

RETINOID-BINDING PROTEINS AND RETINOID-INDUCED DIFFERENTIA-
TION OF EMBRYONAL CARCINOMA CELLS

Uriel Barkai, Mary Lou Gubler and
Michael I. Sherman

Roche Institute of Molecular Biology, Roche
Research Center, Nutley, New Jersey 07110

Embryonal carcinoma (EC) cells are the pluripotent stem
cells of teratocarcinomas. Several lines of evidence have
revealed the close relationship between EC cells and
pluripotent cells of the early embryo (see Martin, 1980);
thus, EC cells hold promise as a model system for studying
the regulation of differentiation. EC cells can be induced
to differentiate in vitro in response to several chemical
agents (see Jetten, 1986 for a recent review). Among
these, retinoids are of considerable interest because of
their potency and because they are naturally-occurring.
Acidic retinoids, such as all-*trans*-retinoic acid (RA) and
13-*cis*-RA, are the most active in inducing EC cell differentiation. Esterified retinoids are generally inactive,
possibly because of difficulties in penetrating the cells
(Gubler and Sherman, 1985). We have found that retinol is
about one order of magnitude less active than all-*trans*-RA
in inducing differentiation of F9 EC cells (Eglitis and
Sherman, 1983), but in the studies of other investigators,
the relative activity of retinol is even lower (Strickland
and Mahdavi; 1978; Jetten et al., 1983; Williams and
Napoli, 1985). Notwithstanding the low potency of retinol
as compared to RA, the former retinoid might play an
important physiological role in promoting differentiation
because its circulating levels are in the micromolar range
(e.g., Smith and Goodman, 1971) whereas RA, when detected in
the circulation, appears to be present at concentrations
which are substantially lower (De Ruyter et al., 1979;
Shidoji and Hosoya, 1980).

Because of the pleiotropic nature of the retinoids, the mechanisms by which they modulate or influence basic cellular processes are still unclear in most instances (discussed by Sherman, 1986). Our laboratory has provided evidence that a cellular binding protein for RA (CRABP) is involved in the promotion of EC cell differentiation by acidic retinoids: (a) all EC lines which respond to RA possess CRABP (Jetten and Jetten, 1979; Matthaei et al., 1983); (b) there is a strong qualitative correlation (with a few notable exceptions) between the ability of retinoids to promote differentiation and to compete with RA for CRABP binding sites (Jetten and Jetten, 1979; Sherman et al., 1983); (c) of seven mutant EC lines that fail to differentiate in response to RA, four have lost most or all of their CRABP activity (Schindler et al., 1981; McCue et al., 1983; Wang and Gudas, 1984); and (d) when CRABP activity is restored to these mutant cells by cell fusion or treatment with sodium butyrate, they are able to differentiate in response to RA (McCue et al., 1984a,b).

McCormick et al. (1984) and Sherman et al. (1985) have reported that CRABP binds specifically to a finite number of sites on or in purified EC nuclei (see also Table 1). When Nulli-SCC1 EC cells incubated with [^{3}H]all-*trans*-RA are subsequently fractionated, about 20% of the radioactivity co-purifies with nuclei (unpublished observations). The label in the nucleoplasm is associated with a 2S component, presumably CRABP, following sucrose density gradient centrifugation (Jetten and Jetten, 1979). Since RA can be extensively metabolized by EC cells (Williams and Napoli, 1985; Sherman et al., 1985; Gubler and Sherman, 1985), and certain RA metabolites might possess at least some biological activity (see Sherman, 1986), we undertook to evaluate the nature of the labeled material associated with purified nuclei following incubation of cultured Nulli-SCC1 cells for 2 hr with [^{3}H]RA. As the HPLC profiles in Figure 1 illustrate, the predominant radioactive peak in the culture medium and the cytosol co-migrates with the all-*trans*-RA marker. The same is true of the extract from purified Nulli-SCC1 nuclei, provided that the cells are fractionated in the presence of an antioxidant. Taken together, these observations suggest that following uptake by cells, intact RA can be translocated to the nuclear compartment and bound to some specific site(s).

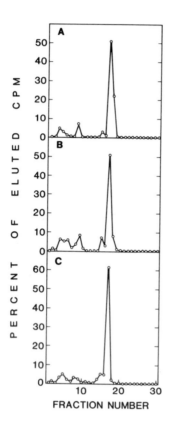

Figure 1. HPLC profile of extracted retinoids following
incubation of Nulli-SCCl EC cells with [³H]RA. Cells were
incubated with [³H]all-*trans*-RA (22 Ci/mmole; final
concentration of 2 µCi/ml) for 2 hr at 37°C. An aliquot of
the culture medium was taken and retinoids were extracted
and analyzed by HPLC (Gubler and Sherman, 1985). The
resultant profile is shown in A. Cells were washed,
collected and fractionated by differential centrifugation
in the presence of the anti-oxidant butylated hydroxy-
anisole (50 µg/ml). B and C are typical of HPLC profiles
obtained from extracts of cytosol and nuclei, respectively.
The latter were purified by repeated cycles of sedimen-
tation through sucrose. In all cases the major peak
(fraction 17) co-eluted from the column with the added
all-*trans*-RA marker and the adjacent small peak at fraction
15 eluted in the position of 13-*cis*-RA.

This nuclear localization of RA raises the possibility that RA can trigger the cascade of events leading to differentiation by some direct influence on transcription.

TABLE 1. Interaction of Holo-retinoid-binding Proteins with Nulli-SCCl Embryonal Carcinoma Cell Nuclei[*]

Binding to Nuclei of	Competed with	Relative % CPM Bound
[^{3}H]retinol-CRBP	-	100
	retinol-CRBP	19
	RA-CRABP	106
[^{3}H]RA-CRABP	-	100
	RA-CRABP	27
	retinol-CRBP	429
	CRBP	83
	retinol	131

[*] Isolated nuclei from Nulli-SCCl EC cells were incubated for 2 hr at 25°C with the indicated [^{3}H]retinoid-labeled binding protein, either alone or in the presence of a 25-fold molar excess of unlabeled homologous binding protein, heterologous binding protein or free ligand. The binding values obtained are expressed relative to those observed in the presence of labeled holo-binding protein alone and are typical of several independent experiments.

Little has been done to establish how retinol promotes differentiation of EC cells. It is unlikely to do so by direct interaction with CRABP since it has little detectable affinity for this binding protein from EC cells

(Jetten and Jetten, 1979). One obvious possibility is that retinol is metabolized to RA by EC cells, but in studies with several EC lines we have consistently failed to observe such a conversion at a detection level of 1% or less (Gubler and Sherman, 1985; Sherman et al., 1985). Williams and Napoli (1985) have recently reported that F9 cells could generate small amounts of RA from retinol; however, the levels they observed appear to be less than 1%, far too low to explain our observations on the relative potency of retinol in inducing differentiation of F9 cells.

EC cells, like most or all others (see Sherman, 1986), possess a binding protein (CRBP) which is structurally related to CRABP but specifically binds retinol rather than RA (Schindler et al., 1981; Matthaei et al., 1983). Chytil and his colleagues (Takase et al., 1979; Liau et al., 1981), and more recently Cope et al. (1984), have demonstrated that holo-CRBP, like holo-CRABP, binds specifically and saturably to liver and testis nuclei: we have demonstrated that this is also the case with holo-CRBP and nuclei from EC cells (Sherman et al., 1985; Table 1). The binding characteristics of holo-CRBP with nuclei are compared to those of holo-CRABP in Table 2. Both the number of estimated nuclear binding sites for the two binding proteins and their binding affinities are similar.

TABLE 2. Properties of the Association of Holo-retinoid-binding Proteins with Nulli-SCC1 Embryonal Carcinoma Cell Nuclei

Holo-binding Protein	Specific Binding Sites/Nucleus	Kd
Retinol-CRBP	2.6×10^5	$3.6 \times 10^{-8} M$
RA-CRABP	1.9×10^5	$2.9 \times 10^{-8} M$

Since retinol and RA promote EC cell differentiation and interact similarly with isolated EC nuclei, we wished to test whether the two retinoid holoproteins associated with the same nuclear sites. Accordingly, we challenged EC nuclei with [^{3}H]retinol or [^{3}H]RA bound to their respective binding proteins and competed with a large molar excess of unlabeled heterologous holo-retinoid-binding protein. We observed that the interaction of [^{3}H]retinol-CRBP was unaffected by the presence of unlabeled RA-CRABP (Table 1). In reciprocal experiments, retinol-CRBP not only failed to compete with [^{3}H]RA-CRABP for nuclear binding sites, but the former binding protein actually potentiated interaction of the latter binding protein with EC nuclei (Table 1). The capacity for potentiation appeared to be a property of the intact holo-binding protein since retinol or apo-CRBP alone had relatively little effect on the amount of [^{3}H]RA-CRABP bound to nuclei (Table 1).

The view that RA, in conjunction with its binding protein, promotes differentiation by a direct effect upon transcription is an attractive one because it eliminates the need to involve, and identify, a second messenger. However, there is as yet no direct support for such a hypothesis and, as discussed elsewhere (Sherman, 1986), there are reports which support the view that in eliciting certain of its pleiotropic effects, RA can act in extra-nuclear sites and without benefit of CRABP. Nevertheless, if RA induction of EC cell differentiation does require nuclear translocation, it is likely from data presented above that RA rather than one of its metabolites is the active agent.

Our observation that there are large numbers of specific nuclear binding sites for RA when delivered by its binding protein is consistent with estimates for nuclei from other cell types (Mehta et al., 1982; Cope et al., 1984) and raises the question of the nature and possible significance of such sites. Clearly, if the role of the RA-CRABP complex in the nucleus is to activate or suppress certain selected genes by direct interaction with them, then one might not expect to find many thousands of specific binding sites. On the other hand, the binding which we are observing might reflect a general, relatively low affinity of the holo-CRABP complex for DNA which, although physiologically insignificant, might be indicative of relevant binding with much greater affinity to a substantially more restricted number of sites. Such an effect has been observed with steroid receptor proteins (see, e.g., Mulvihill et al., 1982). Alternatively, if holo-CRABP is interacting with certain nuclear proteins, as suggested by Cope et al. (1984), gene expression could be selectively influenced if the acceptor proteins possessed regulatory properties. Studies to determine the nature of the nuclear acceptor for RA delivered by its holoprotein must be approached cautiously because the retinoid possesses both hydrophilic and hydrophobic domains and could become distributed in a non-physiological manner following nuclear isolation and fractionation.

Although the interaction of holo-CRBP with EC nuclei closely resembles that of holo-CRABP, the two binding proteins appear not to share sites of interaction at any detectable level. As is the case with holo-CRABP, there is little definitive information on the nature of the inter-action of holo-CRBP with nuclei. Preliminary studies suggest that the holo-CRBP complex with EC nuclei is markedly more susceptible to detergent treatment than is the association of holo-CRABP with these nuclei (U. Barkai, unpublished observations).

The potentiation of the holo-CRABP interaction with EC nuclei by holo-CRBP was unexpected. Recent studies suggest that a similar potentiation can be seen with intact cells: following exposure of EC cells to RA, there is a dramatic increase in specific RA binding sites in the nucleosol, whereas pretreatment with retinol leads to an increase of both retinol and RA binding sites in nucleosolic extracts (U. Barkai, unpublished observations). Our inability to detect production of RA from retinol by EC cells renders it very unlikely that this phenomenon is due solely to such a metabolic conversion. Nevertheless, the potentiation could provide the wherewithal for trace amounts of RA taken up or generated by the cell to have a disproportionate impact on cellular behavior by assuring its transfer to the nuclear compartment.

REFERENCES

Cope FO, Knox KL, Hall RC (1984). Retinoid binding to nuclei and microsomes of rat testes interstitial cells. Nutr Res 4:289-304.
De Ruyter MG, Lambert WE, De Lenheer AP (1979). Retinoic acid: An endogenous compound of human blood. Anal Biochem 98:402-409.

Eglitis MA, Sherman MI (1983). Murine embryonal carcinoma cells differentiate *in vitro* in response to retinol. Exp Cell Res 146:289-296.

Gubler ML, Sherman MI (1985). Metabolism of retinoids by embryonal carcinoma cells. J Biol Chem 260:9552-9558.

Jetten AM (1986). Induction of differentiation of embryonal carcinoma cells by retinoids. In Sherman MI (ed): "Retinoids and Cell Differentiation," Boca Raton: CRC Press, in press.

Jetten AM, De Luca LM (1983). Induction of differentiation of embryonal carcinoma cells by retinol: possible mechanisms. Biochem Biophys Res Commun 114:593-599.

Jetten AM, Jetten MER (1979). Possible role of retinoic acid binding protein in retinoid stimulation of embryonal carcinoma cell differentiation. Nature (London) 278:180-182.

Liau G, Ong DE, Chytil F (1981). Interaction of the retinol/cellular retinol-binding protein complex with isolated nuclei and nuclear components. J Cell Biol 91:63-68.

Martin GR (1980). Teratocarcinomas and mammalian embryogenesis. Science 209:768-776.

Matthaei KI, McCue PA, Sherman MI (1983). Retinoid binding protein activities in murine embryonal carcinoma cells and their differentiated derivatives. Cancer Res 43:2862-2867.

Mehta RG, Cerny WL, Moon RC (1982). Nuclear interactions of retinoic-acid binding protein in chemically induced mammary carcinoma. Biochem J 208:731-736.

McCormick, AM, Pauley S, Winston JH (1984). F9 embryonal carcinoma cells contain specific nuclear retinoic acid acceptor sites. Fed Proc 43:788.

McCue PA, Gubler ML, Maffei L, Sherman MI (1984a). Complementation analyses of differentiation-defective embryonal carcinoma cells. Devel Biol 103:399-408.

McCue PA, Gubler ML, Sherman MI, Cohen BN (1984b). Sodium butyrate induces histone hyperacetylation and differentiation of murine embryonal carcinoma cells. J Cell Biol 98:602-608.

McCue PW, Matthaei KI, Taketo M, Sherman MI (1983). Differentiation-defective mutants of mouse embryonal carcinoma cells: Response to hexamethylenebisacetamide and retinoic acid. Devel Biol 96:416-426.

Mulvihill E, LePennec J-P, Chambon P (1982). Chicken oviduct progesterone receptor: location of specifc regions of high affinity binding in cloned DNA fragments of hormone-responsive genes. Cell 28:621-632.

Schindler J, Matthaei KI, Sherman MI (1981). Isolation and characterization of mouse mutant embryonal carcinoma cells which fail to differentiate in response to retinoic acid. Proc Natl Acad Sci USA 78:1077-1080.

Sherman MI (1986). How do retinoids promote differentiation? In Sherman MI (ed): "Retinoids and Cell Differentiation," Boca Raton: CRC Press, in press.

Sherman MI, Gubler ML, Barkai U, Harper MI, Coppola G, Yuan J (1985). Role of retinoids in differentiation and growth of embryonal carcinoma cells. Ciba Found Symp 113:42-60.

Sherman MI, Paternoster ML, Taketo M (1983). Effects of arotinoids upon embryonal carcinoma cells. Cancer Res 43:4283-4290.

Shidoji Y, Hosoya N (1980). Competitive protein-binding radioassay for retinoic acid. Anal Biochem 104:457-463.

Smith FR, Goodman DS (1971). The effects of diseases of the liver, thyroid and kidneys on the transport of vitamin A in human plasma. J Clin Invest 50:2426-2436.

Strickland S, Mahdavi V (1978). The induction of differentiation of embryonal carcinoma stem cells by retinoic acid. Cell 15:393-403.

Takase S, Ong DE, Chytil F (1979). Cellular retinol-binding protein allows specific interaction of retinol with the nucleus in vitro. Proc Natl Acad Sci USA 76:2204-2208.

Wang S-Y, Gudas LJ (1984). Selection and characterization of F9 teratocarcinoma stem cell mutants with altered responses to retinoic acid. J. Biol Chem 259:5899-5906.

Williams JB, Napoli JL (1985). Metabolism of retinoic acid and retinol during differentiation of F9 embryonal carcinoma cells. Proc Natl Acad Sci USA 82:4658-4662.

Cellular Endocrinology: Hormonal Control of Embryonic
and Cellular Differentiation, pages 215-233
© 1986 Alan R. Liss, Inc.

INDUCTION BY PHYSIOLOGICAL AGENTS OF DIFFERENTIATION OF THE
HUMAN LEUKEMIA CELL LINE HL-60 TO CELLS WITH FUNCTIONAL
CHARACTERISTICS

Theodore R. Breitman, Hiromichi Hemmi, and Masue
Imaizumi

Laboratory of Biological Chemistry, National
Cancer Institute, Bethesda, MD

INTRODUCTION

Recently, there has been interest in the possibility
that "differentiation-inducers" may have utility in the
treatment of some malignancies. This concept is predicated
on the belief that some malignancies are a result of a
block in differentiation which if relieved would result in
a more differentiated and therefore more benign condition.
As a concept for therapy this approach holds the further
promise that induction of differentiation could not only
relieve the tumor burden but also increase the number of
functional cells, that at least for some malignancies, an
absence of is a major complication. HL-60 has been a useful
model system in the search for substances that are active
as inducers of differentiation. HL-60 is induced to differentiate to granulocyte-like cells by incubation with retinoic acid (RA), N,N-dimethylformamide (DMF), and dimethyl
sulfoxide (DMSO) (Breitman et al., 1980, Collins et al.,
1978) or into monocyte/macrophage-like cells by incubation
with 1,25-dihydroxyvitamin D_3 and 12-0-tetradecanoyl phor-
bol-13-acetate (TPA) (Rovera et al., 1979; McCarthy et al.,
1983). Of the many compounds that induce differentiation
of HL-60, RA has probably the most promise of being of use
in the clinic. This is because: it is active at physiological concentrations in vitro (Breitman et al., 1980); has
been shown to induce differentiation of fresh human leukemia cells in primary culture (Breitman et al., 1981;
Honma et al., 1983; Honma et al., 1984); and has been
reported to be effective on patients with some leukemias
(Nilsson, 1984; Flynn et al., 1983). However, while RA as
a sole agent and at pharmacological concentrations of

approximately 1 µM may be a good therapeutic agent, experiments in vitro indicate that combinations of RA and either cyclic AMP inducing agents or lymphokines act synergistically to induce differentiation of HL-60 as well as other myelomonocytic cell lines (Olsson et al., 1982; Breitman et al., 1983; Hemmi and Breitman, 1984). In addition, combinations of RA and a T-cell derived lymphokine (differentiation inducing activity, DIA) synergistically induce differentiation of fresh human leukemia cells in primary culture (Breitman et al., 1983). To the extent that it is possible, results in vitro should suggest treatments in vivo. To this end we have been interested in determining what induction conditions result in the most "normal" mature HL-60. The studies to be presented indicate that combinations of RA and the lymphokine, gamma-interferon, differentiates HL-60 to monocyte-like cells. These cells exhibit immunophagocytosis, increases in F_c receptors, superoxide (O_2^-) production, 5'-nucleotidase activity, nonspecific esterase activity, and antibody-dependent cellular cytotoxicity (ADCC). One of the more important functions of the normal phagocytic cell is its ability to seek-out and kill invading organisms. Our results show that HL-60 induced with a combination of 10 nM RA and DIA mature to cells that show adherence and increases in chemotactic peptide [N-formyl-methionyl-leucyl-phenylalanine (FMLP)] receptors that are functional for both O_2^- production and directed migration. Both the chemotactic peptide receptor concentration and migration were increased markedly by dexamethasone (DEX). We feel that it is important that this differentiation occurs in response to physiological substances and that one of the components of this combination, RA, is at the physiological concentration of approximately 10 nM.

RESULTS

Growth and Adhesiveness of HL-60 During Induction with RA plus DIA

HL-60 cells growing in the presence of both RA and DIA change morphologically from round cells to cells with irregular shapes. This change is time dependent and is observed as early as day 1. By day 2 adhesive cells are observed. At day 4, in cultures grown in the presence of RA and DIA, 35% of the cells are adherent (Table 1).

TABLE 1. The Combination of RA and DIA Promotes Adhesion of HL-60 Cells

Condition	Total cells	Attached cells	% Attached cells
Untreated	10.9	0.18	1.6
10 nM RA	10.3	0.19	1.9
DIA, 80 units/ml	12.7	0.24	1.9
10 nM RA + DIA, 80 units/ml	8.4	2.94	35.0

Cells (2.8×10^5 ml), in a total volume of 5 ml of defined medium (Breitman et al., 1984), were grown in wells of a 6-well dish for 4 days. The medium containing the suspended cells was removed and the surface of the dish was washed gently with PBS. Attached cells were removed with a cell scraper.

Untreated cells and cells growing in the presence of RA alone or DIA alone are not adherent. These results indicate that HL-60 grown in the presence of RA plus DIA mature to cells with a characteristic of monocytes.

FMLP- and TPA-stimulated NBT Reduction of HL-60 Induced by Either RA, DMF, or RA plus DIA

The report of Skubitz et al., (1983) showed that HL-60 induced with DMF had an increased concentration of FMLP receptors while HL-60 induced with RA had no increase and in fact may have had a decrease. In normal human granulocytes both FMLP and TPA stimulate oxidative metabolism with the production of O_2^- as measured by the reduction of ferricytochrome c (Lehmeyer et al., 1979). We reasoned that FMLP-stimulated O_2^- production, as measured by the reduction of NBT, would correlate with the concentration of FMLP receptors on HL-60 induced under different conditions. DMF, in a dose-dependent manner, induces HL-60 to differentiate to cells that reduce NBT in response to either TPA or FMLP (Fig. 1). There is a greater stimulation with TPA than with either 0.1 µM or 1 µM FMLP. A greater stimulation of oxidative metabolism by TPA than by FMLP has also been observed for normal human granulo-

cytes (Lehmeyer et al., 1979). In contrast to DMF, only a
small percentage of RA-induced cells reduce NBT in response
to FMLP even though the population is quite active in
response to TPA (Fig. 2). A peak response to FMLP occurs
with cells induced with approximately 100 nM RA; concentrations of RA greater than 100 nM are inhibitory. An observation which has not been explored further is that there
is a greater response of DMF-induced HL-60 to 10 µM FMLP
than to 1 µM FMLP (Fig. 1) while with RA-induced HL-60
there is a greater response to 1 µM FMLP than to 10 µM
FMLP (Fig. 2).

Fig. 1.   Fig. 2

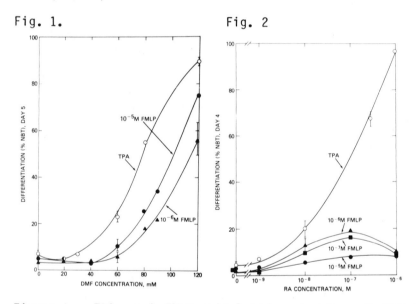

Figure 1.   TPA- and FMLP-stimulated reduction of NBT by
DMF-induced cells.   HL-60 cells were grown for 5 days in
serum-free defined medium containing various concentrations
of DMF.   Cells were then incubated at 37°C for 25 min with
0.5 mg NBT/ml and either 200 ng TPA/ml (o), 1 µM FMLP
(▲), or 10 µM FMLP (●).   The extent of NBT reduction is
expressed as the percentage of formazan positive cells on
cytospin slides.   Symbols with bars are the means ± S.E.M.
of at least 3 experiments.   Symbols without bars are from
one experiment.

Figure 2.   TPA- and FMLP-stimulated reduction of NBT by RA-
induced cells.   HL-60 cells were grown for 4 days in defined
medium containing various concentrations of RA.   Cells were

then incubated at 37°C for 25 min with 0.5 mg NBT/ml and either 200 ng TPA/ml (o), 1 μM FMLP (▲), 10 μM FMLP (●), or 100 nM FMLP (■). The extent of NBT reduction is expressed as the percentage of formazan positive cells on cytospin slides. Symbols with and without bars are as described in the Legend to Figure 1.

The response of DMF-induced and RA-induced HL-60 to FMLP stimulation of NBT reduction appeared at this stage of our study to correlate qualitatively with the reported relative levels of chemotactic peptide receptors. The finding that HL-60, induced with a combination of RA and DIA, actively reduced NBT when stimulated with FMLP indicated that these cells had increased concentrations of FMLP receptors (Fig. 3). In the presence of a physiological concentration of RA (10 nM) there is a DIA concentration-dependent increase in the percentage of cells reducing NBT in response to either TPA or FMLP with the response to TPA being greater than to FMLP. Cells incubated with DIA alone or RA alone were essentially inactive to stimulation by FMLP. Cells incubated with DIA alone responded to TPA with values for differentiation of approximately 8% (Fig. 3).

Fig. 3.

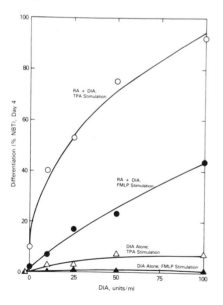

Figure 3. TPA- and FMLP-stimulated reduction of NBT by HL-60 induced with a combination of RA and DIA. Cells were grown for 4 days in defined medium containing 10 nM RA and various concentrations of DIA. Cells were then incubated at 37°C for 25 min with 0.5 mg NBT/ml and either 200 ng TPA/ml or 1 μM FMLP. The extent of NBT reduction is expressed as the percentage of formazan positive cells on cytospin slides.

Quantitation of Formazan Production

In the experiments presented above a qualitative NBT assay was employed that determines the percentage of cells in a population that have a microscopically determined level of cell-associated formazan. This assay does not give information on how active the cells are except in subjective terms. To obtain this information we have recently developed a quantitative NBT test. This assay, as with the more commonly used reduction of ferricytochrome c, gives information of the activity of the total population of cells. The data in Fig. 4 show that HL-60 grown for 4 days in the presence of a combination of 10 nM RA and various concentrations of DIA have a greater capacity to reduce NBT in response to a stimulation by FMLP than either: control cells; cells incubated with RA alone; or cells grown with DIA alone. In addition, exposure of these cells to cytochalasin B immediately prior to the NBT assay results in a marked increase in formazan production. A similar effect of cytochalsin B has been reported on FMLP-stimulated O_2^- production by normal granulocytes (Lehmeyer et al., 1979).

Fig. 4.

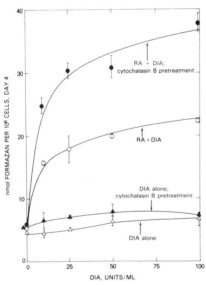

Figure 4. Enhancement by cytochalasin B of FMLP-stimulated production of formazan by HL-60 induced with a combination of RA and DIA. Cells were grown for 4 days in defined medium containing the indicated concentration of DIA with and without 10 nM RA. A portion of each culture was incubated for 20 min with 5 μg cytochalasin B/ml (pretreatment) and then cells (pretreated and non-pretreated) were incubated at 37°C for 25 min with 0.5 mg NBT/ml and 1 μM FMLP. Results are the means ± S.E.M. of 2 experiments.

Expression of FMLP Receptors

The increased response to FMLP of HL-60 cultured in the presence of RA and DIA suggested that these cells had increased concentrations of FMLP receptors. Measurements of the specific binding of FMLP show that HL-60 grown for 4 days in the presence of RA and DIA have a much greater capacity to bind FMLP than untreated cells or cells grown with 300 nM RA (Fig. 5). In separate experiments incubation with DIA alone did not result in an increase of FMLP binding (data not shown). In agreement with the findings of Brandt et al., (1981) and Skubitz et al., (1982) for DMF- and DMSO-induced cells, the addition of 1 μM DEX to the induction medium results in a marked increase of specifically bound FMLP (Fig. 5). From a Scatchard plot analysis (Fig. 6) there are 5400 receptors per cell for cells induced with RA plus DIA and an increase of approximately 5-fold to 26000 receptors per cell for cells induced with added DEX. The calculated K_D values are 19.73 nM and 11.75 nM, respectively. Thus, treatment with DEX results in an increased number of chemotactic peptide receptors with an increased affinity for FMLP.

Fig. 5   Fig. 6

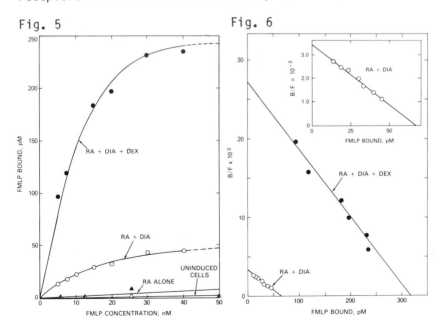

Figure 5. Specific binding of FMLP to HL-60 cells. Cells were grown for 4 days in the absence (**Δ**) or in the presence of either 10 nM RA and DIA (80 units/ml) with (**●**) and without (o) 1 μM DEX or 300 nM RA (**▲**). For each condition there were 7.5 x 10^6 cells per ml.

Figure 6. Scatchard plot analysis of FMLP binding to HL-60 cells. Data from Figure 5 for the conditions of growth in the presence of 10 nM RA and DIA (80 units/ml) with (**●**) and without (**O**) DEX were analyzed with the "LIGAND" computer program (Munson and Rodbard, 1980). The lines were drawn from the computed values for K_D and receptor concentration. The insert is an enlargement of the data for the RA plus DIA condition.

It has been reported that DEX has little effect on DMF-induced or DMSO-induced differentiation of HL-60 assessed by cell morphology (Skubitz et al., 1982; Brandt et al., 1981) or by the ability of the cells to reduce NBT when stimulated by TPA (Skubitz et al., 1982). However, FMLP-stimulated NBT reduction was not examined. As shown by the data in Figure 7, at concentrations of FMLP greater than 100 nM, HL-60 induced in the presence of DEX produced only approximately 1.2-fold more formazan than HL-60 induced in the absence of DEX. In a 2-tailed t test this difference has a p value of 0.05 and is not statistically significant. These results may indicate that a receptor concentration of 5400 or less per cell is required for maximum chemotactic peptide stimulation of O_2^- production.

Fig. 7

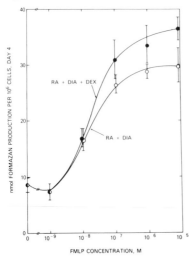

Figure 7. NBT reduction in response to FMLP of HL-60 cells induced for 4 days in the presence of 10 nM RA and DIA (100 units/ml) with (●) and without (o) 1 μM DEX. The incubation time for the NBT reduction assay was 40 min. Each data point is the mean ± S.E.M. of three independent determinations.

Chemotaxis of HL-60

HL-60 induced by RA plus DIA exhibits chemotactic peptide concentration-dependent migration (Fig. 8). Cells induced in the presence of DEX are more active. The percentage of total cells migrating in response to the optimal concentration of 100 nM FMLP increased from 26% for cells induced in the absence of DEX to 47% for cells induced in the presence of 1 μM DEX. This difference has a p value of 0.01 and is considered significant. However, most if not all of the increased response in DEX-treated cells is probably a result of the increased non-directed migration observed in the absence of FMLP (Fig. 8). Untreated cells, cells induced with RA alone (Fig. 8), and cells cultured with DIA alone (data not shown) were essentially unresponsive to FMLP).

Fig. 8

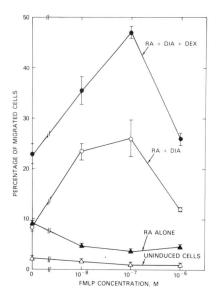

Figure 8. Chemotaxis of HL-60 cells in response to FMLP. Conditions for induction and symbols are the same as those described in the Legend to Figure 6. Each data point is the mean ± S.E.M. of three independent determinations.

Monocytic Differentiation of HL-60 by Gamma-Interferon

We studied the effects of IFN-gamma alone and in combination with 10 nM RA on three functional parameters and four other differentiation markers of mature myelomonocytic cells. IFN-gamma alone at concentrations of 10

units/ml or higher increases the proportion of cells forming EA rosettes (Fig. 9) and at higher concentrations
(1000 units/ml) increases: NBT reduction, phagocytosis
(Fig. 9), the activities of nonspecific esterase and
5'-nucleotidase, the number of cells with a morphology of
monocyte-like cells (Table 2), and ADCC (Fig. 10). The
combination of 10 nM RA and IFN-gamma markedly increases
the extent of all monocytic differentiation markers compared to the effect of each of these agents alone (Figs.
9, 10 and Table 2). Under the same conditions there is no
increase in spontaneous cytotoxicity against either K-562
or MOLT-4 (data not shown). HL-60 treated with 300 nM RA
shows increases in both the percentage of cells reducing
NBT and maturing morphologically to granulocyte-like cells
(Table 2) but exhibits essentially no increase in ADCC or
in the two enzyme markers of monocytes/macrophages (Fig.
10 and Table 2). The viability was approximately 85% in
all conditions.

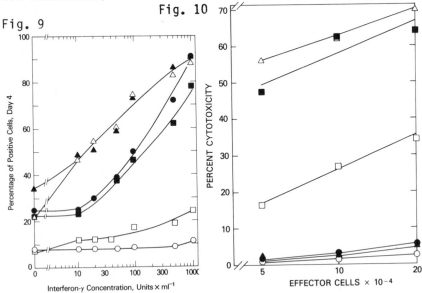

Fig. 10

Fig. 9

Figure 9. Increase in EA rosettes (△,▲); immunoerythro-
phagocytosis (□,■); and NBT reduction (○,●) of HL-60
cells treated with recombinant IFN-gamma alone (open symbols) and in combination with 10 nM RA (closed symbols).

Figure 10. Antibody-dependent cellular cytotoxicity (ADCC)
of HL-60 induced by IFN-gamma and RA. HL-60 cells were

incubated for 4 days with: none (O); 300 nM RA (●); 10 nM RA (▲); 1000 units of IFN-gamma/ml (□); and 1000 units of IFN-gamma/ml plus 10 nM RA (■). Normal human peripheral blood mononuclear cells (△) were used as a positive control. ADCC against chicken red blood cells (CRBC) was assessed by the method of Perlmann et al., (1976).

DISCUSSION

RA induces HL-60 to differentiate to cells with granu-locytic-like morphology and with the ability to express reactions associated with the respiratory burst such as O_2^- production, NBT reduction, and an increased HMPS activity (Breitman et al., 1983). However, while these HL-60 cells actively produce O_2^- in response to TPA (measured by NBT reduction) they are relatively inactive in response to FMLP, a potent chemotactic peptide (Fig. 2). In con-trast, HL-60 induced to differentiate with DMF is active in reducing NBT in response to either TPA or FMLP (Fig. 1). This difference in the response of HL-60 to FMLP was expected from previous studies showing that the number of chemotactic peptide receptors on HL-60 is increased by treatment with DMF or DMSO (Brandt et al., 1981) and does not change or is decreased by RA treatment (Skubitz et al., 1982).

A lower response to FMLP than to TPA is observed for HL-60 induced with increasing concentrations of DMF (Fig. 1). A similar difference in the response to these soluble mediators has been found for normal human granulocytes (Lehmeyer et al., 1979) for which evidence has been pre-sented that it is a consequence of different transduction-al mechanisms operating under different controls and is not due to an activation of different respiratory enzymes (McPhail and Snyderman, 1983). The low response of RA-induced HL-60 to FMLP (Fig. 2) is explained by the very low levels of FMLP binding to these cells (Fig. 5). These results are in agreement with Skubitz et al. (1982) who, in addition, found that RA concentrations greater than 10 nM blocked induction by DMF of FMLP receptors. Therefore, the increase followed by a decrease in the percentage of cells reducing NBT in response to 0.1 μM and 1 μM FMLP (Fig. 2) may be the sum of inductive and inhibitory effects of various RA concentrations. At low concentrations of RA (10 nM) there is primarily induction while at higher con-

TABLE 2. Morphological and Functional Changes of HL-60 Induced by Recombinant Gamma-IFN and RA.

	Myeloid Differential Counts (%)					NBT reduction (%)	Non-specific Esterase (%)	5'Nucleotidase Activity (nmol Pi released/hr/10^6 cells)
	Promyelocyte	Myelocyte	Metamyelocyte	Banded & Segmented Neutrophils	Monocyte			
None	94	4	2	0	0	7	2	0.06
300 nM RA	3	27	32	38	0	97	4	0.04
10 nM RA	73	11	12	4	0	23	1	0.03
IFN-γ, 1000 units/ml	86	5	1	0	8	11	12	3.29
10 nM RA plus IFN-γ 1000 units/ml	3	12	3	0	82	93	90	12.3

HL-60 was cultured in a serum-free defined medium for 4 days.

centration (>100 nM) the inhibitory effect dominates. This inhibitory effect of RA appears to be confined to FMLP receptor-mediated O_2^- production as TPA-stimulation was quite active (Fig. 2). Thus, it appears that HL-60 induced with RA develops the transductional mechanism that can be stimulated by TPA but does not express the transductional mechanism that is stimulated by FMLP because of a deficiency of chemotactic peptide receptors. In a related study Stendahl et al. (1984) have reported recently that RA-induced HL-60, compared to DMSO-induced HL-60, is deficient in receptors for FMLP and in both FMLP-stimulated O_2^- production measured by ferricytochrome c reduction and FMLP-stimulated calcium uptake. In addition, these workers found that 500 nM RA inhibited DMSO-induced increases in these parameters. IgG-mediated phagocytosis and leukotriene B-stimulated calcium uptake were not affected by RA and C3b-mediated phagocytosis was partially decreased by RA. Thus, pharmacological concentrations of RA result in a maturation of HL-60 to cells that are deficient in some characteristics of mature normal phagocytes and HL-60 induced with other agents such as DMF and DMSO. The mechanism by which RA inhibits the development of FMLP receptors is not known.

While induction of HL-60 with RA alone yields cells that are deficient in chemotactic peptide receptor concentration and function, our results indicate that the combination of a T-cell derived lymphokine (DIA) and a physiological concentration of RA (10 nM) induces HL-60 to differentiate to cells with an increased number of FMLP receptors (Figs. 5 and 6). These receptors are functional as shown by FMLP-directed migration (Fig. 8). Pretreatment of these cells with cytochalasin B increased FMLP-stimulated NBT reduction by approximately 1.5-fold (Fig. 4). This effect is seen also with normal human granulocytes (Lehmeyer et al., 1979).

There have been two reports on the effect of DEX on the properties of FMLP receptors expressed on HL-60 induced by DMF or DMSO (Skubitz et al., 1982; Brandt et al., 1981). These studies indicate that DEX induces a 3- to 4-fold increase in receptor number without a significant change of affinity. Our results on RA plus DIA agree with these reports regarding receptor number but indicate that there is a two-fold increase in the affinity of the chemotactic peptide receptor induced in the presence of DEX (Fig. 6).

In normal human monocytes there are two populations of monocytes in regard to chemotactic activity and expression of FMLP receptors: one subpopulation migrates to FMLP and has saturable binding sites for FMLP and the other subpopulation does not migrate and exhibits little chemotactic peptide binding (Falk et al., 1982). In contrast to monocytes, migrating and non-migrating populations of normal human granulocytes show identical binding characteristics for FMLP (Harvath and Leonard, 1982). We have not studied if there are subpopulations with heterogenous chemotactic activity and receptor expression in the monocyte/macrophage-like HL-60 cells induced by RA plus DIA.

Chemotaxis is an integrated function of phagocytic cells, consisting of various properties such as adhesiveness, orientation, presence of chemoattractant receptors, and directed mobility. Several groups have shown that HL-60 induced by DMF and DMSO exhibits an increase of chemotactic activity (Fontana et al., 1980; Niedel et al., 1980; Collins et al., 1979). In this study we have shown that HL-60 cells induced by RA in combination with DIA exhibit not only expression of FMLP receptors but also chemotactic activity (Fig. 8). Furthermore, induction in the presence of DEX increases both the number of receptors and chemotactic activity (Figs. 6 and 8). Alteri and Leonard (1983) found that normal human peripheral monocytes exhibit a maximal chemotactic response at concentrations of 10 nM to 100 nM FMLP. In contrast, the highest chemotactic activity of normal granulocytes is at 1 μM FMLP (Harvath and Leonard, 1982), a concentration that inhibits markedly chemotaxis of monocytes (Alteri and Leonard, 1983). HL-60 induced by RA plus DIA, with and without DEX, exhibited maximal chemotaxis at concentrations of 10 nM to 100 nM FMLP and 1 μM FMLP was inhibitory (Fig. 8). A maximum of 48% of these cells migrated.

One of the more important functions of the normal phagocytic cell is its ability to seek out and kill invading organisms. Our results show that HL-60 induced with a combination of 10 nM RA and DIA mature to cells that show adherence (Table 1) and increases in FMLP receptors that are functional for both O_2^- production and directed migration. We feel that it is important that this differentiation occurs in response to two physiological substances and that one of the components of this combination, RA, is at the physiological concentration of approximately 10 nM

(DeRuyter et al., 1979). The physiological plasma concentration of DIA is unknown but it is probable that this substance(s) plays a role, along with RA and other factors, in normal hematopoiesis.

Guyre et al. (1983) have reported that IFN-gamma at concentration >1 unit/ml increases the number of IgG Fc receptors of the human mononuclear cell lines HL-60 and U-937. These workers showed further that recombinant IFN-alpha and IFN-beta also increased the number of Fc receptors but had an activity that was much lower than that of IFN-gamma. Our present results extend those of Guyre et al. by showing that while IFN-gamma alone increases the proportion of HL-60 cells forming EA-rosettes (an indirect measure of the number of Fc receptors) IFN-gamma alone had little effect on promoting the appearance of other markers of mature myelomonocytic cells (Fig. 9, 10 and Table 2). However, the expression of these parameters was markedly increased when HL-60 was exposed to a combination of IFN-gamma and 10 nM RA, a concentration of RA that alone had essentially no effect on these parameters. With the monocytic cell line U-937, Hattori et al. (1983) have shown that recombinant IFN-alpha and -beta induces an increase of ADCC activity but has no effect on this activity in HL-60 and Tomida et al. (1982) have shown that a combination of 1000 units of either natural IFN-alpha or -beta/ml (alone without effect) and 40 nM RA enhanced the morphological differentiation of HL-60 along the granulocytic pathway. Previous results from this laboratory have shown that differentiation of HL-60 in the presence of 10 nM RA is markedly potentiated by agents including cholera toxin, dibutyryl cAMP, and physiological concentrations of prostaglandin E that increase the intracellular concentration of cyclic AMP (Olsson et al., 1982). It was shown further that HL-60 could be primed to respond to these agents, including DIA, by incubation with 10 nM RA alone. In the microenvironment of the developing myelomonocytic cell the interplay between RA (derived ultimately from the diet) and prostaglandin E or lymphokines including the interferons may be one of the important controls of maturation.

Acute myelogenous leukemia has been viewed as a disease involving a block in the normal maturation of myeloid cells. Thus, it is possible that some leukemia cells do not mature either because they have a decreased ability to respond to exogenous differentiative factors or because the production of specific gene products obligatory for differentiation is altered. It is now clear, at least for some human myelomonocytic cell lines, that this block in maturation is not permanent and that incubation with physiological agents promotes end-terminal differentiation. These findings have generated interest in the induction of differentiation as an alternative approach to the treatment of some leukemias. In previous studies it was shown that fresh cells from patients with acute promyelocytic leukemia are induced to differentiate in primary culture by RA (Breitman et al., 1981) and that combinations of RA and DIA were even more effective (Breitman et al., 1983). The finding in this study that DIA is also associated with recombinant IFNs mean that the availability of DIA is not a problem for clinical studies. Recombinant technology should also allow for the construction of new DIAs having greater specificities and/or less toxic side effects.

REFERENCES

Alteri E and Leonard EJ (1983). N-formylmethionyl-leucyl-[^{3}H]phenylalanine binding, superoxide release, and chemotactic responses of human blood monocytes that repopulate the circulation during leukapheresis. Blood 62:918-923.

Brandt SJ, Barnes KC, Glass DB, Kinkade JM, Jr (1981) Glucocorticoid-stimuulated increase in chemotactic peptide receptors on differentiating human myeloid leukemia (HL-60) cells. Cancer Res 4:4947-4951.

Breitman TR, Collins SJ, Keene BR (1981). Terminal differentiation of human promyelocytic leukemia cells in primary culture in response to retinoic acid. Blood 57:1000-1004.

Breitman TR, Keene BR, Hemmi H (1983). Retinoic acid-induced differentiation of fresh leukaemia cells and the human myelomonocytic leukaemia cell lines, HL-60, U-937, and THP-1. Cancer Surveys 2:263-291.

Breitman TR, Keene BR, Hemmi H (1984). "Methods for Serum-free Culture of Neuronal and Lymphoid Cells." New York: A. Liss, pp 215-236.

Breitman TR, Selonick SE, Collins SJ (1980) Induction of differentiation of the human promyelocytic leukemia cell line (HL-60) by retinoic acid. Proc Natl Acad Sci USA 77:2936-2940.

Collins SJ, Ruscetti FW, Gallagher RE, Gallo RC (1978) Terminal differentiation of human promyelocytic leukemia cells induced by dimethyl sulfoxide and other polar compounds. Proc Natl Acad Sci USA 75:2458-2462.

Collins SJ, Ruscetti FW, Gallagher RE, Gallo RC (1979) Normal functional characteristics of cultured human promyelocytic leukemia cells (HL-60) after induction of differentiation by dimethyl sulfoxide. J Exp Med 149:969-974.

DeRuyter MG, Lambert WE, DeLeenheer AP (1979) Retinoic acid: An endogenous compound of human blood. Unequivocal demonstration of endogenous retinoic acid in normal physiological conditions. Anal Biochem 98:402-409.

Falk W, Harvath L, Leonard EJ (1982). Only the chemotactic subpopulation of human blood monocytes expresses receptors for the chemotactic peptide N-Formylmethionyl-leucyl-phenylalanine. Infection and Immunology 36:450-454.

Flynn PJ, Miller WJ, Weisdorf DJ, Arthur DC, Brunning R, Branda RF (1983). Retinoic acid treatment of acute promyelocytic leukemia: in vitro and in vivo observations. Blood 62:1211-1217.

Fontana JA, Wright DG, Schiffmann E, Corcoran BA, Deisseroth AB (1980). Development of chemotactic responsiveness in myeloid precursor cells: Studies with a human leukemia cell line. Proc Natl Acad Sci USA 77:3664-3668.

Guyre PM, Morganelli PM, Miller R (1983). Recombinant Immune Interferon Increases IgG Fc receptors on cultured human mononuclear phagocytes. J Clin Invest 72:393-397.

Harvath L, Leonard EJ (1982). Two neutrophil population in human blood with different chemotactic activities: Separation and chemoattractant binding. Infect Immun 36:443-449.

Hattori T, Pack M, Bougnoux P, Chang Z-L, Hoffman T (1983). Interferon-induced differentiation of U-937 cells. Comparison with other agents which promote differentiation of human myeloid or monocyte-like cell lines. J Clin Invest 72:237-244.

Hemmi H, Breitman TR (1984). Monocytic differentiation of human myelomonocytic leukemia cell lines induced by T-lymphocyte derived differentiation inducing activity. Tissue Culture (Japan) 10:185-190.

Honma Y, Fujita Y, Kasukabe T, Hozumi M, Sampi K, Sakurai M, Tsushima S, Nomura H (1983). Induction of differentiation of human acute non-lymphocytic leukemia cells in primary culture by inducers of differentiation of human myeloid leukemia cell line HL-60. Eur J Cancer Clin Oncol 19: 251-261.

Honma Y, Fujita Y, Kasukabe T, Hozumi M, Sampi K, Sakurai M., Tsushima S, Nomura H. (1984). Differentiation in vitro of human myelogenous leukemia cells from patients in relapse. Gann 75:518-524.

Lehmeyer JE, Snyderman R, Johnston RB, Jr (1979). Stimulation of neutrophil oxidative metabolism by chemotactic peptides: Influence of calcium ion concentration and cytochalasin B and comparison with stimulation with phorbol myristate acetate. Blood 54:35-45.

McCarthy DM, Sah Miguel JF, Freake HC, Green PM, Zola H, Catovsky D, Goldman JM (1983). 1,25-Dihydroxyvitamin D_3 inhibits proliferation of human promyelocytic leukemia (HL-60) cells and induces monocyte-macrophage differentiation in HL-60 and normal human bone marrow cells. Leukemia Res 7:51-55.

McPhail LC, Snyderman R (1983). Activation of the respiratory burst enzyme in human polymorphonuclear leukocytes by chemoattractants and other soluble stimuli. J Clin Invest 72:192-200.

Munson PJ, Rodbard D (1980). Ligand: A versatile computerized approach for characterization of ligand-binding systems. Anal Biochem 107:220-239.

Niedel J, Kahane I, Lachman L, Cuatrecasas P (1980). A subpopulation of cultured human promyelocytic leukemia cells (HL-60) displays the formyl peptide chemotactic receptor. Proc Natl Acad Sci USA 77:1000-1004.

Nilsson B (1984). Probable in vivo induction of differentiation by retinoic acid of promyelocytes in acute promyelocytic leukaemia. Brit J Haemat 57:365-371.

Olsson IL, Breitman TR, Gallo RC (1982). Priming of human myeloid leukemic cell lines HL-60 and U-937 with retinoic acid for differentiation effects of cyclic adenosine 3':5' monophosphate-inducing agents and a T-lymphocyte-derived differentiation factor. Cancer Res 42:3928-3933.

Perlmann H, Perlmann P, Hellstorm U, Hammarström S (1976). "In Vitro Methods in Cell-Mediated Antitumor Immunity." New York, Academic Press, pp 496-510.

Rovera G, Santoli D, Damsky C (1979). Human promyelocytic leukemia cells in culture differentiate into macrophage-like cells when treated with a phorbol diester. Proc Natl Acad Sci USA 76:2779-2783.

Skubitz KM, Zhen Y, August JT (1982). Dexamethasone synergistically induces chemotactic peptide receptor expression in HL-60 cells. Blood 59:586-593.

Stendahl O, Andersson T, Coble BI, Dahlgren C, Lew D (1985).
    "Retinoids: New Trends in Research and Therapy, Retinoid
    Symp., Geneva 1984." Basel, Karger pp 260-264.
Tomida M, Yamamoto Y, Hozumi M (1982). Stimulation by
    interferon of induction of differentiation of human pro-
    myelocytic leukemia cells. Biochem Biophys Res Commun
    104:30-37.

Cellular Endocrinology: Hormonal Control of Embryonic
and Cellular Differentiation, pages 235–242
© 1986 Alan R. Liss, Inc.

TWO DISTINCT EVENTS IN LINEAGE ESTABLISHMENT OF A BIOPOTENTIAL HEMOPOIETIC CELL LINE

Edward S. Golub and Teresita Pagan

Department of Biological Sciences, Purdue
University, West Lafayette, Indiana 47907

INTRODUCTION

A very useful way of looking at cellular differentiation is as a series of branch-point choices. Each
choice brings the cells along an ever narrowing establishment of lineage while simultaneously closing off the
chance to follow other lineages. Hemopoiesis is a good
differentiating system to study because there are enough
decisions involved that one can, in theory, enter the
system at any one of several points. All of the differentiated cells of the blood are the progeny of
multipotent hemopoietic stem cells. Stem cells, by
definition (Hall, 1983) are in almost vanishingly small
concentration but increase in number as they differentiate
and progress along their decision making route. While
this is a very efficient strategy for the system to have
evolved, it seems to indicate that evolution has been
indifferent, so far, to the needs of biologists. In
blood cell formation for example, the frequency of the
stem cell is very low ($ca 10^{-4}$) and the frequency of the
committed progenitor cells only slightly higher (10^{-3}).
Their direct study therefore becomes impossible without
means of isolation and enrichment (Golub, 1982). The
use of cloned lines such as HL-60 (Collins et al, 1978)
allows the investigator to use adequate numbers of cells
in reasonable synchrony to study some of the differentiative events.

HL-60 is a powerful tool to study lineage establishment
in the hemopoietic system because it is a cell which still

has one last branch point decision to make. This cell line
is a human promyelomonocytic leukemic line which can be
chemically induced to undergo differentiation along either
the granuloid or monocytic pathways. It can be used in a
manner similar to Friend erythroleukemia transformed
cell lines to study the biochemical events associated with
the movement along an established differentiation pathway,
but because it is a cell frozen at a junction point it
affords the extra added intellectual value of allowing
examination of one of the most important questions in all
of biology, viz, what are the events which occur when a cell
reaches a decision point and establishes a lineage. The
caveat of course is that since the decision attendent upon
lineage establishment is one which is regulatory, a cell
which has an altered regulatory control of its proliferation
may also have an altered differentiative control as well.

Since differentiation is the selective use of genes or
sets of genes as the cell has progressed along its path
the goal ultimately becomes to use these tumor lines to
analyze the genes and their regulation. The great power
of molecular biology has been turned in a very short time to
the question of the control of a gene which is being used
but the questions we are addressing are of another level of
complexity. We are attempting to determine what events
allow or force a cell to use a given gene or block of genes.
The question obviously has no easy answer and will not be
answered by that lightning bolt experiment we all dream of.
In this paper we will present some of the work which has
been going on in our laboratory in an attempt to ask, not
how does HL-60 choose which of its two pathways of differentiation, but rather, what can we do to get at the
biochemical locus of that choice? We have opted to use a
series of inducing agents which are probably not of
physiological significance (and hence we call them surrogate
inducers) and variants of HL-60 which do not respond to
one or more of them.

RESULTS AND DISCUSSION

Surrogate Inducers;

Several chemical agents have been reported to induce
differentiation of HL-60 (see Gargus, et al, 1985). Table 1
lists the inducers used in the experiments reported
here.

Table 1. Surrogate Inducers

Acid	Dose	Pathway
Retinoic Acid (RA)	10^{-5}M	G
1,25 OH vit D3 (D3)	10^{-6}M	G/M
phorbol ester (TPA)	10^{-8}M	M
ouabain	3μM	G
A23187	3μM	G
EGTA	2.5mM	G

(G=granulocyte, M=monocyte)

The important point about the surrogate inducers is that while the molecules themselves may not be physiologically significantly their point of action in the differentiative pathway probably is. Differentiation in HL-60 is induced along one of two lines by these agents, toward granulocytes or monocytes (Breitman et al, 1980, Murao et al, 1983). The terminally differentiated cells can be clearly distinguished by morphology but intermediate stages are less easily distinguished. For this reason the use of biochemical markers is essential. For granulocytes the ability to reduce nitroblue tetrazolium, NBT, is the marker of choice (Collins, et al 1978). Under some conditions of the assay and in some clinical states cells of the monocyte lineage may exhibit NBT reduction, but in the absence of unique surface markers or gene probes this is the best indicator of this lineage. The monocyte lineage is identified by the presence of the enzyme nonspecific esterase (ES). It must be recalled that these markers are not absolute but serve as reasonably reliable biochemical indicators of lineage establishment. In our hands RA inducer cells with only granulocytes morphology which are all NBT$^+$. TPA induces only with monocyte morphology. These cells are all ES$^+$ and NBT$^-$. For most inducers there is no overlap, but as will be seen below, some inducers cause both markers to be expressed.

Kinetics of the Inductive Events;

Figure 1 shows the kind of results obtained when various of the surrogate inducers are added to cultures of HL-60 grown in the presence of 20% FCS. In the top panel the inducers were added at time 0 and the percent granulocytes (NBT positive cells) were assayed at the indicated

times. It can be seen that there are two classes of
inducers. One set causes the appearance of differentiating
cells by 12 hours while the other causes cells to begin to
express the differentiation marker at day 2.

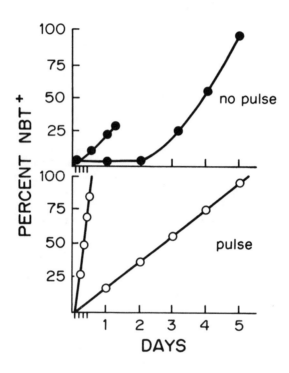

Figure 1. Kinetics of granulocyte
induction in HL-60 showing two classes
of reactions. See text for details.

The inducers of the fast reactions are ouabain and
A23187, agents which have an effect on ions. RA and D3
induce the slow reactions. The ouabain data can be compared
to data from Friend erythroleukemia experiments by Bernstein
and his coworkers (1976) who have shown that this agent,
which inhibits $NA^+/K^+ATPase$ induces erythroid differentiation.
In HL-60 Gargus et al (1985) have shown that cells induced
to granulocytes with DMSO show a ouabain-sensitive K^+

efflux (t1/2 = 14 hr). In Figure 1 we show that ouabain
induces rapid differentiation in HL-60. The net result
of all of this should be the conclusion that K^+ efflux is
a signal to move down the granulocyte pathway. However
Gargus et al (1985) have shown that intracellular levels of
K^+ and Na^+ are not significantly different in DMSO induced
and uninduced cells. This must mean that these cations do
not act as direct signals because we still do not know if
the ouabain induction is linked indirectly to Ca^{++}. It
is known that amiloride prevents erythroid induction in
Friend cells but that the Ca ionophore A23187 overcomes
this inhibition (Levenson et al 1981). This is significant since both the ionophore and ouabain induce granulocyte
differentiation in HL-60 (Table 1 and Figure 1) but this
induction is not sensitive to amiloride (Golub and Pagan,
to be published). We are currently examining the free
intracellular Ca^{++} levels using Quin-2 in collaboration
with Ken Robinson as well as the total intracellular K^+
and Na^+ after ouabain and A23187 induction.

Variants of HL-60;

Given that there are slow and fast reactions in the
induction of one of the two pathways which HL-60 can follow,
it is tempting to reason that the two pathways are linked.
One way of testing the notion that the two classes of
temporal events are in fact sequential events is by the
use of variants. The argument would be strengthened, though
of course not proven, if variants which did not respond to
RA also did not respond to the ion-affecting agents. We
have accumulated a series of variants, cloned them and looked
for the coordinate loss of ability to be induced by the
surrogate inducers (Golub and Pagan, in preparation). It
can be seen in Table 2 that in two of three variants there
is coordinate loss of both fast and slow inducers. The
exception is the variant H-1 which is able to respond to
RA but not ouabain or A23187. If the slow reaction
triggers the fast one, then a loss of RA reactivity while
the ouabain reactivity is retained would be expected. The
fact that it is the RA activity which is retained would
tend to argue that the two reactions may not be linked unless
an alternative explanation for the inability to respond
to the fast inducers can be found. Using the notion that
a good theory is worth retaining we are seeking such an
explanation.

Table 2. Responses of Variants of HL-60 to Surrogate Inducers

Line	DMSO	RA	D3	TPA	Ouabain	A23187	EGTA
H	G	G	G/M	M	G	G	G
P	G	-	G	M	-	-	-
R	G	-	G/M	-	-	-	-
H-1	G	G	M	M	-		

(H is considered the wild type)

Effect of Colony Stimulating Factor;

It is generally agreed that the natural inducing molecule for granulocyte/monocytes is colony stimulating factor, CSF. There are CSF which induce only granulocytes (G-CSF), only monocytes (M-CSF) or both (GM-CSF). The genes for both human and murine GM-CSF have recently been cloned (Gough et al 1984, Wong et al 1985). Metcalf (1980) has shown that GM-CSF when added to single cells at high concentration induces granulocyte differentation but at low concentration induces monocytes. The purified product of a cloned gene for human GM-CSF was provided to us by Dr. Chris Henney of Immunex Corp., Seattle and we have been able to show that this product induces differentiation of HL-60. The results, however, are different than those obtained on normal cells by Metcalf. As seen in Table 3 treatment of HL-60 with GM-CSF results in differentiation into both granulocytes and monocytes as determined by the two enzyme markers used here. Similar results are also seen with D3. The important point is that each cell must be expressing both markers because there are over 90% NBT[+] and 90% ES[+] cells with GM-CSF.

Table 3. Comparison of GM-CSF and D3 Induction in Variants of HL-60

Variant	GM-CSF	D3
H	G/M	G/M
P	-/-*	G
R	G/M	G/M
H-1	M	M

*no NBT or ES reaction but the initial morphological changes seen with this inducer in the other lines are present.

Like RA and D3, GM-CSF is a slow inducer, in fact, the curve obtained in a pulse experiment is superimposable upon the slow curve in Figure 1. We are currently determining if the receptors for the two are the same. But these results raise a very important question. If the two markers we are using are indeed indicators of two distinct lineages then HL-60 may be unable to use the 'switch mechanism' which normal cells use. The variants P and H-1 apparently use only one of the avenues available at the switch point. If these assumptions are correct, these variants will become powerful tools to probe the decision point. With David Asai we are currently looking for surface markers as indicators of lineage establishment and should unique protein surface molecules be found, we will attempt to isolate the genes in which they are encoded.

SUMMARY

HL-60, a human myelomonocytic cell line can be induced to differentiate along either granulocyte or monocyte pathways and therefore is a good model to study lineage establishment. We have shown that there are two classes of reactions in the establishment of the granulocytic line distinguishable by their kinetics. The fast reaction occurs in hours and is induced by ouabain or A23187, agents which effect ions. The slow reactions occur at a constant rate over a period of 5 days and are induced by the surrogate inducers RA and D3 but also by the natural inducer GM-CSF. GM-CSF induces the enzyme markers which we use to characterize both granulocytes and monocytes in the same cell. If these markers are indeed unique to each of the lines this means that HL-60 has both gene programs initiated by GM-CSF and D3. Variant lines which do not respond to one or more of the inducers can be used to analyze this point since variants which are induced only to granulocytes or only to monocytes by GM-CSF have been isolated.

Acknowledgements;

This work was supported by National Science Foundation Grant DCB 8411716. We thank Dr. E. Huberman for kindly providing us with the wild type HL-60 and the TPA-resistant variant (designated R in this paper), Dr. Milan Uskokovic of Hoffmann-LaRoche for the generous gift of the 1,25OH vit D3, and Dr. Chris Henney for the generous gift of GM-CSF.

REFERENCES

Bernstein A D, Hunt D M, Critchley V, Mak T (1976).
Induction by ouabain of hemoglobin synthesis in cultured
Friend erythroleukemia cells. Cell 9:375-381.
Breitman T R, Selonick S E, Collins S J (1980). Induction
of differentiation of human promyelocytic leukemia cell
line (HL-60) by retinoic acid. Proc Natl Acad Sci (USA)
77:2936-2940.
Collins J, Ruscetti F W, Gallagher R E, Gallo R C (1978).
Terminal differentiation of human promyeloctic leukemia
cells induced by dimethyl sulfoxide and other polar
compounds. Proc Natl Acad Sci (USA) 75:2485-2462.
Gargus J J, Adelberg E A, Slayman C W, (1985). Coordinated
changes in potassium fluxes as early events in the
differentiation of the human promyelocyte line HL-60.
Soc Gen Physiol Series 39:179-191.
Golub, E S (1982) In vitro approaches to hemopoiesis.
Cell 28:687-688.
Gough N M, Gough J, Metcalf D, Kelso A, Grail D, Nicola
N A, Burgess A W, Dunn A R (1984). Molecular cloning of
cDNA encoding a muring haematopoietic growth regulator,
granulocyte-macrophage colony stimulating factor. Nature
309:763-767.
Hall A K, (1983). Stem cell is a stem cell is a stem cell.
Cell 33:11-12.
Levenson R D, Housman D, Cantley L (1980). Amiloride
inhibits murine erythroleukemia cell differentiation:
evidence for a Ca^{2+} requirement for commitment. Proc
Natl Acad Sci (USA) 77:5948-5952.
Mager D, and Bernstein A (1978). Early transport changes
during erythroid differentiation of Friend leukemic
cells. J Cell Physiol 94:275-286.
Metcalf D (1980). Clonal analysis of proliferation
differentiation of paired daughter cells: action of
granulocyte-macrophage colony-stimulating factor on
granulocyte-macrophage precursors. Proc Natl Acad Sci
(USA) 77:5327-5330.
Murao S, Gemmel M A, Callaham M F, Anderson N L, Huberman
E (1983). Control of macrophage cell differentiation in
human promyelocytic HL-60 leukemia cells by 1,25-
dihydroxyvitamin D3 and phorbol-12-myristate-13-acetate.
Cancer Res 43:4989-4996.
Wong G G, Witek J S, Temple P A, Wilkens K M, Leary A C,
Luxenberg D P, Jones S S, Brown E L, Kay R M, Orr E C,
Shoemaker C, Golde D W, Kaufman R J, Hewick R M, Wang E
A, Clark S C (1985). Human GM-CSF: Molecular cloning
of the complementary DNA and purification of the
natural and recombinant proteins. Science 228:810-815.

Section 4. COMMITMENT AND EXPRESSION OF DIFFERENTIATED FUNCTIONS

Cellular Endocrinology: Hormonal Control of Embryonic
and Cellular Differentiation, pages 245–264
© 1986 Alan R. Liss, Inc.

THE ROLE OF PROGENITOR CELLS IN CELLULAR DIFFERENTIATION, CELLULAR SENESCENCE AND NEOPLASTIC TRANSFORMATION

Sarah A. Bruce, Scott F. Deamond, Shuji Nakano,
Toshimitsu Okeda, Ali M. Saboori, Paul O.P. Ts'o,
Hiroaki Ueo and Yasushi Yokogawa

Division of Biophysics, School of Hygiene and Public
Health, The Johns Hopkins University, Baltimore,
Maryland 21205

INTRODUCTION

As a source of fully differentiated, functional cells required for the normal development and maintenance of an organism, stem cells and progenitor cells obviously play an important role in normal cellular differentiation. However, the involvement of these cells in aging and cancer is less well defined. One approach to this question is to utilize cellular senescence and neoplastic transformation as in vitro models of aging and cancer respectively, in order to determine the role of stem cells and progenitor cells and their differentiation in these processs.

Although in vitro cellular senescence (i.e. the limited proliferative capacity of cultured normal cells) was first described nearly thirty years ago (Swim and Parker, 1957; Hayflick and Moorhead, 1961), the mechanism of cellular senescence is still unknown. It has been proposed alternatively to be the accumulation of error or genetically programmed cell death or cell differentiation (Holliday, 1984; Hayflick, 1982; Bell, et al., 1978). In addition, although in vitro senescence is considered to be a cellular model of organismal aging (Hayflick, 1965; 1984), the exact relationship between in vitro senescence and in vivo aging is unknown. Senescent cells in culture are not necessarily equivalent to cells aged in vivo (Schneider and Mitsui, 1976) which suggests that the relationship between senescence and aging may not be direct. Nonetheless, these two phenomena are related as shown by the inverse correlation between in vitro proliferative capacity and in vivo donor age (Schneider and Mitsui, 1976; Bruce, et al., 1986). A better understanding of the mechanism of senescence (in particular its relationship to differentiation) may lead to a clarification of the relationship between in vitro senescence and in vivo aging as well as a better understanding of the role of reduced stem cell function in aging in vivo.

With regard to the relationship between neoplasia and differentiation, one obvious question is the relative susceptibility to carcinogen-induced neoplastic transformation of cells at different stages of differentiation or development. It is unlikely that post-mitotic (e.g. senescent), terminally differentiated cells are significantly affected by carcinogen-induced damage because if the damaged cell does not proliferate the carcinogen damage cannot be manifested as a tumor. However, it is not known whether cells along the continuum between a pluripotent or unipotent stem cell and a lineage-committed, actively differentiating cell show differences in susceptibility to carcinogen-induced neoplastic transformation.

In this report we summarize our recent studies on the mechanism(s) of cellular senescence, the relationship between in vitro senescence and in vivo aging, and the relative susceptibility to neoplastic transformation of cells at various stages of development, differentiation and aging.

EXPERIMENTAL SYSTEM AND STRATEGY FOR IN VITRO CELLULAR STUDIES OF NEOPLASTIC TRANSFORMATION, SENESCENCE AND DIFFERENTIATION

One approach to understanding two or more interrelated phenomena is to study them simultaneously in a single experimental system in which the phenomena under study occur and can be monitored and manipulated. One such system for the study of neoplastic transformation, cellular senescence and cellular differentiation is the Syrian hamster cell culture system. The choice of this system for these studies is based on the following properties of Syrian hamster mesenchymal (fibroblastic-like) cells in culture. Firstly, normal diploid primary cell strains of Syrian hamster origin exhibit cellular senescence with a very low rate of spontaneous conversion to permanent cell lines (Bruce, et al., 1986). Secondly, low passage Syrian hamster cells can be neoplastically transformed in vitro by exposure to chemical carcinogens. This property along with the low background rate of spontaneous transformation of these cells led to the development of Syrian hamster cells from 13 day gestation fetuses as a model system for in vitro neoplastic transformation studies (Heidelberger, et al., 1983). Thirdly, several lineages of mesenchymal cell differentiation (e.g. adipocyte and muscle cell differentiation) occur spontaneously at a high frequency in both primary cell cultures and established cell lines derived from 9 day gestation Syrian hamster embryos. In addition, as an animal model, the entire system can be manipulated at both the organismal and cellular level. Furthermore, pre-embryonic (e.g. morula, blastocyst), embryonic and fetal cells plus all ages and types of adult tissue are available as sources for primary cultures of normal diploid cells.

Our strategy is to investigate the entire system from early development to old age by isolating cell cultures at different developmental stages and ages. These cell cultures are then passaged, manipulated with growth factors, hormones, carcinogens, phorbol ester tumor promoters, or other agents and analyzed with regard to senescence, differentiation and susceptibility to neoplastic transformation (Figure 1). An eventual aim is to correlate the in vitro cellular response to an in vivo cellular and organismic response.

We have thus far studied mesenchymal cell cultures derived from tissues ranging from 9 day gestation embryos to 24 month aged adults (Table 1). Nine day gestation material is used because it is the earliest stage at which the embryo can be clearly distinguished and separated from the maternal tissue. By 9 days gestation in the Syrian hamster, all the major organ systems are developed which suggests that 9-10 days is the end of embryonic development (organogenesis) in this species and that the remainder of the 15.5 days gestation is fetal or maturational development (Boyer, 1968; Bruce, et al., 1984). Based on these observations, we designate cell strains isolated from ≤ 9-10 days gestation

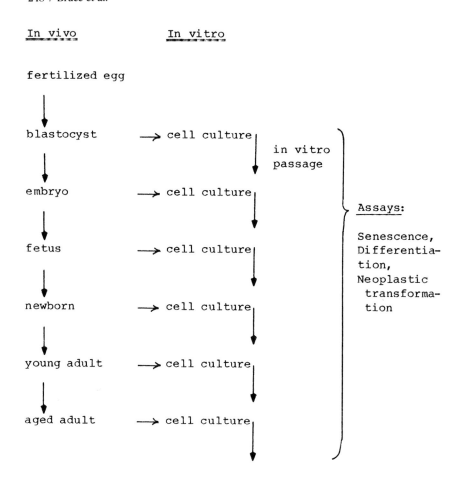

Figure 1. An overall scheme presenting an in vitro/in vivo strategy for the study of development, differentiation and aging.

as embryonic (E) and ≥ 11 days gestation as fetal (F) (Table 1). Since embryonic development is characterized by differentiation and fetal development by growth and maturation, the distinction between embryonic and fetal cell strains may have a direct bearing on our studies on the differentiation, senescence, and spontaneous and induced neoplastic transformation of these cell types. The final

Table 1.   In Vitro Cell Cultures Analyzed

Cell designation	Source	
	tissue	age
E9	whole embryo	9 days gestation
FC13	fetal carcass	13 days gestation[a,b]
FE13	fetal extremities	13 days gestation[a]
FD13	fetal dermis	13 days gestation[a]
ND3	neonatal dermis	3 days postpartum
AD6	adult dermis	6 months
AD24	adult dermis	24 months[c]

a   Gestation in the Syrian hamster is 15.5 days.
b   FC13 cells are equivalent to SHE cells used in neoplastic
    transformation experiments (see Heidelberger, et al.,
    1983).
c   Average life span and maximum life span of male LVG
    Syrian hamsters are 18.5 and 28 months respectively
    (Bruce, et al., 1986).

time point in our studies is 24 months of age at which time
the hamster is considered to be aged. Based on 84 natural
deaths in our own Syrian hamster aging colony, the average
mean in vivo life span for males of this species (strain
LVG) is 18.5 months and the maximum in vivo life span is
28.0 months under conventional animal housing conditions
(Bruce, et al., 1986).

IN VITRO CELLULAR SENESCENCE OF SYRIAN HAMSTER MESENCHYMAL
CELL CULTURES

Primary cultures of normal diploid Syrian hamster
dermal fibroblasts of fetal, neonatal, young adult and aged
adult origin have been isolated and compared with regard to
their in vitro proliferative capacity (Bruce, et al., 1986).
Greater than 95% of these replicate Syrian hamster cultures,
regardless of the age of the tissue of origin, exhibited
cellular senescence characterized by a limited in vitro
proliferative life span similar to that described for human

diploid fibroblast cell cultures (Hayflick and Moorhead, 1961; Hayflick, 1965). All Syrian hamster cell cultures exhibited an initial phase of rapid proliferation followed by a progressive reduction in proliferative rate. The overall pattern of senescence of the cells from fetal, neonatal, young adult and aged adult tissue was similar in terms of proliferative changes indicated by a reduction in saturation density, cloning efficiency and ^{3}H-thymidine labeling index and by an increase in population doubling time and cell volume. However, the maximum cumulative population doubling level (cumPDL) attained at senescence was characteristic for each type of cell culture: fetal, 28.6; neonatal, 18.7; young adult, 13.8; aged adult, 11.1 cumPDL. Thus, the in vitro proliferative capacity of Syrian hamster dermal fibroblasts of fetal to aged adult origin is inversely related to the in vivo age of the donor tissue in a manner similar to that described for human fibroblasts by Martin, et al. (1970) and Schneider and Mitsui (1976).

More recently, we have analyzed the proliferative capacity and senescence pattern of 9 day gestation embryonic (E9) cells. Most E9 cell cultures exhibit cellular senescence and the pattern of alterations in morphology and proliferation is similar to fetal and adult cells. However, E9 cells require higher (20% versus 10%) serum supplementation throughout their in vitro life span, grow more slowly than fetal cells, and achieve a lower average maximum cumPDL (15.3) as compared to fetal cells. This reduced in vitro proliferative capacity of E9 cells relative to fetal cells can in part be explained by the reduced plating efficiency (i.e. efficiency of attachment at each subculture) of E9 cells (~50%) relative to fetal cells (>85%), but may also be related to our incomplete understanding of the culture requirements of cells from this stage of development. E9 cells are also distinct from fetal and adult cells with regard to the frequency of spontaneous escape from senescence which is >4-fold higher in E9 cells (20%) compared to fetal and adult cells (<5%) (Okeda, et al., 1984; Bruce et al., 1986). Lastly, as will be discussed in the following section, E9 cells are also unique with regard to the types of cell differentiation which they exhibit.

CELLULAR DIFFERENTIATION OF CULTURED SYRIAN HAMSTER CELLS

Adipocyte and Muscle Cell Differentiation

As described in the previous section, cellular senescence is one pathway which cultured Syrian hamster cells can follow. In addition, cell differentiation pathways, such as adipocyte and muscle cell differentiation, can be observed in these cell cultures. Notably, however, these two examples of mesenchymal lineage cell differentiation have only been observed in primary and established cell cultures derived from 9 day gestation embryonic tissue (E9 cells) and not in cultures derived from 13 day gestation fetal or older tissue. This difference in the differentiation potential in vitro is presumably related to an in vivo developmental change at 9-10 days gestation coincident with the interface between embryonic development (organogoenesis) and fetal or maturational development in the Syrian hamster (see above).

Adipocyte differentiation occurs spontaneously and at high frequency (>50%) in confluent normal diploid E9 cell cultures, which appear fibroblast-like in morphology during exponential growth. The lipid-laden cells which develop have been identified as mature adipocytes by lipid-specific staining with Oil-Red O, electron microscopy and a <10-fold acummulation of triglyceride (Ueo, et al., 1982; Bruce, et al., 1984). A non-proliferative state, resulting from either confluence or senescence, is required for adipocyte differentiation. Clonal analysis of passage 1 E9 cells shows that >50% of the colonies contain adipocytes which indicates that a majority of the cells are preadipocytes or undifferentiated mesenchymal cells that become committed to the adipocyte lineage in culture. E9 cells are unique in their high frequency of adipocyte differentiation. There is a rapid decline in the frequency of adipocyte-containing colonies in cultures generated from 10-12 days gestation tissue, and no adipocyte differentiation is observed in cell cultures from 13 day gestation fetal carcass or dermis, neonatal dermis or adult dermis. One spontaneously established, clonal aneuploid cell line (E9/1) which exhibits up to 100% adipocyte differentiation in clonal assay has been isolated from E9 primary cell strains.

Muscle cell differentiation, as indicated by myoblast fusion into striated contractile myotubes is also observed in primary and low passage Syrian hamster E9 cell cultures and to a lesser degree in 13 day gestation fetal cell cultures. In addition, several established lines have been derived from E9 cells which have retained the capacity for muscle cell differentiation. One such established cell line, E9/11 PDD, was derived from a primary culture of E9 cells by continuous treatment with the tumor promoter phorbol-12,13-didecanoate (PDD) at 0.1 µg/ml (Okeda, et al., 1984). These cells were maintained in the presence of PDD for >100 population doublings and during that time they exhibited low frequencies of both adipocyte differentiation and muscle cell differentiation (as indicated by myoblast fusion and altered patterns of creatine phosphokinase isozymes). At PDL 145, these cell cultures exhibited a typical, stellate fibroblastic morphology and an aneuploid chromosome number and the frequency of muscle cell differentiation was 15% in clonal assay. After PDL 145, when PDD was removed from the mass culture, the cells displayed a significant morphological change from a stellate morphology to a more elongated morphology, and by PDL 180 the culture was morphologically homogeneous. By PDL 215, a significant diploid chromosomal mode of 44 had appeared although there were still aneuploid cells in the population. By PDL 257, 86% of the cells were diploid and the karyotype appeared to be the normal Syrian hamster karyotype based on chromosome number and banding pattern. Concurrent with the observed change in morphology and selection for a diploid cell type, the frequency of muscle cell differentiation increased dramatically from 15% at PDL 145 to 98% at PDL 300. A number of diploid clones have been isolated from the mass culture which exhibit various frequencies of myoblast fusion up to 100% (Yokogawa, et al., 1985).

We conclude from these observations that E9 cell cultures contain unipotent mesenchymal progenitor cells which are either preadipocytes or premyoblasts. In addition, the presence of multipotent mesenchymal progenitor cells in primary and low passage E9 cell cultures is indicated by the presence of clonal colonies which contain two or more morphologically and/or histochemically distinct cell types. We are currently attempting to isolate the morphologically undistinguished progenitor cells prior to their differentiation to morphologically, histochemically or biochemically distinct end points.

Contact-insensitive (CS⁻) Cells

   Primary and low passage Syrian hamster cell cultures
also contain a transient subpopulation of
contact-insensitive (CS⁻) cells (Nakano and Ts'o, 1981).
CS⁻ cells are detected by their ability to proliferate and
form a colony on a preformed, irradiated monolayer of
contact-sensitive (CS⁺) cells (cell mat assay). The
frequency of these CS⁻ cells in 13 day fetal cell cultures,
quantitated as cloning efficiency on cell mat, declines from
10-20% at passage 1 to <0.001% by passage 6 (PDL 15-20)
(Ueo, et al., 1986). It is unlikely that these cells are
lost by negative selection because the frequency of
CS⁻ cells declines even when the cultures are grown
continuously on cell mats, a condition that selects for
CS⁻ cells. Furthermore, isolation and reanalysis of cells
in cell mat colonies shows that the cell mat colonies
contain both CS⁻ cells (up to 20%) and CS⁺ cells. We
conclude from these observations that CS⁻ cells are lost by
conversion to CS⁺ cells. We have proposed that this
conversion may represent an early stage of differentiation
which is characterized by an altered control of
proliferation which is acquired prior to the appearance of a
terminally differentiated phenotype (Nakano and Ts'o, 1981;
Ueo, et al., 1986).

MANIPULATION OF DIFFERENTIATION AND SENESCENCE OF SYRIAN
HAMSTER CELLS IN CULTURE

Phorbol Ester Tumor Promoters

   Tumor promoters have been reported to inhibit
mesenchymal cell differentiation in several cell culture
systems including the 3T3 preadipocyte cell line (Diamond,
et al., 1977) and chick myoblasts (Cohen, et al., 1977) and
chondrocytes (Pacifici and Holtzer, 1977). Similarily, both
adipocyte and muscle cell differentiation in Syrian hamster
primary and established cell cultures are inhibited by
treatment with PDD or 12-O-tetradecanoyl phorbol-13-
acetate (TPA) at 0.1 μg/ml. In addition, the loss of the
CS⁻ cells present in primary Syrian hamster fetal cell
cultures is also retarded by continuous exposure of mass
cultures to PDD. We conclude from this observation that
tumor promoters can at least partially inhibit (i.e. retard)
the conversion of CS⁻ cells to CS⁺ cells in a manner similar

to the inhibition of the conversion of pre-adipocytes to adipocytes, myoblast to myotubes, etc.

As part of a study investigating the relationship between senescence and differentiation, we examined the effect of tumor promoters on the senescence pattern of Syrian hamster cells. Continuous treatment of Syrian hamster fibroblastic cell cultures from passage 1 with tumor promoters can result in an extension of the proliferative life span of the cells (Ueo, et al., 1986). However, the magnitude of the response is related to the developmental stage or age of the tissue source. Fetal and neonatal cells treated with 0.1 µg/ml PDD exhibit a 60-120% increase in cumPDL at senescence. Similarly treated young adult cells show a reduced response (<30% increase in cumPDL) while PDD-treated aged adult cells generally show no extension in life span (Bruce, et al., 1983). This age-related difference in the magnitude of life span extension with PDD appears to be related to the frequency of CS$^-$ cells at passage 1 when PDD treatment is initiated. In these experiments, the highest initial frequency of CS$^-$ cells was exhibited by fetal cells and the lowest frequency was exhibited by aged adult cells. In addition, this response to PDD decreases with passage and loss of the CS$^-$ subpopulation. If PDD treatment is initiated at midpassage when the cultures contain <0.001% CS$^-$ cells, no effect on life span is observed. Although PDD can extend the proliferative life span of fetal, neonatal and young adult cells, no increase in the frequency of escape from senescence has been observed with these cells after PDD treatment.

The effects of tumor promoters on E9 cells are distinct from the effects of these compounds on fetal to adult cells. Continuous treatment of E9 cells from passage 1 results in an increase in the frequency of escape from senescence and conversion to established cell lines which eventually lose their requirement for the presence of tumor promoters for continued proliferation. In contrast to a frequency of 20% escape from senescence in control E9 cultures, 75% of PDD-treated E9 cell cultures escape senescence. The permanent E9 cell lines derived either spontaneously or by treatment with promoters fall into one of two categories: (i) preneoplastic or neoplastic cell lines, or (ii) non-neoplastic, progenitor-like cell lines that have

retained the capacity for adipocyte or muscle cell
differentiation at frequencies up to 100% in clonal assays
(Okeda, et al., 1984; Yokogawa, et al., 1985). All
spontaneously established fetal or adult cell lines that
have arisen thus far fall only into the first category. The
second category appears to be unique to E9 cell lines and is
presumably related to the fact that only E9 cell strains
exhibit adipocyte and muscle cell differentiation.

Two conclusions can be drawn from the promoter studies.
Firstly, exposure of Syrian hamster cell cultures to a
single agent, the tumor promoter PDD, results in an
inhibition (or at least a retardation) of the growth and/or
differentiation pathway these cells normally follow, i.e.
adipocyte differentiation, muscle cell differentiation,
conversion of CS^- cells to CS^+ cells and cellular
senescence. Secondly, in comparison to fetal or adult
cells, cells from 9 days gestation are unique in their
capacity for adipocyte and muscle cell differentiation and
are far more sensitive to external perturbation. It was of
interest to determine whether these effects on senescence
and differentiation of these cells was unique to tumor
promoters or whether other growth promoters/regulators, such
as polypeptide growth factors, had similar effects.

Epidermal Growth Factor (EGF) and Fibroblast Growth Factor
(FGF)

Similar to the effect of tumor promoters on the
senescence of E9 cells, continuous treatment from passage 1
of E9 cells with 10 ng/ml EGF or 50 ng/ml FGF increased
significantly the frequency of escape from senescence (Table
2). The effect of FGF was slightly greater than that of EGF
presumably because of the fibroblastic nature of these
cells. FGF-treated E9 cells generally showed an increased
growth rate from the beginning of treatment as compared to
control cells and escaped senescence with a minimal crisis
period. Further, those FGF-treated E9 cultures which did
senesce exhibited an extension of proliferative capacity
indicated by an elevated maximum cumPDL at senescence
relative to control cultures. In contrast, EGF neither
stimulated the initial growth rate of E9 cells nor extended
the in vitro proliferative life span of cultures which did
senesce. Further, EGF-treated established cell lines
frequently exhibited a very long crisis period (30-50 day)

characterized by a minimal growth rate. These E9 cell lines derived by treatment with growth factors also fall into one of two catagories (preneoplastic/neoplastic cell lines or non-neoplastic, progenitor cell lines) as described above.

Continuous treatment of fetal cells (FC13 or FE13 cells) with EGF or FGF resulted in a similarly increased frequency of escape from senescence (Table 2). As with E9 cells, FGF is more effective on F13 cells than is EGF in terms of initial growth stimulation and frequency of escape from senescence. All growth factor-treated fetal cell lines appear to be in neoplastic progression. They do not exhibit adipocyte or muscle cell differentiation, and with passage in vitro, many have acquired anchorage independent growth and, in some cases, tumorigenicity (Saboori, et al., 1985).

Preliminary data on the effect of 10 ng/ml EGF on adipocyte and muscle cell differentiation in established Syrian hamster E9 cell lines show that EGF inhibits the formation of mature adipocytes and retards the acquisition of contractility by colonies of fused myoblasts. The effect of EGF and FGF on the loss of the CS^- subpopulation is currently under investigation.

RELATIONSHIP BETWEEN CS^- CELLS AND PROGENITOR CELLS

Undifferentiated progenitor cells are morphologically undistinguished. Thus, their presence is only surmised from their subsequent conversion into overtly differentiated cell types (e.g. adipocytes, myotubes, etc.) that can be identified morphologically, histochemically or biochemically. Thus, in order to isolate and characterize undifferentiated progenitor cells, some property of these cells needs to be identified on which to base an isolation procedure.

We are currently investigating whether the CS^- phenotype is a valid marker for undifferentiated progenitor cells. There are several reasons to believe that progenitor cells are CS^-. Firstly, CS^- cells are present in primary and low passage cultures and are lost during in vitro passage presumably by conversion to CS^+ cells. Secondly, the size of the CS^- subpopulation at passage 1 is inversely related to donor age with the highest frequency being observed in 13 day gestation fetal cell cultures and

TABLE 2.   Effect of Growth Factors on the Frequency
            of Escape from Senescence of Syrian
            Hamster Embryonic and Fetal Mesenchymal
            Cell Cultures

Cell type[a]	Percentage of cultures that escaped senescence (number in parentheses indicates total number of flasks analyzed)		
	Control	EGF (10 ng/ml)	FGF (50 ng/ml)
E9	20% (16)	50% (10)	67% (6)
FC13, FE13	0% (24)[b]	35% (17)	42% (12)

[a] See Table 1
[b] No spontaneous escape from senescence was observed
among the control flasks from these experiments.
We have previously reported a frequency of ~3%
among a total of 148 replicate flasks of fetal to
aged adult origin (Bruce, et al., 1986).

the lowest frequency being observed in adult cell cultures.
Thirdly, the initial size of the CS⁻ subpopulation is
directly related to the maxcumPDL which the mass culture
achieves at senescence. This is true both for different
preparations of fetal cells (which show some variation in
the frequency of CS⁻ cells at passage 1) and in comparing
fetal cell cultures with adult cell cultures. Lastly the
frequency of CS⁻ cells is directly related to the
responsiveness of cultures to tumor promoter-induced
extension of in vitro proliferative life span. The
observation that CS⁻ cells are present in fetal tissue and
in primary culture and are lost by conversion to another
cell type during in vivo development and aging, and during
in vitro proliferation suggests that these cells are
progenitor-like cells. Current experiments are aimed at
isolating pure populations of these cells in order to

determine more precisely the role of these cells in differentiation, senescence and aging.

RELATIVE SUSCEPTIBILITY OF THE CS⁻ SUBPOPULATION IN SYRIAN HAMSTER CELL CULTURES TO NEOPLASTIC TRANSFORMATION

To determine whether the above described transient CS⁻ cells are more sensitive to carcinogenic and/or mutagenic perturbation, the susceptibility to neoplastic transformation and somatic mutation induced by N-methyl-N'-nitro-N-nitrosoguanidine (MNNG) was examined in clonally isolated cell cultures containing various proportions of CS⁻ cells (4% - 0.02%). The frequencies of MNNG-induced morphological transformation, focus formation and neoplastic transformation were 20-40 fold higher in CS⁻ enriched cultures (4%) compared to CS⁻ depleted cultures (0.02%). In contrast, the frequency of MNNG-induced somatic mutation at the Na^+/K^+ ATPase locus was similar among cultures varying in their proportion of CS⁻ cells. These data show that the transient CS⁻ cells in primary Syrian hamster cell cultures are more susceptible to neoplastic transformation although equally susceptible to induced point mutation when compared to CS^+ cells (Nakano, et al., 1985). By extension of the above stated hypothesis, these observations suggest that less differentiated progenitor-like cells (e.g. CS⁻ cells) are more susceptible to neoplastic transformation than are their more differentiated progeny (e.g. CS^+ cells).

Preliminary experiments comparing the susceptibility of fetal, young adult and aged adult dermal fibroblast mass cultures to carcinogen-induced neoplastic transformation show an inverse correlation between transformation frequency and donor age which may be related to the lower initial frequency of CS⁻ cells in adult cell cultures compared to fetal cell cultures. This apparent decrease in susceptibility of mesenchymal cells with increased donor tissue age may be associated with the age-related incidence of sarcomas which, in contrast to carcinomas, are most prevalent in childhood (Silverberg and Lubera, 1983).

DISCUSSION AND CONCLUSION

Our current working hypothesis to explain the above described observations is outlined in Figure 2. Pluri- or

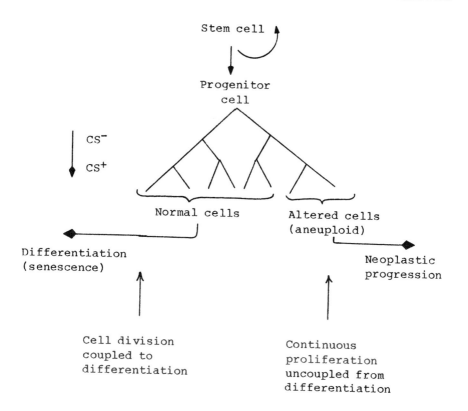

Figure 2. Working hypothesis on the relationship between differentiation, proliferation and neoplasia.

unipotent stem cells divide asymmetrically to produce their own replacement and a progenitor cell with some degree of commitment to a given differentiation lineage. Subsequently, the progenitor cells become fully committed to a specific lineage and may undergo symmetric division as part of clonal expansion. After a characteristic number of divisions, proliferation is reduced (possibly through altered cell contact or density-dependent inhibition) and overt differentiation begins. In this situation, cell division is coupled to differentiation as originally suggested by the work of Sachs and colleagues in the myeloid leukemia system (Lotem and Sachs, 1981). However, in some of the progeny of the progenitor cell, this coupling can be disrupted and these cells continue to proliferate. In our studies, these cells are generally aneuploid, but it is unclear whether the aneuploidy is a cause or an effect. The acquisition of aneuploidy is most likely the result of a stochastic event (non-disjunction, endoreduplication, recombination, etc.). This initial genome disruption overrides, at least transiently, the cell's genetic commitment to a given differentiation lineage which would otherwise lead to reduced proliferation and overt differentiation. In this case, cell division and differentiation have become uncoupled. Additional errors in chromosome segregation or other forms of genome instability could then lead to neoplastic progression. However, within this sequence, selection can still occur for a diploid chromosome complement (such as in the diploid E9/11 PDD premyoblast cells) or some other chromosome complement (such as in the aneuploid E9/1 preadipocyte cells) that permits the genetic commitment to differentiation to be reexpressed.

Another important consideration in these studies is the difference between the embryonic (E9) cells and the fetal or older cells. Embryonic cells are 4-5X more likely to become spontaneously established cell lines when compared to fetal and adult cells and this frequency is substantially increased by treatment with tumor promoters or growth factors. It is unclear whether the tumor promoters and growth factors increase this frequency of conversion to established cell lines simply by lengthening the culture's proliferative phase thereby enhancing the chance of spontaneous conversion to aneuploidy, or whether they have a more direct effect. Regardless of the mechanism, this observation suggests that the 9 day gestation embryonic genome is less stable than that of cells at later developmental stages and ages both in terms of structure and control of function. If less differentiated cells from early developmental stages cells do have less stable genomes, it is likely they would be more susceptible to external genomic perturbations such as carcinogens.

Lastly, our observation on the presence in primary and low passage culture of a subpopulation of progenitor-like cells, the number of which and the rate of loss of which are directly related to the proliferative capacity of the mass culture, suggests a relationship between senescence and differentiation. Although the identification of a biochemical marker of the differentiation of these cells

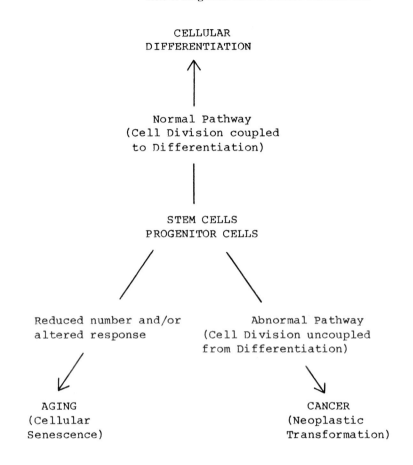

Figure 3. Working hypothesis on the relationship between cellular differentiation, carcinogenesis and aging.

during the life span of the culture is required as further evidence, we tentatively conclude that the loss of proliferative capacity by cultured Syrian hamster fibroblastic cells is part of a differentiation sequence. In this case, the question of the relationship between in vitro senescence and in vivo aging arises again. In vitro cellular senescence may not be directly related to aging in that all cellular changes which occur during in vitro senescence do not necessarily parallel cellular changes which occur during in vivo aging. However, the proliferative capacity of a culture appears to be a reflection of the frequency of progenitor-like cells in primary culture which is presumably directly related to the frequency of these cells in the variously aged tissue from which a primary culture is derived. This then could explain the inverse correlation between in vitro proliferative capacity and in vivo donor age that has been documented both in the Syrian hamster system and in the human fibroblast system. By extension, this conclusion suggests that, at least for skin fibroblasts, aging in vivo may be related to a loss of progenitor cells either in terms of decreased number or decreased response to a proliferation stimulus.

Based on the above described observations, we conclude that progenitor cells play a central role in aging and carcinogenesis as well as in normal differentiation and that progenitor cells may be the basis of the interrelationship among these phenomena (Figure 3).

REFERENCES

Bell E, Marek LE, Levinstone DS, Merrill C, Sher S, Young IT, Eden M (1978). Loss of division potential in vitro: aging or differentiation?. Science 202: 1158-1163.

Boyer CC (1968). Embryology. In: The Golden Hamster, eds Hoffman RA, Robinson PG, Magalhaes H, Iowa State Univ Press, Ames, pp 73-89.

Bruce S, Deamond S, Ueo H., Ts'o P (1983). Age-related differences in promoter-induced extension of in vitro life span of Syrian hamster cells. J Cell Biol 97: 346a.

Bruce SA, Gyi KK, Nakano S, Ueo H, Zajac-Kaye M, Ts'o POP, (1984). Genetic and developmental determinants in neoplastic transformation. In: Biochemical Basis of Chemical Carcinogenesis, eds Greim H, Jung R, Kramer M, Marquardt H, Oesch F, Raven Press, New York, pp 159-174.

Bruce S, Deamond SF, Ts'o POP (1986). In vitro senescence of Syrian hamster mesenchymal cells of fetal to aged adult origin. Inverse relationship between in vivo donor age and in vitro proliferative capacity. Mech Ageing Devel, in press.

Cohen R, Pacifici M, Rubinstein N, Biehl J, Holtzer H (1977). Effect of tumour promoter on myogenesis. Nature 266: 538-540.

Diamond L, O'Brien TG, Rovera G (1977). Inhibition of adipose conversion of 3T3 fibroblasts by tumor promoters. Nature 269: 247-249.

Hayflick L (1965). The limited in vitro lifetime of human diploid cell strains. Exp Cell Res 37: 614-636.

Hayflick L (1982). Ageing and death of vertebrate cells. In: Lectures on Gerontology, vol 1, On the Biology of Ageing pt A, ed Viidik A, Academic Press, London, pp 59-98.

Hayflick L (1984). Intracellular determinants of cell aging. Mech Ageing Devel 28: 177-185.

Hayflick L, Moorhead PS (1961). The serial cultivation of human diploid cell strains. Exp Cell Res 25: 585-621.

Heidelberger C, Freeman AE, Pienta RJ, Sivak A, Bertram JS, Casto BC, Dunkel VC, Francis MW, Kakunaga T, Little JB, Schectman LM (1983). Cell transformation by chemical agents - A review and analysis of the literature. Mut Res 114: 283-385.

Holliday R (1984). The unsolved problem of cellular ageing. In: Cellular Ageing, Monographs in Developmental Biology, vol 17, ed Sauer HW, Karger, Basel, pp 60-77.

Lotem J, Sachs L (1982). Mechanisms that uncouple growth and differentiation in myeloid leukemia cells: Restoration of requirement for normal growth-inducing protein without restoring induction of differentiation-inducing protein. Proc Natl Acad Sci USA 79: 4347-4351.

Martin GM, Sprague CA, Epstein CJ (1970). Replicative life-span of cultivated human cells. Lab Invest 23: 86-92.

Nakano S, Ts'o POP (1981). Cellular differentiation and neoplasia: Characterization of subpopulations of cells that have neoplasia-related properties in Syrian hamster embryo cell cultures. Proc Natl Acad Sci USA 78: 4995-4999.

Nakano S, Ueo H., Bruce SA, Ts'o POP (1985). A contact-insensitive subpopulation in Syrian hamster cell cultures with a greater susceptibility to chemically induced neoplastic transformation. Proc Natl Acad Sci USA 82: 5005-5009.

Okeda T, Ueo H, Bruce SA, Bury MA, Ts'o POP (1984). Tumor promoters and epidermal growth factor increase the frequency of conversion of Syrian hamster embryonic cell cultures to permanent cell lines. J Cell Biol 99: 337a.

Pacifici M, Holtzer H (1977). Effects of a tumor-promoting agent on chondrogenesis. Am J Anat 150: 207-212.

Saboori A, Deamond SF, Bruce SA (1985). Epidermal growth factor and fibroblast growth factor increase the frequency of conversion of Syrian hamster embryonic and fetal cells to permanent cell lines. J Cell Biol 101: 351a.

Schneider EL, Mitsui Y (1976). The relationship between in vitro cellular aging and in vivo human age. Proc Natl Acad Sci USA 73: 3584-3588.

Silverberg E, Lubera (1983). A review of American cancer society estimates of cancer cases and deaths. CA - A Journal for Clinicians 33: 2-25.

Swim HE, Parker RF (1957). Culture characteristics of human fibroblasts propagated serially. Am J Hygiene 66: 235-243.

Ueo H, Bruce SA, Gyi KK, Nakano S, Ts'o POP (1982). Effects of phorbol esters on cellular differentiation of adipocyte and contact-insensitive cells in Syrian hamster cell cultures. J Cell Biol 95: 58a.

Ueo H, Bruce SA, Nakano S, Ts'o POP (1986). Tumor promoters retard the loss of a transient subpopulation of cells in low passage Syrian hamster cell cultures - Effect on in vitro proliferative lifespan of the culture. J Cell Physiol, in press.

Yokogawa Y, Okeda T, Bruce SA (1985). Isolation of a diploid myoblast cell line from Syrian hamster embryos. J Cell Biol 101: 170a.

Cellular Endocrinology: Hormonal Control of Embryonic
and Cellular Differentiation, pages 265-275
© 1986 Alan R. Liss, Inc.

DIFFERENTIATED BOVINE PARATHYROID CELLS CULTURED FOR MORE
THAN 140 POPULATION DOUBLINGS SHOW BOTH PARATHYROID HORMONE
SYNTHESIS AND GROWTH REGULATION BY CALCIUM ION CONCENTRATION

Maria Luisa Brandi, Lorraine A. Fitzpatrick, Susan
Fedak, Gerald D. Aurbach, and Hayden G. Coon

Section on Endocrine Regulation, Metabolic Diseases
Branch, National Institute of Arthritis, Diabetes,
and Digestive and Kidney Diseases (M.L.B., L.A.F.,
S.F., G.D.A.), and Laboratory of Genetics, National
Cancer Institute, (H.G.C.), National Institutes of
Health, Bethesda, MD 20892.

Although many have attempted to develop differentiated,
serially replicating cultures of parathyroid cells, none has
succeeded until now. As usual with differentiated cell
strains, some short term success was reported, but long term
cultures have failed (LeBoff et al., 1983; MacGregor et al.,
1983) usually because the cultures became overgrown by
"fibroblasts". Today, such problems immediately prompt
development of media low in serum or of hormonally defined
serum-free medium. The pioneering efforts of Sato and his
colleagues (Sato, 1975, Barnes et al., 1984) suggest
supplementing a basal medium with hormones and growth
factors until survival and/or growth appears. (Note that
this strategy differs from replacing serum by alternately
lowering its concentration and then attempting to recover
lost mitotic activity by supplementation with growth
factors.) By now enough of these results have been
collected so that it is possible to make fairly good a
priori guesses as to which hormones and growth supplements
might be needed for a particular cell type. One often
starts with a very complex medium, containing crude extracts
(such as saline extracts of brain or pituitary) and then
seeks to simplify the mixture until a fully successful
(ideally fully defined) medium is found. These efforts seem
to evolve towards highly cell-type specific formulations
which offer the benefit of discouraging potential competing
cell types such as fibroblasts. Often it is possible to

culture difficult or refractory cell types in this way, and
the common thread running through many of these attempts has
been the demonstration that mammalian sera at concentrations
of from 1% to 20% (or more) are frankly toxic to many cells
and especially to most epithelial cells. In this
communication we present an example of these generalities in
the culture of parathyroid hormone (PTH) secreting cells,
probably representing the chief cells, of the bovine
parathyroid gland. Many of the results reported here have
previously been published elsewhere (Brandi et al., 1986).

Primary cultures were made by mincing dissected
parathyroid gland tissue from adult cattle and dissociating
these fragments in collagenase as previously described
(Brandi et al., 1985). Since the bovine parathyroid (BPT)
cells attached poorly or not at all to plastic tissue
culture plates in serum-free medium, collagen or fibronectin
coatings were tried. BPT cells attach and spread
satisfactorily on these substrata, but it was also found
that precoating culture plates with serum was equally as
effective. Three ml of newborn calf serum were pipetted
into 100 mm tissue culture plastic petri dishes, allowed to
stand for a few hours and then aspirated (leaving <0.3 ml
residue/plate). The coated plates were stored overnight at
37°C in the incubator. Precoating of plates with serum
proved easier and less costly than coating with collagen
and/or fibronection and was adopted as routine. Figure 1
illustrates that all of the coating methods yield the same
50 fold increase in cell number within eight days of culture
(one medium change).

The nutrient medium used was a modified F12
(Ambesi-Impiombato et al., 1980) which was supplemented with
several hormones, growth factors and brain extracts as
follows: insulin (10 ug/ml), hydrocortisone (3.5 ng/ml),
Tri-iodothyronine [T3] (25 pg/ml), epidermal growth factor
(100 ng/ml), transferrin (5 ug/ml), retinoic acid (15
ng/ml), putrescine (30 ug/ml), selenous acid (5 ng/ml),
galactose (200 ug/ml), Ca++ (0.3 mM), Mg++ (0.5 mM), bovine
hypothalamic extract [BHE] (150 ug/ml), bovine pituitary
extract [BPE] (5 ug/ml). This medium, called GSmF12, was
used without serum to replace the medium twice weekly.

Transferrin, insulin, selenous acid, T3, and
hydrocortisone were added as basic to serum-free culture.
Galactose has been used with a positive trophic effect in

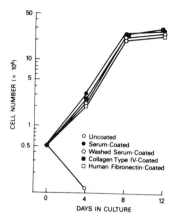

Figure 1. Growth curves of bovine parathyroid cells in plastic tissue culture dishes treated as indicated. Serum coating was used in most of the experiments described but it is apparently needed only for initial cell attachment.

rat small intestine cultures (Planas et al., 1981). The pituitary extract was used because the pituitary contains a variety of growth factors plus a factor reported to stimulate parathyroid secretion in vitro (Latman, 1980). The hypothalamus contains mitogenic factors for endothelial cells, keratinocytes, melanocytes and pituitary cells. Vitamin A and its analogs have been implicated in the control of epithelial cell growth and differentiation. In addition it has been reported to increase the release of PTH from bovine parathyroid fragments (Chertow et al., 1974). A high concentration of putrescine was used in view of a report that fibroblast growth is impeded under these conditions (Stoner et al., 1980). Cells maintained in a medium selectively lacking epidermal growth factor, BPE, or BHE showed a progressive impairment of cell growth. Increasing the Ca++ concentration, from 0.3 mM to 1.0 mM, caused a marked reduction of cell growth in GSmF12 medium (i.v.). In medium lacking epidermal growth factor, BPE, BHE, and containing 1.0 mM Ca++, cell proliferation ceased.

In primary cultures the BPT cells attached as small groups and formed a uniform monolayer between the 10th and 14th day of culture. The cell population appeared as

homogeneous epithelial cells with prominent nucleoli and
highly granulated cytoplasm (Figure 2). As with many
epithelial cell strains, occasionally dome-like structures
were noted. For the first 3 months of culture, doubling
times ranged from 18-22 hrs. Gradually, however, growth
rate slowed and by 5 months the population doubling times
had reached 58 to 60 hrs, as shown in Figure 3. The
saturation density attained at the 150th generation was
approximately half that of the 15th generation. Altogether
the BPT cells underwent 140-150 population doublings in 32
weekly passages. At about generation 140 signs of
senescence were apparent: the growth rate slowed, the cells
had become enlarged, often showing multiple nuclei and
numerous cytoplasmic extensions. The total number of
mitoses was reduced and growth was no longer uniform over
the culture dish. During the first 50-75 population
doublings the cells remained diploid. By the 150th
population doubling, however, 17% of metaphases were
hypotetraploid (5 of 30 metaphases had >95 chromosomes, 21
were diploid and 4 hypodiploid). The accumulation of
heteroploid cells in the population, without "spontaneous"
cell transformation might account for the slowed growth
rates interpreted as signs of senescence. It should prove
illuminating to culture some of the diploid cells as clones
from the higher passages to determine whether they generate
heteroploid cells more rapidly than at early passages.

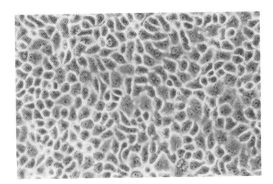

Figure 2. Phase contrast photomicrograph of a confluent culture of bovine parathyroid cells between passages 5 and 10.

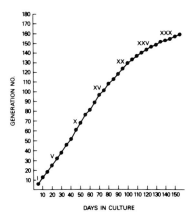

Figure 3. The cumulative growth curve of the bovine
parathyroid cells described in this work.

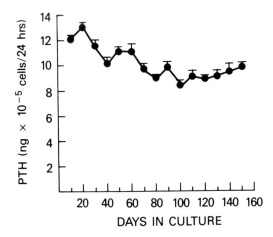

Figure 4. Parathyroid hormone (PTH) released in the medium
at different times throughout the culture history of the
bovine parathyroid cells. The determinations were performed
as described in Brandi et al., 1986.

The BPT cells we have studied show none of the now classic signs of transformation to become a "permanent cell line." They do, however, divide a prodigiously large number of times in vitro and such a cell strain, producing 140 or more cell generations could with the use of a judicious freezing strategy supply enough cells for any conceivable use. The differentiated characteristics of parathyroid cells continued unabated and at high levels throughout the passage history of the BPT cells (e.g., Figure 4).

It is obviously crucial to identify parathyroid hormone [PTH] in characterizing parathyroid cells. Using a mid-region specific radioimmunoassay we showed that growth rate and PTH production increased in parallel throughout the 7 days of a typical passage (Figure 5). Indirect immunofluorescence showed that >96% of the cells contained immuno-reactive PTH throughout all passages studied (Figure 6). Throughout 150 population doublings we observed a constant relation between cell number and the amount of radioimmunologically determined PTH in the medium, indicating a remarkable stability of the differentiated phenotype over extended periods. This relationship held even after the population growth rate had begun to decrease between population doublings 140 and 150 (Figure 5).

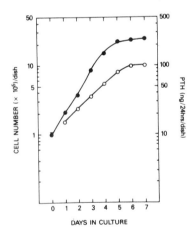

Figure 5. PTH production increases in parallel with cell number during the standard 7 day passage. The results shown are for passage V; similar results were found in X, XV and XX.

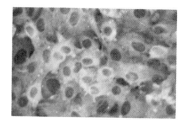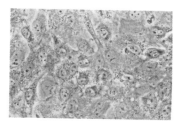

Figure 6. Immunofluorescence photomicrograph using rhodamine-labeled rabbit-anti-goat antibody following incubation with goat anti-bovine parathyroid hormone (left panel). In the right panel the same field appears with phase contrast.

We utilized the procedure of Silve et al., 1985, [rat osteosarcoma cells (Rodan et al., 1983) show increased intracellular cAMP response to PTH] to test the biological activity of PTH released into the medium. The cultured parathyroid cells indeed released a substance with biological activity into the medium throughout the culture lifetime of the BPT cells (Table 1). This fact taken together with the radioimmunoassay data provide stong evidence that these cells secrete PTH.

In the parathyroid gland the actions of calcium are complex: it affects growth (Raisz 1963), cyclic nucleotide phosphodiesterase (Brown 1980), hormone peptidase activity (Habener et al., 1975), PTH mRNA synthesis (Russel et al., 1983), and hormone secretion (Shoback et al., 1984).

TABLE 1. Bioactivity of PTH Released into the Medium of Bovine Parathyroid Cell Cultures

Day	PTH (pg-eq/ml)
30	27.3 ± 1.70
60	61.1 ± 2.36
150	33.7 ± 1.30

Results represent the mean (±SD) for triplicate samples expressed as pg-equivalent of human PTH (1-34). There was no detectable hormone in media incubated without cells.

In vivo, calcium negatively regulates the rate of PTH secretion. With BPT cells we also found a calcium-dependent suppression of PTH release, albeit with lower sensitivity to calcium than found in freshly isolated bovine cells (Figure 7). In the BPT cultures PTH suppression was half-maximal at approximately 2.2 mM Ca++ compared to 1.0 mM in the freshly dispersed cell model. We do not have an explanation for this finding, which may reflect the complex effects of Ca++ or the effects of our added growth factors on growth, hormone biosynthesis, degradation and secretion.

Low blood Ca++ causes parathyroid hypertrophy in vivo (Arnaud, 1973). Thus, it was anticipated that the optimum calcium concentration for cell growth might be lower than 1.1 mM. As shown in Figure 8a, a sharp optimum was found for tritiated thymidine (dT) uptake by BPT cells at 0.3 mM. At concentrations of calcium above 0.3 mM there was a precipitous drop with increasing calcium concentration. Regulation of dT incorporation by calcium ion concentration is a striking attribute of BPT cells. One might, however, legitimately worry that increasing Ca++ beyond the approximately 1.0 mM commonly found in cell culture media would inhibit dT incorporation in any cell strain. We have tested this possibility with FRTL-5, a differentiated thyroid cell strain from rat thyroid. The results, shown in Figure 8b, document that increasing Ca++ even to 4.0 mM has no effect on dT incorporation in these cells from the thyroid.

Prostaglandin E1, a well known stimulator of PTH secretion in freshly isolated bovine parathyroid cell preparations, increased cAMP accumulation and PTH release from BPT cells. The incubation of prostaglandin E1 with BPT cells caused cAMP accumulation up to 10-fold and PTH release up to 2-fold in a dose dependent fashion (Figure 9). We take this response as further evidence of the similarity of the BPT cell strain to the freshly isolated gland cell systems that have heretofore been used extensively.

We believe that the BPT cell system offers an excellent model for the study of factors that control parathyroid cell growth. These cell strains appear to be an ideal system for investigation of the PTH gene and the factors that regulate its expression. Study of parathyroid cells in vitro should help our understanding of the clinical problem of primary parathyroid hyperplasia and primary hypoparathyroidism.

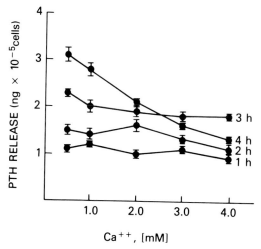

Figure 7. Calcium ion regulation of PTH release into the culture medium at different incubation times. Cells were grown to confluence in 1 cm (24 well) plates and tested in triplicate. After 4 hrs incubation the effect of Ca++ concentration on PTH is clear. Incubation medium: Eagle's medium (containing 20 mM Hepes, 500 KIU/ml aprotinin, 0.3% BSA fraction V, 0.5 mM magnesium, pH 7.4).

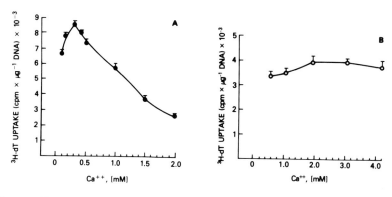

Figure 8. Incorporation of tritiated thymidine (dT) at different concentrations of Ca++ which have a marked effect on bovine parathyroid cells (panel A) but no effect on a similar glandular, epithelial cell from the thyroid, FRTL-5, (panel B). Details of the methods are described in Brandi et al., 1986.

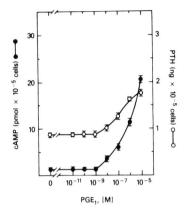

Figure 9. Prostaglandin E1 induced cAMP accumulation and PTH
release after 15 and 90 minute incubations respectively.
The incubations were carried out in the presence of a phosphodiesterase inhibitor: 0.5 mM 3-isobutyl-1-methyl xanthine. A
similar effect was observed at passages III, XII and XV.

REFERENCES

Ambesi-Impiombato FS, Parks LAM, Coon HG (1980). Culture of
hormone-dependent functional epithelial cells from rat
thyroids. Proc Natl Acad Sci USA 77: 3455–3459.
Arnaud CD (1973). Hyperparathyroidism and renal failure.
Kidney Int 4: 89–95.
Au W, Raisz LG (1965). Effect of vitamin D and dietary calcium
on parathyroid activity. Am J Physiol 209: 637–642.
Barnes DW, Sirbasku DA, Sato GH (1984) (eds). "Cell Culture
Methods for Molecular and Cell Biology." New York: Alan R.
Liss, vols 1–4.
Brandi ML, Fitzpatrick LA, Coon HG, Aurbach GD (1986). Bovine
parathyroid cells: cultures maintained for more than 140
population doublings. Proc Natl Acad Sci USA. In the press.
Brown EM (1980). Calcium regulated phosphodiesterase in bovine
parathyroid cells. Endocrinology 107: 1998–2003.
Chertow BS, Williams GA, Kiani R., Stewart KL, Hargis GK,
Flayter RL (1974). The interactions between vitamin A,
vinblastine, and cytochalazin B in parathyroid hormone
secretion. Proc Soc Exp Biol Med 147: 16–19.

Habener JF, Kemper B, Potts GT (1975). Calcium-dependent intracellular degradation of parathyroid hormone: a possible mechanism for the regulation of hormone stores. Endocrinology 97: 431–441.

Latman NS (1980). Pituitary stimulation of parathyroid hormone secretion: evidence in cattle for a parathyroid stimulating hormone. J Exp Zool 212: 313–322.

LeBoff MS, Rennke HG, Brown EM (1983). Abnormal regulation of parathyroid cell secretion and proliferation in primary cultures of bovine parathyroid cells. Endocrinology 113: 277–284.

MacGregor RR, Sarras MP, Houle A, Chon DV (1983). Primary monolayer culture of bovine parathyroids: effects of calcium, isoproterenol and growth factors. Mol Cell Endocrinol 3: 313–328.

Planas JM, Moreto M, Bolufer J (1981). Galactose and leucine transport in the developing small intestine. Experientia 37: 864–865.

Raisz LG (1983). Regulation by calcium of parathyroid growth and secretion in vitro. Nature 197: 1115–1116.

Rodan SB, Insogna KL, Vignery AM, Stewart AF, Broadus AE, D'Souza SM, Bertolini DR, Mundy GR, Rodan GA (1983). Factors associated with humoral hypercalcemia of malignancy stimulate adenylate cyclase in osteoblastic cells. J Clin Invest 72: 1511–1515.

Russell J, Lettieri D, Sherwood LM (1983). Direct regulation by calcium of cytoplasmic messenger ribonucleic acid coding for pre-proparathyroid hormone in isolated bovine parathyroid cells. J Clin Invest 72: 1851–1855.

Sato GH (1975). The role of serum in cell culture. In Litwack G (ed): "Biochemical Actions of Hormones." New York: Academic Press, pp 391–409.

Silve C, Santora A, Spiegel A (1985). A factor produced by cultured rat Leydig tumor (Rice 500) cells associated with humoral hypercalcemia stimulates adenosine 3',5'-mono-phosphate production via the parathyroid hormone receptor in human skin fibroblasts. J Clin Endocrinol Metab 60: 1144–1147.

Shoback DM, Thatcher J, Leombruno R, Brown EM (1984). Relationship between parathyroid hormone secretion and cytosolic calcium concentration in dispersed bovine parathyroid cells. Proc Natl Acad Sci USA 81: 3113–3117.

Stoner GD, Harris CC, Meyers GA, Trump BF, Connor RD (1980). Putrescine stimulates growth of human bronchial epithelial cells in primary culture. In Vitro 16: 399–406.

Cellular Endocrinology: Hormonal Control of Embryonic
and Cellular Differentiation, pages 277–285
© 1986 Alan R. Liss, Inc.

TSH-EGF COOPERATION IN THE FRTL5 THYROID CELL GROWTH
STIMULATION

Bianca M. Veneziani, Donatella Tramontano and
Francesco S. Ambesi-Impiombato

Centro di Endocrinologia ed Oncologia Sperimentale del CNR c/o Dipartimento di Biologia e Patologia Cellulare e Molecolare, II Policlinico,
Via S. Pansini, 5 - 80131 - Naples, Italy.

INTRODUCTION

Cell functions are under physiological control of an
array of hormones or hormone-like effectors. Ligand-recep-
tor recognition at the cell surface triggers intracellular
response both cytoplasmic and nuclear, leading to modulation of cell differentiation and proliferation.

In multicellular organisms, a highly ordered coordination is achieved through embryological differentiation
and through maintainance of cellular differentiated phenotype in the adult animal.

We propose to consider the control of cell proliferation as an aspect of differentiation and tissue-specific
gene expression: it is also acquired during development,
maintained under physiological conditions and lost under
pathological conditions i.e. during transformation and
tumorigenesis. This contention is supported by the following observations: a) hormones with known trophic effects
were found to posses also mitogenic activity. TSH for
example regulate thyroid follicular cells in vivo by
stimulating differentiated functions such as thyroglobulin
synthesis, iodide uptake and thyroid hormone secretion.
More recently a mitogenic role of this hormone has been
demonstrated in vitro on primary follicles (Nitsch and
Wollman, 1980), isolated cells in primary culture (Winard
and Kohn, 1975; Roger et al., 1984) and long term strains
(FRTL, FRTL5) (Ambesi-Impiombato et al., 1980; Ambesi-
Impiombato et al., 1982). b) Similarities between growth

factors, growth factors receptors and oncogenes (Robbins et al., 1983; Downward et al., 1984) have been reported. These strong analogies suggest that cell transformation leads to dedifferentiation and unregulated cell proliferation, by subverting physiological control mechanisms.

In this view controlled cell proliferation may be regarded as part of the more comprehensive phenomenon of cell differentiation. In the differentiative program for each cell the command for proliferation rate is also included and genetically controlled. The mechanisms by which regulation is subverted during tumorigenesis, anaplasia, and other pathological conditions are now beginning to be elucidated by a more detailed knowledge of the biochemistry of the various hormones, growth factors and oncogene products. Cell culture systems offer the unique advantage of permitting such studies to be made outside the organism without unknown and/or uncontrollable cell-cell interactions. Particularly the use of serum-free or hormonally defined media is critical in controlling the experimental enviroment.

Our system of differentiated thyroid cells has proven very useful for the investigation of some aspects of cell proliferation and differentiation in vitro.

MATERIALS AND METHODS

The FRTL5 cell strain (Ambesi-Impiombato et al., 1982) was grown in Coon's modified Ham's F12 medium (mF12) supplemented with 5% calf serum (mF12+5CS) (GIBCO USA) and a mixture of six hormones (6H) (Ambesi-Impiombato et al., 1980).

The growth medium was substituted with serum-free medium without thymidine (mF12-T) after 3 days from plating in Costar 24-well dishes at concentrations of 1×10^5 cells/well in mF12+5CS. mF12-T was supplemented with 0.25% bovine serum albumine (BSA), different concentrations of thyrotropin (TSH) (National Hormones and Pituitary Program, USA) and epidermal growth factor (EGF) (SIGMA or Collaborative Research) as specified. Cells were maintained in such media for 36 hours.

Triplicate samples were washed three times in the well and incubated for 5 hours in mF12-T+0.25% BSA added with (^{3}H)thymidine (1 μCi/ml) (Amersham, Spec. Act. 70-90 Ci/mmole). After incubation cells were washed 3x with buffered saline and 3x with 10% trichloroacetic acid (TCA). The TCA precipitate was solubilized in 500 ul 1N NaOH for 15 min at 37°C. The TCA-precipitated, solubilized material was transferred in vials, 5 ml scintillation liquid (Insta-gel, Packard) was added and radioactivity was measured to quantitate (^{3}H)thymidine incorporation in DNA, expressed in cpm/10^5 cells.

RESULTS AND DISCUSSION

Thyroid cells grown as already reported (Ambesi-Impiombato et al., 1982) and maintained in the conditions described in the Methods section were divided in aliquots. To some of the cells hormones were withdrawn. After three days of starvation (no hormone added, referred to as 0H) serum was substituted with 0.25% BSA to reduce the presence of undefined components and at the same time EGF, EGF+TSH, and none (control) were added to separate groups of cells. Morphological observations in phase contrast performed three days after the addition (Fig. 1) confirmed the presence of altered morphology and lack of cell growth in the 0H cells and recovery of normal morphology and growth after TSH readdition. The presence of EGF alone and EGF+TSH did not show any significant morphological modification if compared to control cells (0H and TSH readdition respectively).

The effect of EGF alone on FRTL5 cell growth was studied by ^{3}H-thymidine incorporation experiments. EGF concentrations ranging from 0.1 pg/ml to 100 ng/ml did not stimulate significantly DNA synthesis over controls (Table 1). This result differs from what reported for other systems (Roger and Dumont, 1982; Westermark et al., 1985). The lack of stimulation by EGF alone on FRTL5 cells may be accounted for by species differences (Fischer rat in our system), or by cultural characteristics (genetically homogenous continously growing cell strain in our case) or by different conditions (lack of serum, presence of 0.25% BSA, absence of the other hormones in our cultures). Additional experiments are needed to explain this differences.

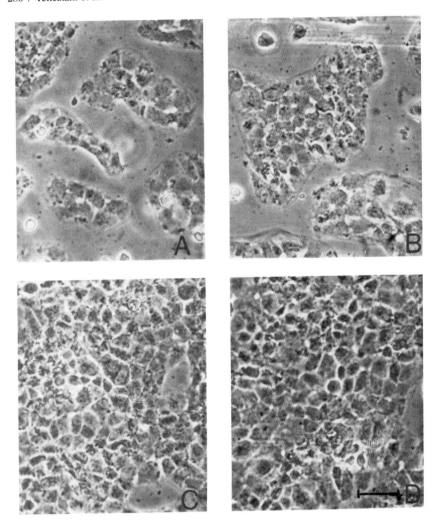

Fig 1. Phase contrast microphotography of FRTL5 cells in OH (without hormones)(A), and after 3 days readdition EGF (B), TSH (C) and EGF+TSH (D). Bar=50μm.

Table 1. Effect of EGF on ^{3}H-thymidine incorporation on FRTL5 cells.

EGF addition	$cpm/10^5$ cells*
NONE (control)	951$\pm$244
0.1 pg/ml	1084$\pm$119
1 pg/ml	752$\pm$90
10 pg/ml	1015$\pm$212
100 pg/ml	901$\pm$40
1 ng/ml	1039$\pm$208
10 ng/ml	725$\pm$42
100 ng/ml	2088$\pm$278

* Mean $\pm$ SD.

When a constant dose of EGF (50 ng/ml) was added to varying doses of TSH, the concentration dependence of the mitogenic effect of TSH was shifted to lower values by more than two log unit. The cooperative effect of EGF and TSH was evident, as stimulation of DNA synthesis in terms of ^{3}H-thymidine incorporation, only at submaximal doses of TSH (Fig. 2).

Similarly to the previous experiment, cells were mantained in 5CS and OH for three days. After the starvation, serum was substituted with 0.25% BSA and at the same time the hormone and growth factor were added.

The maximal effect of EGF, i.e. the maximal increase over TSH alone was observed at 10^{-10} M TSH, but the EGF stimulation was evident between 5×10^{-10} and 10^{-9} M TSH. At higher doses of TSH (10^{-8} M) the EGF effect was no longer present. EGF stimulation on FRTL5 DNA synthesis occurred at TSH concentrations considered physiological in all animal species including humans. It is possible that EGF could modulate physiologically thyroid follicular cell proliferation in vivo. Under pathological conditions involving higher TSH levels, the EGF effect could become negligible. Additional experiments on the EGF and TSH combined effect on FRTL5 thyroid differentiated functions are in progress in our laboratory to further clarify the role of EGF in this respect.

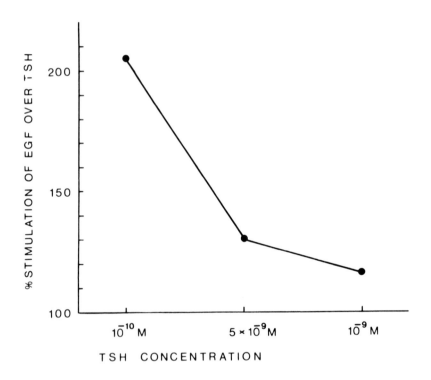

Fig. 2. Effect of 50 ng/ml EGF on increasing amounts of TSH. The percentage of EGF overstimulation has been calculated for each point.

In a different set of experiments, the kinetics of the EGF effect was evaluated. The experimental conditions were chosen to obtain maximal EGF overstimulation: after the usual three days starvation, EGF (50ng/ml) and TSH (10^{-10}M) were added. ^{3}H-thymidine incorporation was performed at 12 and 24 hours (Fig.3).

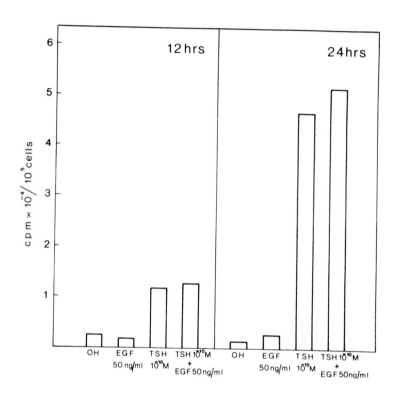

Fig. 3. Time effect of EGF and TSH addition on FRTL5 cells.

The EGF stimulation was already present at the shorter time interval from the additions (12 hrs) and was significantly increased at the longest time interval (24 hrs). A time period between 36 and 48 hrs was needed however to reach maximal EGF overstimulation levels comparable to the previous experiments. Such time lenght is compatible with complex surface and intracellular phenomena such as receptor-mediated stimulation of enzymatic activities leading to nuclear events culminating in DNA synthesis.

The presence of EGF mitogenic stimulation in normal, differentiated follicular cells in culture is important and warrants further studies on the mechanism of action of growth factors. The TSH requirement for the obtainment of EGF effect, or in essence the cooperativity of the EGF-TSH stimulation in our cell system, is also very promising in studies of hormone-growth factor cooperation and interaction. Because of the characteristics of our cell system, parallel investigation of growth and differentiation control will be possible. The site of EGF-TSH interaction (receptor, cytoplasmic, nuclear) is an interesting and challenging goal for further research in cellular endocrinology.

ACKNOWLEDGMENTS

We wish to thank Dr. S.M. Aloj for critical review of the manuscript and Michele Mastrocinque for skilful technical assistance. Work partially supported vy a grant of the Italian National research Council, Special Project "Oncology".

REFERENCES

Ambesi-Impiombato FS, Parks LAM, Coon HG (1980). Culture of hormone-dependent functional epithelial cells from rat thyroids. Proc Natl Acad Sci USA 77: 3455-3459.
Ambesi-Impiombato FS, Picone R, Tramontano D (1982). Influence of hormones and serum on growth and differentiation of the thyroid cell strain FRTL. Cold Spring Harbor Conference on Cell Proliferation. 9: 483-491.
Bachrach LK., Eggo MC, Mak WW, Burrow GN (1985). Epidermal growth factor modulation of differentiated function in cultured thyroid cells. In Eggo MC, Burrow GN (eds): "Thyroglobulin-The Prothyroid Hormone", New York: Raven

Press, Vol.2 pp 263-270.

Downward J, Yarden Y, Mayes E, Scrace G, Totty N, Stock-well P, Ullrich A, Schlessinger J, Waterfield MD (1984). Close similarity of epidermal growth factor receptor and v-erb-B oncogene protein sequences. Nature 307: 521-527.

Nitsch L, Wollman SH (1980). Thyrotropin preparations are mitogenic for thyroid epithelial cells in follicles in suspension culture. Proc Natl Acad Sci USA 77: 2743-2747.

Robbins KC, Antoniades HN, Devare SG, Hunkapiller MW, Aaronson SA (1983). Structural and immunological simila-rities between simian sarcoma virus gene product(s) and human platelet- derived growth factor. Nature 305: 605-608.

Roger PR, Dumont JE (1982). Epidermal growth factor con-trols the proliferation and the expression of differen-tiation in canine thyroid cells in primary culture. FEBS Letters 144: 209-212.

Roger PR, Dumont JE (1984). Factors controlling prolifera-tion and differentiation of canine thyroid cells cultu-red in reduced serum conditions: effect of thyrotropin, cyclic AMP and growth factors. Molecular and Cellular Endocrinology 36: 79-93.

Westermark K, Karlsson FA, Ericson LE, Westermark B (1985). Epidermal growth factor: a regulator of thyroid growth and function in vitro. In Eggo MC, Burrow GN (eds): "Thyroglobulin-The Prothyroid Hormone", New York: Raven Press, Vol.2 pp 255-262.

Winand RJ, Kohn LD (1975). Thyrotropin effects on thyroid cells in culture. J. Biol. Chem. 250: 6534-6540.

Cellular Endocrinology: Hormonal Control of Embryonic and Cellular Differentiation, pages 287–296
© 1986 Alan R. Liss, Inc.

MUSCLE REGENERATION REVISITED: GROWTH FACTOR

REGULATION OF MYOGENIC CELL REPLICATION

by

Richard C. Strohman and Elissavet Kardami

Department of Zoology, University of California,
Berkeley, CA 94720. U.S.A.

INTRODUCTION

Muscle fiber regeneration takes place through a cycle which includes destruction of old fibers followed by replication of muscle stem cells, satellite cells, which fuse to form new myotubes within the confines of the original basal lamina (see review by Campion,1984). Satellite cells have been identified as single, bipolar, largely dormant cells localized outside of the muscle fiber plasma membrane but within the muscle fiber basal lamina (Mauro, 1961). Activation of satellite cells has been observed on injury to the muscle either in vivo or in vitro (Bischoff,1980; Konigsberg et al.,1975). The new muscle formed from satellite cells recapitulates embryonic development in the sense that the early regenerating muscle expresses embryonic isoforms of myosin subunits prior to the final expression of a fully adult myosin isoform phenotype (Matsuda et al.,1983; Whalen et al.,1985).

While the satellite cell is clearly the source of muscle regenerating power (Schultz,1985), there is very little known about factors and conditions regulating replication of these cells. What accounts for their dormancy? What is involved in their activation on injury? How is this activation correlated with other aspects of regeneration such as new nerve growth or the development of new blood vessels? Of course, in the case of connective tissue and capillary endothelial cell growth there has been extensive evidence for the involvement of growth factors which serve to regulate these cell populations in a highly specific manner (Gospodarowicz et al, 1984; Maciag et al., 1984; Shing et al.,1984). That a similar factor is involved for satellite cell regulation is highly probable and there have been several studies on the effects of FGF and EGF on myogenic cell replication in vitro (Hauschka et al., 1985; Linkhardt et al., 1982; Allen et al., 1984). In addition, there has been one report of a growth factor from crushed muscle which stimulates satellite cell division in vitro (Bischoff, 1981). Aside from these in vitro studies there appears to be very little research dealing with satellite cell growth regulation.

Our interest in this question began several years ago when we realized that certain slow muscles like the ALD in the chicken yielded greater numbers of satellite cells than other (fast) muscles (Matsuda et al., 1983). We were able to show that the chicken ALD muscle also contained significantly higher levels of a growth factor which stimulated myogenesis in vitro. On analysis, this factor was shown to be transferrin (Tf) and much to our suprise we found that Tf was heavily localized in the muscle extracellular space (Matsuda et al., 1984). At the same time, we could show that extracts of the chicken ALD were also active in stimulating growth in rat cells and since Tf is class specific in its activity (Ii et al., 1982), we had to assume that a growth factor in addition to Tf was also localized in the muscle extracellular space. In the last two years we have identified this additional factor (Kardami et al., 1985). This factor isolates together with a family of peptides of MW = 14-17,000 daltons and it may be extensively purified by heparin-sepharose chromatography (Kardami et al., 1985). This material is quite similar to and may be identical with FGF and we have tenatively called it chicken muscle growth factor (CMGF). CMGF, in nanogram amounts, stimulates myogenic cell division and delays muscle cell fusion in vitro. It thereby ultimately stimulates myosin accumulation in myotubes although its growth stimulus is restricted to its action as a mitogen; it has no effect on multinucleated myotubes.

Whatever its relationship to FGF, the major questions that have emerged have to do with CMGF localization within the muscle itself. What is the mechanism by which this growth factor is accumulated in muscle? Is accumulation in vivo related to the affinity of CMGF to heparin in vitro? If so, does binding of growth factor to extracellular matrix components like heparin serve in some way to mediate or regulate satellite cell replication. In this review we will summarize recent experiments dealing with these questions and attempt to relate our results to the larger issue of muscle regeneration.

TRANSFERRIN IS ACCUMULATED IN MUSCLE EXTRACELLULAR SPACE

The slow ALD muscle of adult chickens normally yields a larger number of satellite cells than can be derived from an equal weight of fast pectoralis major (PM) muscle (Matsuda et al., 1983). On investigation of this result it was discovered that ALD muscle also yielded an extract containing growth promoting activity when tested on primary chicken myogenic cell cultures. This activity could be isolated from normal PM muscles as well but in extremely reduced amounts. Curiously, while normal PM muscles provided low yields of growth activity, PM muscles from dystrophic chickens provided extracts high in myogenic cell growth stimulation activity (Matsuda et al., 1984).

The growth promoting activity in these muscle extracts was identified as transferrin (Tf) which could be shown to be accumulated in normal ALD and in dystrophic PM muscles (Matsuda et al., 1984). Tf was not synthesized by muscle as determined by direct injection of ^{35}S-methonine into muscle and we assumed that Tf was accumulated from the blood. Some mechansim for accumulation must be present since we could show, for example, that while high Tf levels were found in dystrophic but not in normal PM, the blood levels in the two different animals were identical. Furthermore, the accumulating mechanism must be related to molecules of the muscle extracellular space since Tf could be shown by immunocytochemical means to be localized almost exclusively in muscle interstitial space (Matsuda et al., 1984).

MUSCLE AND NERVE ALSO ACCUMULATES A NON-Tf GROWTH FACTOR

On further testing we became aware that our muscle extracts were also active on rat muscle cell cultures. Since Tf was known to be class specific (Ii et al., 1982), it was clear that our chicken muscle extracts contained a growth factor other than Tf. This factor has been partially purified from normal chicken ALD muscle, from dystrophic PM muscle and from sciatic nerves of adult normal chickens (Kardami et al., 1985). It has many properties in common with FGF and we have tentatively named it chicken muscle growth factor or CMGF.

TABLE 1

STIMULATION OF MYOGENESIS IN VITRO BY Tf-DEPLETED
MUSCLE AND NERVE EXTRACTS[a]

Additions	ug protein/culture
1.Control, no additions.	60
2.ALD Muscle extract.	165
3.Tf-depleted ALD extract.	120
	ug myosin heavy chain /culture
4.Control, no additions.	35
5.Sciatic Nerve extract.	52
6.Tf-depleted sciatic extract.	48

[a]All extracts were added to the cultures at a final concentration of 0.3mg/ml. Values for protein and MHC accumulation are averages over 4 replicate plates and the mean variation was +- 10%. Extracts were prepared as previously described (Matsuda et al., 1984). Tf was removed by passage of extracts over anti-Tf columns. Measurements were made on day 7 of culture at which time myogenic cell fusion was complete and myotubes were extensive.

All of the above experiments were done in complete medium containing 10% horse serum and 1.5% embryo extract. The embryo extract is known to contain Tf and most probably very small amounts of the growth factor we are in fact extracting from ALD muscle and sciatic nerve. We have demonstrated that the Tf levels in embryo extract are not saturating with respect to optimal myogenic cell growth (Kardami et al., 1985). If we add Tf (about 20 ug/ml) together with our extracts then total protein and MHC accumulation is elevated beyond that found for extracts alone. It seems clear therefore that Tf and the growth factor activity from ALD muscle and from sciatic nerve are acting synergistically in promoting myogenesis in vitro. CMGF has no effect on protein or MHC accumulation if it is added to cultures after cell fusion indicating that its growth promoting effect is due entirely to its role as a mitogen for myogenic cells.

MUSCLE GROWTH FACTOR IS PURIFIED BY CHROMATOGRAPHY ON HEPARIN-SEPHAROSE

The growth promoting activity of ALD extracts has been subjected to purification by chromatography on heparin-sepharose columns (Kardami et al., 1985). One gram (total protein) of total extract at 8mg/ml was applied to a heparin-sepharose column at room temperature in 0.6M NaCl. The washing and elution was done following methods published for other growth factors purified by heparin-sepharose chromatography (Shing et al., 1984). The fraction eluting from the column at 1.0M NaCl had no growth-promoting activity when tested in myogenic cell cultures. The 2.0M NaCl fraction however was extremely active as shown in Table 2.

The 2M NaCl fraction from the heparin column is active in the nanogram range. The stimulation in DNA synthesis as measured by ^{3}H-thymidine uptake takes place against a background of growth in the presence of serum and saturating levels of Tf. In addition, the stimulation is abolished by treatment of the CMGF with acid (0.2M HCl for 2 hrs), with trypsin (0.1mg/ml for 2 hrs), or by heating to 70°C for 15 minutes.

When the 2M NaCl fraction from heparin-sepharose is analyzed by SDS/PAGE the most apparent material is a

family of peptides with an apparent MW of between
14-17,000 daltons. Over 98% of the protein in muscle
extracts does not bind to heparin so that an extensive
purification of CMGF is obtained in a single
binding-elution cycle om heparin-sepharose columns. Other
higher MW components are present in the 2M eluate but
these high MW peptides are also seen in fractions eluting
between 0.9M and 1.1M NaCl which contain no myogenic
growth stimulating activity. We have therefore
tentatively identified these peptides of MW 14-17,000
daltons as CMGF.

TABLE 2
CMGF PURIFIED BY HEPARIN-SEPHAROSE CHROMATOGRAPHY
STIMULATES MYOGENESIS IN VITRO[b]

Additions,treatments.	^{3}H-T uptake,CPM
1. Control, no additions.	77000
2. 1 ng/ml CMGF	93000
3. 2 ng/ml CMGF	101000
4. 3 ng/ml CMGF	115000
5. 4 ng/ml CMGF	107000
6. 2 ng/ml CMGF, trypsin	80000
7. 2 ng/ml CMGF, heat treatment	82000
8. 2 ng/ml CMGF, acid treatment	85000

	MHC accumulation, ug/dish	
	day 5	day 8
9. 2ng/ml CMGF added on day 1 together with Tf.	15	40
10. CMGF only	9	28

[b]CMGF twice chromatographed on heparin-sepharose was added
to the cultures at concentrations indicated. Cultures
were grown in 10% horse serum and 20 ug/ml Tf, MEM. DNA
synthesis levels were measured at 48 hours of culture.

Work in progress is aimed at purification of these
peptides to homogenity under conditions which preserve

biological activity. At present, the characterization of CMGF that we have provided so far indicates a strong similarity of CMGF to FGF. Both have very similar molecular weight, bind to heparin, are inactivated by heat and acid and delay myogenic cell fusion when added to muscle cultures.

MYOGENESIS IN VITRO IS INHIBITED BY HEPARIN

The ability of CMGF to bind heparin naturally led to the suggestion that heparin would inhibit normal myogenesis by binding to CMGF found in serum and embryo extract. This expectation was born out by experiments shown in Table 3. Heparin and heparin sulfate both completely inhibited myogenesis at about 100 ug/ml. At the same time, hyaluronic acid and chondrotin sulfate at similar concentrations were without effect.

TABLE 3

EFFECTS OF HEPARIN ON MYOGENESIS IN VITRO[c]

Additions to cells.	MHC accumulation ug/35 mm culture
1. Control, no additions.	35
2. 90ug/ml heparin.	less than 5
3. 0.5 mg/ml ALD extract	65
4. heparin and ALD extract together	52
	Total protein accumulation. ug/35 mm culture
5. Control, no additions.	130
6. 100 ug/ml heparin	30
7. 100 ug/ml hylauronic acid or chondrotin sulfate	150

[c]Additions were made on day 1 of culture. Protein and MHC measurements were usually made on day 5. Cells were grown in complete medium consisting of MEM, 10% horse serum and 1.5% embryo extract.

Thus the heparin inhibition is somewhat specific and this result strengthens the possibility that CMGF present in complete medium is bound by added heparin and is unable to stimulate myogenic cell growth. The heparin effect is clearly reversed by adding ALD extract.

SPECULATION ON SATELLITE CELL ACTIVATION DURING MUSCLE FIBER REGENERATION

We have tested purified CMGF for ability to stimulate myogenesis in rat and mouse cultures. Satellite cells from adult muscle are cultured and preliminary results make it clear that CMGF stimulates myogenic cell growth and delays fusion just as in chicken cultures. All indications point to CMGF as a component that is concentrated in normal tonic muscles and in nerve. The question remains, "What is the function of a sequestered growth factor in muscle and nerve in vivo?" We can only speculate at the moment. Our working hypothesis is that CMGF is, similarily to Tf, bound in the extracellular spaces of muscle tissue to heparin components of the extracellular matrix and/or basal lamina. During damage to the muscle and perhaps during excessive or chronic stimulation, CMGF is released from ECM binding sites to activate satellite cells. Part of a normal inflammatory response in tissue is invasion by lymphocytes which contain a heparinase activity (Naparstek et al., 1984). This model of muscle growth control may be tested both in vivo and in vitro and may provide us with a basis for a renewed attack on the problem of muscle regeneration.

REFERENCES

Allen, R.E., Dodson,M.V., & Luiten,L.S. (1984). Regulation of skeletal muscle satellite cell proliferation by bovine pituitary fibroblast growth factor. Exp.Cell Res. 152:154-160.

Bischoff, R. (1981). Activation and proliferation of muscle satellite cells on isolated fibers J. Cell Biol. 91:342a.

Bischoff,R. (1980). Plasticity of the myofiber-satellite cell complex in culture. In Plasticity Of Muscle. Ed. Dirk Pette. pp.119-129 W.DeGruyter, Berlin,New York.

Campion, D. (1984). The muscle satellite cell: A review. Inernat Rev Cytol 87:225-251.

Gospodarowicz, D., Cheng, J., Lui, G., Baird, A., and Bohlent, P. (1984). Isolation of brain fibroblast growth factor by heparin-Sepharose affinity chromatography:Identity with pituitary fibroblast growth factor. Proc. Nat. Sci. USA. 81:6963-6967.

Hauschka,S., Lim,R., Clegg,C., Chamberlain,J., Bulinski,C., Linkhardt,T. (1985). in Gene Expression In Muscle. eds. Strohman, R.C. & Wolf,S. pp113-122. Adv. Exp. Biol. & Med. Vol. 182. Plenum Press. New York.

Ii, I., Kimura, I., and Ozawa, E. (1982). A myotrophic protein from chick embryo extract: its purificaation,identity to transferin, and indispensibility for avian myogenesis. Dev. Biol. 94:366-377.

Kardami,E., Spector,D., & Strohman, R.C. (1985). Selected muscle and nerve extracts contain an activity which stimulates myoblast proliferation and which is distinct from transferrin. Dev. Bio. In press.

Kardami,E., Spector,D., & Strohman,R.C. (1985). Myogenic growth factor present in skeletal muscle is purified by heparin affinity chromatography. Proc.Natl.Acad.Sci.USA. In press.

Konigsberg,U., Lipton,B., & Konigsberg,I.R. (1975). The regenerative response of single mature muscle fibers isolated in vitro. Dev.Biol. 45:260-275.

Linkhardt,T.A., Clegg,C.H., Lim,R.W., Merril,J., Chamberlain, J.S. & Hauschka, S.D. (1982). In, Molecular and Cellular Control of Muscle Development. Eds. M.L. Pearson & H. Epstein. Cold Spring Harbor Laboratories, New York.

Maciag, T., Mehlman, T., Friesel, R. and Schreiber, A. (1984). Heparin binds endothelial cell growth factor, the

principal endothelial cell mitogen in bovine brain.
Science 225:932-935.

Matsuda, R., Spector, D. H., Strohman, R. C. (1983).
Regenerating adult chicken skeletal muscle and satellite
cell cultures express embryonic patterns of myosin and
tropomyosin isoforms. Dev. Biol. 100:478-488.

Matsuda, R., Spector, D., and Strohman, R. C. (1984).
There is a selective accumulation of a growth factor in
chicken skeletal muscle. I. Transferrin accumulation in
adult ALD. Dev. Biol. 103: 267-275.

Matsuda, R., Spector, D H., Micou-Eastwood, J., and
Strohman, R. C. (1984). There is a selective accumulation
of a growth factor in chicken skeletal muscle. II.
Transferrin accumulation in dystrophic fast muscle. Dev.
Biol. 103:276-284.

Mauro, A. (1961). Satellite cells of skeletal muscle
fibers. J. Biophys. Biochem. Cytol. 9:493-495.

Naparstek,Y., Cohen,I.R., Fuks,Z. & Vlodasky,I. (1984).
Activated T-lymphocytes produce a matrix degrading heparin
sulfate endoglycosidase. Nature (London) 310:241-244.

Schultz,E. (1985). Satellite cells in
normal,regenerating and dystrophic muscle. In,Gene
Expression In Muscle. Eds.R.C. Strohman & S. Wolf.
pp.73-84. Adv. Exp. Biol.& Med. Vol.182. Plenum Press.
New York.

Shing, Y., Folkman,Sullivan,Butterfield,Murray, and
Klagbrun, M. (1984). Heparin affinity: Purification of a
tumor-derived capillary endothelial cell growth factor.
Science 223:1296-1299.

Whalen,R.G.,Butler-Browne,G.S.,et al. (1985). Myosin
iszyme transitions in developing and regenerating rat
muscle. In, Gene Expression In Muscle. Ed. R.C.Strohman &
S.Wolf.pp249-258 Adv. Exp. Biol.& Med. Vol.182. Plenum
Press. New York.

Cellular Endocrinology: Hormonal Control of Embryonic
and Cellular Differentiation, pages 297–306
© 1986 Alan R. Liss, Inc.

HORMONAL REGULATION OF GLUTAMINE SYNTHETASE IN THE RETINA:
ROLE OF CELL INTERACTIONS

A. A. Moscona

Department of Molecular Genetics and Cell Biology,
The University of Chicago, Cummings Life Science
Center, Chicago, Illinois 60637

INTRODUCTION

    Cell and tissue interactions play an essential role in
embryonic morphogenesis, gene expression and differentiation,
and in post-natal developmental processes. Long-range
interactions refer to communication between distant cells
by means of hormones or hormone-like effectors. Short-range
interactions include contact-dependent communication between
aposed cells, isotypic or heterotypic, or between cells and
extracellular matrix. Composite interactions involve synergistic effects of both long-range and short-range communication. Clarification of these mechanisms is crucial to
understanding of embryonic development and of various
pathologies including neoplasias and congenital malformations.
This article describes a case of composite interactions:
the joint role of corticosteroid hormone and cell contact in
the induction of glutamine synthetase in neural retina.

    Glutamine synthetase (GS) catalyzes the amidation of
glutamate to glutamine. In neural tissues (including retina)
GS is a constituent of the "small glutamate compartment"
(Van den Berg, 1970). Glutamine is used by certain neurons
for production of neurotransmitter amino acids, glutamate
and GABA. Retina GS is an octamer with subunit molecular
weight of 42,000 daltons (Sarkar et al., 1972). This
article concentrates on regulation of GS in the retina of
chicken embryo since this system has been studied in detail
(for reviews see Moscona et al., 1980; Moscona, 1983).

    In mature avian retina the level of GS is very high,

*whereas during early stages of embryonic development its
level is very low (basal, constitutive). It starts to rise
sharply on the 16th day of embryonic development, following
increase of corticosteroid hormones in the circulation which
elicit GS induction in the retina. By that time, the retina
had completed its growth and overall histogenesis and is in
final stages of functional maturation. In 4-5 days, the
level of GS activity rises 100-fold and reaches a high
plateau soon after hatching which is maintained thereafter
(Moscona and Linser, 1983).*

LOCALIZATION OF GS IN GLIA CELLS

*The avian neural retina consists of several classes of
neurons and one type of glia, Müller glia cells. Neurons
are arranged in layers; Müller cells extend across the whole
width of the retina, send numerous arborizations and are in
close juxtaposition with multiple neurons. Which cells
contain GS? This question was answered by immunostaining
retina with monospecific anti-GS antibodies and examining
the cells for antibody binding by immunofluorescence. Anti-
GS antibodies react only with Müller glia cells; the enzyme
is present in all Müller cells, throughout the cell body
and arborizations. Therefore, GS in avian retina is
exclusively a Müller glia enzyme (Linser and Moscona, 1979;
Moscona and Degenstein, 1981), as it is also in mammalian
retina (Linser et al., 1984). This conclusion was confirmed
by other tests (Linser and Moscona, 1981); it is consistent
with earlier suggestions that the "small glutamate compartment" (in which GS is an important constituent) is localized
in glia cells.*

PRECOCIOUS INDUCTION OF GS

*As mentioned above, GS in the retina begins to rise
sharply on the 16th day of development following elevation
in the embryo of inducing corticosteroid hormones. What
makes this system particularly attractive for investigation
of regulatory mechanisms is the fact that GS can be induced
precociously several days ahead of normal time by prematurely
exposing the retina to cortisol (in vivo or in vitro). Thus,
when retina tissue isolated from 10-day embryo is incubated
in cortisol-containing culture medium, the hormone very
rapidly elicits accumulation of GS mRNA, resulting in
synthesis and accumulation of GS in the Müller cells (Linser
and Moscona, 1979; Moscona and Degenstein, 1981); within*

24 hrs the enzyme level increases 10 to 15-fold (Moscona, M. et al., 1972). Therefore, Müller glia cells become induction-competent and responsive to cortisol long before the hormone is produced in the embryo. In fact, GS can be induced as early as on the 8th day of development. At that time, inducibility is low; however, it increases progressively and rapidly with embryonic age, i.e., the rate of GS accumulation and the amount induced in a 24 hr period are significantly greater in retina from older than from younger embryos (Moscona, M. et al., 1972). On the other hand, at still earlier ages GS is not inducible (Moscona, M. and Moscona, 1979). Therefore, competence for GS induction is acquired at a specific, early age; subsequently, inducibility of competent cells increases as retina histogenesis and cell differentiation progress.

CORTISOL RECEPTORS AND GS INDUCTION

In considering possible mechanisms for this age-dependent increase of GS inducibility an obvious candidate is cortisol action. The hormone binds to cytosolic receptor molecules; the complexes translocate into the nucleus where they associate with DNA and elicit differential gene expression resulting in GS synthesis (Sarkar and Moscona, 1974; 1975; 1977). We investigated whether the onset and the age-dependent increase of GS inducibility coincided with appearance and accumulation of cortisol-binding molecules.

Surprisingly, a strikingly different situation was discovered (Koehler and Moscona, 1974; Saad and Moscona, 1985). The level of cortisol-binding molecules in the retina is high already on the 6th day of development and increases to a peak by the 9th day; then, their amount gradually de-clines to a low level that persists in adult retina. (There is a transient, small increase on the 16-17th day; its significance is not known). Hence, in developing retina there is an _inverse_ relationship between increase in GS inducibility with cortisol, and decrease in cortisol-binding molecules. We examined if functional properties of cortisol receptors change with embryonic age (cortisol-binding affinity; saturation equilibrium, dissociation kinetics, effectiveness of hormone translocation into nuclei). No significant differences were found that could explain the progressive increase of GS inducibility (Saad and Moscona, 1985).

These results demonstrated that changes in total amount of cortisol-binding molecules are not the primary factor in the developmental regulation of GS inducibility. It follows that inducibility is determined at the genome level and reflects differences in gene responsiveness to the hormonal inducer. We have suggested that Müller cells become induction-competent due to intrinsic activation of the gene complex that encodes for GS synthesis (Moscona, M. and Moscona, 1979); and that the subsequent age-dependent increase of GS inducibility results from yet another aspect of retina development: progressive cell organization and association of glia cells with specific neurons. We have proposed that the GS gene complex in induction-competent Müller glia is responsive to induction with cortisol only when these cells are contact-associated with specific neurons; as these contact-associations arise and develop, GS inducibility increases. Before further discussing this matter, another point concerning cortisol receptors should be considered.

The estimated amount of cortisol-binding molecules in retina of 12-day embryo is in the range of 1,600 per cell (assuming equal distribution in all cells, which may not be the case); in 8-day retina it is 5,000 per cell (Sarkar and Moscona, 1977). GS is the only known major gene product induced by cortisol in the retina, but may not be the only product. Assuming a one-to-one reaction between cortisol-receptor complex and target gene, the total amount of cortisol receptors per cell is in great excess at all ages, considering the likely number of target genes. Probably only a minute portion of these molecules actually functions in cortisol-mediated gene regulation. The fact that the amount of these molecules is highest in early embryonic retina is puzzling, especially since a definitive hormone-secreting adrenal cortex is not yet present. The possibility arises that, at early stages of retina development these molecules perform functions that are not specifically related to their affinity for cortisol. It is possible that they are involved in some early processes of retina cell differentiation or growth. As such processes become completed the total amount of these molecules declines to about 16% of the early maximum. Even so, only a small fraction of this residual amount would be specifically involved in cortisol-mediated gene regulation. The function of the rest is not known. These are important, unresolved questions and they deserve to be investigated. It would certainly be useful to have detailed information about developmental changes in level of cortisol receptors in other embryonic tissues, and in inducibility of gene products regulated by cortisol.

CELL CONTACT AND GS INDUCTION

The possibility that cell contact is required for GS induction first arose when the enzyme could not be induced in dispersed retina cells (Moscona, 1968; Morris and Moscona, 1970). Cells dissociated from induction-competent retina (10 or 12-day embryos) maintained in suspension or plated monodispersed in cortisol-containing medium, showed no significant increase in GS level. Induction could not be detected by measuring enzyme activity, or by immunostaining cells with anti-GS antibodies (Linser and Moscona, 1982). However, if the dissociated cells were aggregated (by rotation in flasks), and restored retinotypic associations, GS could be induced (Morris and Moscona, 1971; Linser and Moscona, 1979). Immunostaining of such cell aggregates with anti-GS antibodies showed GS induction and expression in those glia cells that had re-established contact with neurons (Linser and Moscona, 1979). In other experiments, GS was induced in retina tissue to a high level, then the cells were dissociated and were maintained in cortisol-containing medium; the dispersed cells did not maintain the high level of GS. Therefore, both GS induction and its continued expression require cell contact.

Conclusive evidence that glia-neuron contacts are prerequisite for GS induction was obtained in cell cultures which were set up so that neurons formed small clusters on top of patches of glia cells. The medium contained cortisol. Detailed immunocytochemical examination of individual glia cells revealed that only those that were in contact with neurons expressed induced GS; those separated from neurons even by a small distance, showed no induction (Linser and Moscona, 1983).

The finding that cortisol can induce GS in Müller cells only if they contact-interact with neurons raises further questions. Which type(s) of neurons participate in this composite interaction? Perhaps glutamatergic and GABAergic neurons, since they are main users of glutamine (the product of GS activity). Considering that, in the retina Müller glia are simultaneously juxtaposed with a number of different neurons, multiple heterotypic cell contacts may be required to capacitate glia cells for GS induction.

The exact rationale for glia-neuron contact in this case remains to be clarified. Our _working hypothesis_ is that, contact with neurons elicits in glia cell-membrane a signal which is relayed to the GS gene complex and capacitates it for induction with cortisol (Moscona and Linser, 1983; Moscona, 1983) (Fig. 1).

RETINA

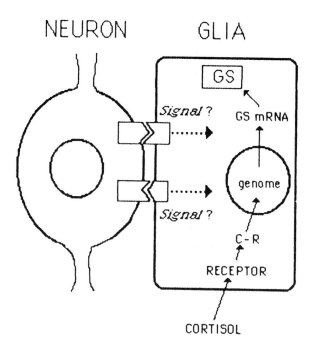

Figure 1. Diagram of GS induction with cortisol in Müller glia: requirement for membrane signal generated by ligand-mediated contact with neuron(s).

According to present evidence, this signal is not some substance that freely diffuses from the neurons; it is probably not transmitted by way of gap junctions, since characteristic gap junctions have not been detected between glia and neurons in induction-competent avian retina. Our assumption is that the capacitating signal originates in the

glia cell membrane as a consequence of adhesion to neurons.
Specific cell adhesion is mediated by interactions of cell
ligands (Moscona, 1980), and involves particular topological
dispositions of the ligands (and other membrane molecules)
on the cell surface. When glia cell is contact-associated
with specific neuron(s), its ligand interactions and topo-
graphy are signaled internally capacitating it for GS
induction with cortisol (Fig. 1). When retina tissue is
dissociated, these conditions are altered; therefore, separated glia cells are not inducible.

Extending this model to early development of the retina
suggests that the age-dependent increase of GS inducibility
in competent Müller cells results from progressive establishment of specific and definitive contact-associations
with various neurons. When this process is completed, GS is
maximally inducible.

CONCLUDING REMARKS

The details of the above hypothesis remain to be tested.
However, the principle of double regulation of GS induction
in Müller glia cells by synergistically acting long-range
(hormonal) and short-range (cell contact) interactions is
now well established. It seems unlikely that such a mechanism is unique to Müller cells; the principle of composite
interactions probably applies to still other systems
regulated by hormones or hormone-like effectors.

The above model may have broader implications. Failure
of mechanisms that mediate specific cell contacts (due to
genetic or environmental factors) resulting in detachment
or mis-attachment of cells, might reduce cell responsiveness
to specific inducers and, hence, impair normal cell differentiation or phenotype stability. In embryonic systems,
this could result in congenital disorders. In adult tissues,
persistent disruption of normal cell contacts and cell
deprivation of contact-interactions, might lead to change of
phenotype and propensity for neoplastic transformation
(Moscona and Linser, 1983). It has been found that, if
dissociated Müller cells are maintained in a dispersed state
and are continually deprived of normal contact-interactions
with neurons, their phenotype changes drastically and they
transform into another cell type (Moscona et al., 1983).
Such results reaffirm the need for increased attention to
contact-interactions and to contact-mechanisms of cells in

studies on cell regulation in normal and pathogenic states.

REFERENCES

Koehler DE, Moscona AA (1975). Corticosteroid receptors in
the neural retina and other tissues of the chick embryo.
Arch Biochem Biophys 170:102-113.
Linser P, Moscona AA (1979). Induction of glutamine synthetase in embryonic neural retina: localization in Müller
fibers and dependence on cell interactions. Proc Natl
Acad Sci USA 76:6476-6480.
Linser P, Moscona AA (1981). Induction of glutamine synthetase in embryonic neural retina: its suppression by the
gliatoxic agent α-aminoadipic acid. Develop Brain Res
1:103-119.
Linser P, Moscona AA (1982). Cell interactions in embryonic
neural retina: role in hormonal induction of glutamine
synthetase. In Brown IR (ed): "Molecular Approaches to
Neurobiology," New York: Academic Press, pp 179-193.
Linser P, Moscona AA (1983). Hormonal induction of glutamine
synthetase in cultures of embryonic retina cells: requirement for neuron-glia contact interactions. Develop Biol
96:529-534.
Linser P, Sorrentino M, Moscona AA (1984). Cellular
localization of carbonic anhydrase-C in developing and
mature neural retina of the mouse. Develop Brain Res
13:65-71.
Morris JE, Moscona AA (1970). Induction of glutamine synthetase in embryonic retina: its dependence on cell interactions. Science 167:1736-1738.
Morris JE, Moscona AA (1971). The induction of glutamine
synthetase in aggregates of embryonic neural retina cells:
correlations with differentiation and multicellular
organization. Develop Biol 25:420-444.
Moscona AA (1968). Induction of retinal glutamine synthetase in the embryo and in culture. Accademia Nazionale
dei Lincei 104:237-256.
Moscona AA (1980). Embryonic cell recognition: cellular and
molecular aspects. In Cohen EP, Köhler H (eds):
"Membranes, Receptors and the Immune Response," New York:
Alan R. Liss, Vol 42, pp 171-188.
Moscona AA (1983). On glutamine synthetase, carbonic anhy-
drase and Müller glia in the retina. In Osborne N,
Chader G (eds): "Progress in Retinal Research," Oxford
and New York: Pergamon Press, Vol 2, pp 111-135.

Moscona AA, Brown M, Degenstein L, Fox L, Soh BM (1983). Transformation of retinal glia cells into lens phenotype: expression of MP26, a lens plasma membrane antigen. Proc Natl Acad Sci USA 80:7239-7243.

Moscona AA, Degenstein L (1981). Normal development and precocious induction of glutamine synthetase in the neural retina of the quail embryo. Develop Neurosci 4:211-219.

Moscona AA, Linser P (1983). Developmental and experimental changes in retinal glia cells: cell interactions and control of phenotype expression and stability. Curr Topics Develop Biol 18:155-188.

Moscona AA, Linser P, Mayerson P, Moscona M (1980). Regulatory aspects of the induction of glutamine synthetase in embryonic neural retina. In Mora J, Palacios R (eds): "Glutamine: Metabolism, Enzymology and Regulation," New York: Academic Press, pp 299-313.

Moscona M, Frenkel N, Moscona AA (1972). Regulatory mechanisms in the induction of glutamine synthetase in the embryonic retina: immunochemical studies. Develop Biol 28:229-241.

Moscona M, Moscona AA (1979). The development of inducibility for glutamine synthetase in embryonic neural retina: inhibition by BrdU. Differentiation 13:165-172.

Saad AD, Moscona AA (1985). Cortisol receptors and inducibility of glutamine synthetase in embryonic retina. Cell Differentiation 16:241-250.

Sarkar PK, Fischman DA, Goldwasser E, Moscona AA (1972). Isolation and characterization of glutamine synthetase from chicken neural retina. J Biol Chem 247:7743-7749.

Sarkar PK, Moscona AA (1974). Binding of receptor-hydrocortisone complexes to isolated nuclei from embryonic neural retina cells. Biochem Biophys Res Commun 57:980-986.

Sarkar PK, Moscona AA (1975). Nuclear binding of hydrocortisone-receptors in the embryonic chick retina and its relationship to glutamine synthetase induction. Am Zool 15:241-247.

Sarkar PK, Moscona AA (1977). Glutamine synthetase induction in embryonic neural retina: interactions of receptor-hydrocortisone complexes with cell nuclei. Differentiation 7:75-82.

Van den Berg CJ (1970). In Lajtha A (ed): "Handbook of Neurochemistry," New York: Plenum Press, Vol III, pp 355-379.

ACKNOWLEDGMENTS

The work described here has been supported by research grants: PCM8408585 from the National Science Foundation; and 1-983 from the March of Dimes-Birth Defects Foundation. The dedicated technical assistance of Linda Degenstein and Lyle Fox are gratefully acknowledged.

Cellular Endocrinology: Hormonal Control of Embryonic
and Cellular Differentiation, pages 307-318
© 1986 Alan R. Liss, Inc.

ENVIRONMENTAL REGULATION OF DIFFERENTIATED STATES OF THE
PIGMENTED EPITHELIAL CELL: A UNIQUE CULTURE SYSTEM FOR
STUDYING MOLECULAR MECHANISMS OF CELL DIFFERENTIATION

Goro Eguchi

Department of Developmental Biology, National
Institute for Basic Biology, Nishigonaka 38,
Myodaijicho, Okazaki

INTRODUCTION

Since it was demonstrated by Eguchi and Okada (1973)
using clonal culture technique that the progeny of pigmented epithelial cells (PECs) dissociated from 8- to 9-day-
old chick embryos can express lens phenotype, similar evidences have been accumulated enough to suggest that such a
dormant capacity to switch the original phenotype into
lens-like cells might be widely conserved in vertebrate
PECs (Reviews, Clayton, 1978, 1982; Eguchi, 1976, 1979,
1986; Okada, 1980, 1983; Yamada, 1982). The culture system
of this cell type, therefore, has been thought to be a useful experimental model for analyzing mechanisms controlling
cellular metaplasia, transdifferentiation, at both cellular
and molecular levels. From such a view point, it has been
attempted in my laboratory using PECs from chick embryos to
establish an efficient in vitro system in which transdifferentiation of PECs can be easily regulated, and also in
which homogeneous population of cells at various differentiated states can be obtained.

Transdifferentiation of PECs into lens phenotype was
found to be efficiently enhanced by phenylthiourea (PTU)
contained in the medium (Eguchi, 1976; Eguchi and Itoh,
1982; Eguchi et al., 1982). On the contrary, PECs stably
maintain their original differentiated state when cultured
on artificial collagen substrata (Eguchi, 1979; Yasuda,
1979). In addition, both testicular hyaluronidase (HUase)
and ascorbic acid (AsA) efficiently promote expression of
lens phenotype in cultures of neural retinal cells (Itoh,

1976, 1978). On the basis of these studies, my colleagues and I have eventually succeeded in establishing a unique culture system of PECs of chick embryos by introducing dialyzed fetal bovine serum (dFBS), PTU, HUase and AsA as agents controlling cellular environments in vitro. This system is able to provide a homogenous cell population at each step of transdifferentiation from PECs to lens phenotype in addition to the production of dedifferentiated PECs (dePECs), which can readily express either lens or pigment cell specificities.

In this paper I briefly review recent studies conducted in my laboratory to approach the regulatory mechanisms of transdifferentiation of PECs of chick embryos.

TRANSDIFFERENTIATION OF PECs IN VITRO

PECs dissociated from retinas of 8- to 9-day-old chick embryos grow actively when cultured with Eagle's MEM supplemented with fetal bovine serum (FBS). These PECs in cultures can maintain their original phenotype as pigment cells through at least two passages of culture. However, completely dedifferentiated PECs, which no longer express melanogenic properties, appear usually at the end of second subcultivation. These dedifferentiated cells still continue to grow and finally develop into lentoid bodies, spherical aggregates of fully differentiated lens cells with a full complement of lens specific proteins (crystallins), 60-90 days after the primary inoculation. Evidence for the expression of lens phenotype by retinal PECs has been obtained in clonal cultures (Eguchi and Okada, 1973).

ENVIRONMENTAL CONTROL OF DIFFERENTIATED STATES OF PECs

PECs in the eye in situ settle on a supportive collagenous substratum and are in close contact with each other to form a cohesive monolayered epithelium. Under such conditions in vivo and in vitro, the differentiated state of PECs is stably maintained and their growth potential is repressed. In fact, expression of lens phenotype by PECs in culture was effectively suppressed by an artificial collagen substratum applied to plastic culture dishes prior to seeding PECs (Eguchi, 1979; Yasuda, 1979). From these observations, it was speculated that surface properties of PECs might be modified during the process of transdifferentiation by environmental factors which affect both cell adhesion and motility.

Phenylthiourea (PTU), a potent inhibitor of melanin synthesis, was found to enhance the lentoid differentiation in cultures of PECs (Eguchi, 1976). This substance was also found to promote cell membrane permeability for divalent cations by chelating Cu^{2+} ions (Masuda and Eguchi, 1984). PECs were readily depigmented as they grew when cultured in standard medium containing PTU (PTU medium). These dedifferentiated PECs (dePECs) constituting the confluent cell sheet in PTU medium no longer produce melanosomes, continue to grow without showing contact inhibition of growth, and eventually form multicellular layers from which lentoids develop (Fig. 1).

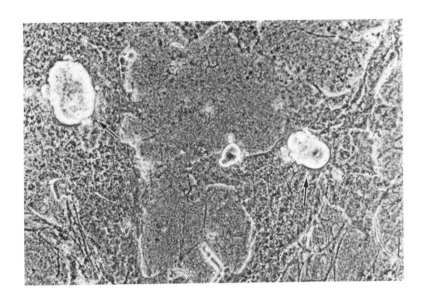

Fig. 1. A phase micrograph of primary cultures of PECs maintained for 25 days with medium containing PTU (0.1 mM). Lentoids indicated by arrows are developing from multilayered areas in the culture. (X50).

Based on the following assumption that PTU affects the stability of the differentiated state of PECs by altering cell-surface properties, PECs dissociated freshly from chick embryos were cultured for 20 days in PTU medium. The depigmented circular area of the cellular monolayer was cut out with a stainless-steel tube of ca 2.0 mm in diameter. After treatment with Dispase II, these disks detached from the plastic substratum without losing cell-to-cell junction and turned into a tiny vesicles. These vesicles were then cultured on soft agar with PTU medium. All of 48 vesicles cultured for 5 days develop into lentoids consisting of well-differentiated lens fibers surrounded by epithelium. This important result strongly suggests that the enhancing effect of PTU on expression of lens phenotype by PECs can be amplified by controlling the microenvironment of dePECs (Eguchi and Itoh, 1982; Eguchi, et al., 1982).

In order to modify the microenvironment of PECs cultured in vitro testicular hyaluronidase (HUase) has been introduced into the culture system to selectively decompose intercellular matrices. The application of this enzyme to our culture system was based on the finding by Itoh, who demonstrated that HUase remarkably promoted expression of lens cell phenotype in cultures of neural retinal cells of chick embryos (Itoh, 1978).

PECs maintained in standard medium for a week were transferred to PTU medium (PTU; 0.5 mM) containing HUase (50 to 500 U/ml medium). Lentoid differentiation was markedly amplified by addition of HUase to PTU medium, depending upon the concentration of this enzyme. In contrast, HUase alone inhibited the expression of lens phenotype by PECs, although induced the loss of differentiated properties of them. Semiquantitative estimation of the number of lentoids developed in a unit area of the culture revealed that the efficiency of expression of lens phenotype in PTU medium containing HUase in optimum concentrations was amplified more than 50-fold when compared with control cultures maintained in PTU medium (Eguchi and Itoh, 1982; Eguchi et al., 1982; Itoh and Eguchi, 1981, 1982, 1986a).

ESTABLISHMENT OF THE BIPOTENT DEDIFFERENTIATED STATE OF PECs IN VITRO

I has been clearly demonstrated by Itoh (1976) that expression of both lens and pigment cell phenotype in cultures of neural retinal cells can be remarkably enhanced by supplementing Eagle's MEM with dialyzed fetal bovine serum (dFBS) and ascorbic acid (AsA). Based on this discovery, we have applied AsA and dBFS in place of non-dialyzed serum to test the effect of them on transdifferentiation of PECs. When PECs were cultured in medium (EdFPH medium) which was prepared by supplementing MEM with dFBS (6 to 8%), PTU

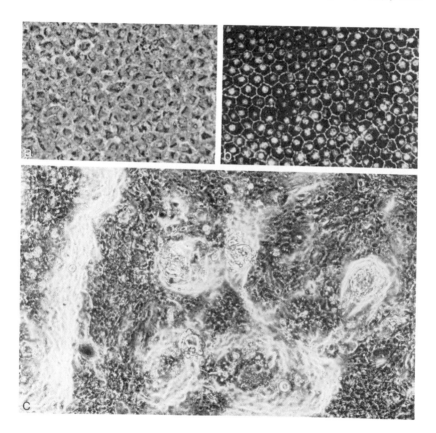

Fig. 2. Phase microscopic images of various differentiated states expressed by chick embryonic PECs depending on their culture conditions. a: Dedifferentiated PECs (dePECs) in a confluent culture showing large cytoplasmic processes (dark spots) (X125). b: Redifferentiated PECs from dePECs. Subconfluent dePECs cultured with EdFPH medium were transferred in EdFA medium and cultured for 12 days (X200). c: A typical feature of lentoid differentiation in cultures of dePECs, which were seeded at an extremely high cell density (4 X 10^6 cells per 3.5 cm dish) and maintained for 10 days in EdFPHA medium. Lentoids (L) have developed throughout the culture (X40).

(0.5 mM), and HUase (250 U/ml medium), the cells dedifferentiated rapidly, grew vigorously, and eventually formed
compact, multilayered cell sheets within about 2 weeks
(Eguchi, 1986; Eguchi and Itoh, 1982; Eguchi et al., 1982;
Itoh and Eguchi, 1982, 1986b). The dedifferentiated state
of these dePECs could be maintained by culturing with successive transfers using EdFPH medium (Itoh and Eguchi,
1986b). In contrast, dePECs readily expressed lens phenotype when cultured at especially high cell density (4 X 10^6
cells per 3.5-cm dish) and maintained with EdFPH medium
containing AsA (0.15 mM). Almost all the dePECs began to
express lens phenotype very synchronously, forming numerous
transparent lentoids within about 15 days (Fig. 2). On the
contrary, sister population of dePECs (cf. Fig. 2a) expressed pigment cell phenotype when cultured in the same medium
without both PTU and HUase (Fig.2b). Quantitative measurement of δ-crystallin content revealed that more than 50% of
the total protein of cultures at the final stage of lentoid
differentiation is δ-crystallin,the major specific protein
for the developing chick lens (Eguchi and Itoh, 1982;
Eguchi,et al.,1982; Itoh and Eguchi, 1986b). These results
show that the dePECs thus established is at least bipotent
and the expression of either of two different phenotypes
can be readily manipulated by artificially controlling cellular microenvironments.

GENE EXPRESSION BY PECs IN THE PROCESS OF
TRANSDIFFERENTIATION

Using our established culture system (Fig. 3) we have
attempted to describe the transcriptional patterns of genes
which should be specifically expressed by both lens cells
and pigment cells, as the first step to approach the molecular mechanisms which control the transdifferentiation.
Recent results on the transcription of δ-crystallin gene in
the process of transdifferentiation of the PECs in vitro
are highly relevant not only to characterize the bipotent
dedifferentiated state also to understand modulation of
cell phenotype in terms of gene expression.

A large number of dePECs were collected after at least
two additional subcultivations with EdFPH medium. These
cells were dissociated and cultured under two different
conditions (Fig. 3). Expression of lens phenotype in cultures with EdFPHA medium began to be observed within a
week, whereas redifferentiation of pigment cells was achi-

eved much faster. Cells were harvested at each state in
these processes for analyses of transcripts of δ-crystallin
genes.

Poly(A)$^+$RNAs were extracted from cells harvested from
cultures and isolated by binding to oligo(dT)-cellulose.
They were separated by electrophoresis on 0.1% agarose gels
and then blotted onto a nylon filters according to Agata et

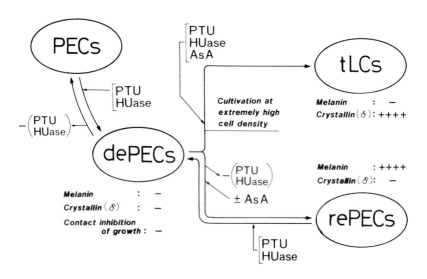

Fig. 3. Schematic representation of the culture system in
which transdifferentiation of PECs from chick embryos can
be manipulated. Pigmented epithelial cells (PECs) maintain their differentiated properties in Eagle's MEM supplemented with dialyzed fetal bovine serum (6 to 8%) and
ascorbic acid (0.15mM) (EdFA medium). They dedifferenti-
ate readily when cultured with EdFA medium containing
phenylthiourea (PTU: 0.5mM) and testicular hyaluronidase
(HUase; 250 U/ml medium) but not AsA (0.15 mM) (EdFPH
medium). Dedifferentiated cells (dePECs) express lens
cell phenotype (tLCs) when cultured at especially high
cell density with EdFPH medium supplemented with AsA
(0.15mM). In addition, the same population of dePECs
readily expresses pigment cell phenotype (rePECs) under
condition of culture which lack both PTU and HUase.

al.(1983).The RNAs thus blotted were hybridized with a ^{32}P-labeled PstI fragment of cloned δ-crystallin cDNA (pBδ11) (Yasuda et al., 1984).

Transcripts hybridizing with δ-crystallin cDNA were detected in RNAs extracted from dePECs. A clear band at the level of 9.5 kb corresponding to a precursor RNA of δ-crystallin mRNA was found in dePECs RNAs. However, no mature mRNA was detected in the transcripts of dePECs. In contrast, RNAs extracted from cultures maintained in EdFPHA medium, the condition permissive for lens phenotype expression, for 2 weeks were found to contain only small amount of the 9.5 kb transcript, in addition to large amount of mature mRNA for δ-crystallin (Agata and Eguchi, 1984; Eguchi, 1986). The rapid disintegration of the 9.5 kb transcript was observed in dePECs when placed in the conditions permissive for redifferentiation to pigment cells. We have also demonstrated that δ-crystallin mRNA accumulated gradually, when they are exposed at high cell density to EdFPHA medium, permissive for expression of lens phenotype. Neither δ-crystallin mRNA nor the 9.5 kb transcript was detected in both freshly dissociated PECs from 8- to 9-day-old chick embryos and redifferentiated cells (rePECs in Fig. 3) from dePECs.

These results suggest that (1) the δ-crystallin gene is transcribed but not processed to the mature mRNA for δ-crystallin in dePECs; (2) transcripts of δ-crystallin gene detected in the dePECs are rapidly processed to mature mRNA for δ-crystallin soon after exposure of these cells to conditions permissive for expression of lens phenotype; and (3) transcripts of δ-crystallin gene detected in dePECs are readily decomposed during redifferentiation of dePECs into pigment cells.

CONCLUDING REMARKS

The evidence accumulated through cell culture works since 1973 (Eguchi, 1976, 1979, Okada, 1980,1983; Clayton, 1978, 1982; Yamada, 1982) permit us to assume that the population of PECs capable of transdifferentiation is widely conserved in vertebrates including human, at least in the embryonic period. However, the multipotential nature is repressed or stabilized in physiological conditions in situ.

A unique and useful culture system has been now established. In this system a pure population of dePECs can be easily produced and maintained. With this system, we are able to investigate cellular characteristics of dePECs, which are in the multipotent dedifferentiated state.

It is of interest that these dePECs exhibit properties characteristic to neoplastic cells. DePECs can continue to grow even at confluence to form multicellular layers with significant alteration of cell surface properties, and exhibit high glycolytic activity in place of consumption of oxygen (unpublished observations). These dePECs with such properties as observed in neoplastic cells are multipotent (at least bipotent) cells with the ability to express either lens phenotype or pigment cell phenotype. It has been emphasized that the environmental factors which can alter the cell-cell as well as cell-substratum contacts by modifying cell surface properties must be responsible for the regulation of the differentiated state of PECs in vitro (Eguchi and Itoh, 1982, Eguchi et al., 1982; Itoh and Eguchi, 1986b). In this respect, a disruption of normal cell contact has been also emphasized as a cue for the expression of lens cell phenotype by retinal glia cells in vitro (Moscona et al., 1983).

The effort to elucidate the molecular mechanisms of transdifferentiation in terms of the regulation of gene expression has been started in my laboratory. The culture system established by us fulfills conditions permit us to collect a large number of bipotent cells and of cells in the process of commitment to express either lens or pigment cell phenotype. Our Northern blot analysis showed that the δ-crystallin gene, specially expressed in avian lens cells in situ, is transcribed in bipotent dePECs, although the transcripts are not processed. In addition to δ-crystallin gene, we have attempted to clone genes of melanosome structural proteins, which are specifically expressed in pigment cells, using monoclonal antibodies against melanosome core proteins (unpublished), in order to conduct analyses similar to those for the δ-crystallin gene.

Finally, it should be emphasized that our culture system of PECs is highly useful for conducting such analyses as introduced briefly in this chapter. Further studies of molecular and cellular mechanisms of transdifferentiation using this system will provide the fundamental information which is required for more deeply understanding the molecu-

lar basis of the phenotypic instability of differentiated
tissue cells and also of cell commitment in differentiation
of the multipotent undifferentiated cells.

ACKNOWLEDGEMENTS

I greatly acknowledge the following people for their
great contribution to the recent works reviewed in this
paper; Drs. Y. Itoh (Aichi Medical University), K. Agata,
R. Kodama, Y. Karasawa, and M. Mochii (from my laboratory).
My sincere thanks are also due to Drs. K. Yasuda and H.
Kondoh (Kyoto University) who kindly provided δ-crystallin
cDNA and gave us invaluable advice. The work in my laboratory reviewed here was supported by Grants-in-Aid for Basic
Cancer Research, Specific Project Research, and for General
Research from the Ministry of Education, Science and Cul-
ture to G. E.

REFERENCES

Agata K, Eguchi G (1984). δ-crystallin gene is transcribed
in multipotent dedifferentiated pigmented epithelial
cells. Dev Growth Differ 26:385.(Abstract)
Agata K, Yasuda K, Okada TS (1983). Gene coding for a lens
protein, δ-crystallin, is transcribed in non-lens tissues
of chick embryos. Dev Biol 100:222-226.
Clayton RM (1978). Divergence and convergence in lens cell
differentiation: Genetic regulation in the vertebrate
lens fiber cells. In Loydo BI, Potten CS, Cole RJ (eds):
"Stem Cells and Tissue Homeostasis, " London/New York:
Cambridge Univ Press, pp.115-180.
Clayton RM (1982). Cellular and molecular aspects of
differentiation and transdifferentiation of ocular tissue
in vitro. In Yeoman MM, Truman DES(eds): "Differentia-
tion IN Vitro, "Cambridge: Cambridge Univ Press,
pp.83-120.
Eguchi G (1976). "Transdifferentiation" of vertebrate
cells in in vitro cell culture. In "Embryogenesis in
Mammals (Ciba Foundation Symposium 40), " Amsterdam:
Elsevier, pp. 241-258.
Eguchi G (1979). "Transdifferentiation" in pigmented
epithelial cells of vertebrate eyes in vitro. In Ebert
JD, Okada TS (eds): "Mechanisms of cell change, "New
York: John Wiley & Sons, pp.273-291.
Eguchi G (1986). Instability in cell commitment of

vertebrate pigmented epithelial cells and their
transdifferentiation into lens cells. In Okada TS,
Moscona AA (eds): "Current Topics in Developmental
Biology 20," Orlando Fla: Academic Press, pp.21-37.
Eguchi G, Itoh Y (1982). Regeneration of lens as a
phenomenon of cellular transdifferentiation: Regulability
of the differentiated state of the vertebrate pigment
epithelial cells. Tran Ophthalmol Soc UK 102:374-378.
Eguchi G, Okada TS (1973). Differentiation of lens tissue
from the progeny of chick retinal pigment cells cultured
in vitro: A demonstration of a switch of cell types in
clonal cell culture. Proc Natl Acad Sci USA 70:1495-1499.
Eguchi G, Masuda A, Karasawa Y, Kodama R, Itoh Y (1982).
Microenvironments controlling the transdifferentiation of
vertebrate pigmented epithelial cells in in vitro culture. Adv Exp Med Biol 54:157-162.
Itoh Y (1976). Enhancement of differentiation of lens and
pigment cells by ascorbic acid in cultures of neural
retinal cells of chick embryos. Dev Biol 54:157-168.
Itoh Y (1978). Promotion of growth lens and differentiation by hyaluronidase in cultures of neural retinal cells
of chick embryos. Zool Mag Tokyo 87:370 (in Japanese).
Itoh Y, Eguchi G (1981). Regulation of transdifferentiation of pigmented retina cells into lens cell. Dev Growth
Differ 23:396. (Abstract)
Itoh Y, Eguchi G (1982). Characterization of various cell
states in transdifferentiation of pigmented epithelial
cells. Devel Growth Differ 24:396. (Abstract)
Itoh Y, Eguchi G (1986a). Enhancement of expression of
lens phenotype in cultures of pigmented epithelial cells
by hyaluronidase in the presence of phenylthiourea. Cell
Differ 17: (in press).
Itoh Y, Eguchi G (1986b). In vitro analysis of cellular
metaplasia from pigmented epithelial cells to lens phe-
notypes: A Unique model system for studying cellular
and molecular mechanisms of "transdifferentiation". Dev
Biol 117: (in press).
Masuda A, Eguchi G (1984). Phenylthiourea enhances Cu^{2+}
cytotoxicity in cell culture: Its mode of action. Cell
Struct Funct 9:25-35.
Moscona AA, Brown M, Degenstein L, Fox L, Soh BM (1983).
Transformation of retinal glia cells into lens phenotype:
Expression of MP26, a lens plasma membrane antigen. Proc
Natl Acad Sci USA 80:7239-7243.
Okada TS (1980). Cellular metaplasia or transdifferentia-
tion as a model for retinal cell differentiation. In

Moscona AA, Monroy A, Hunt HK (eds): "Current Topics in Developmental Biology 16," Orlando Fla: Academic press, pp.349-390.

Okada TS (1983). Recent progress in studies of the transdifferentiation of eye tissue vitro. Cell Differ 13: 177-183.

Yamada T (1982). Transdifferentiation of lens cells and its regulation. In McDevitt (ed): "Cell Biology of the Eye," Orlando Fla: Academic press, pp. 193-242.

Yasuda K (1979). Transdifferentiation of "lentoid" structures derived from pigmented epithelium was inhibited by collagen. Dev Biol 68:618-623.

Yasuda K, Nakajima N, Isobe N, Okada TS, Shimura Y (1984). The nucleotide sequence of a complete chicken δ-crystallin cDNA. EMBO J 3:1397-1402.

Cellular Endocrinology: Hormonal Control of Embryonic
and Cellular Differentiation, pages 319–332
© 1986 Alan R. Liss, Inc.

HORMONAL AND ENVIRONMENTAL REGULATION OF RESPIRATORY MUCUS
CELL DIFFERENTIATION

Reen Wu and Mike J. Whitcutt

Department of Anatomy, School of Veterinary
Medicine, University of California, Davis,
California 95616, (R.W.), and W. Alton Jones
Cell Science Center, Lake Placid, New York
12946 (M.J.W.)

INTRODUCTION

Respiratory tract epithelia are recognized to play an
important role in the pulmonary defense. The epithelial
cells secrete the viscoelastic substances, mucus, whose
major protein component is the glycoprotein mucin (Reid and
Clamp, 1978). Inhaled pollutants and particles are entrapped
and dissolved by the mucus, which is then moved to the
larynx by the action of ciliated epithelial cells and removed from the airway system by swallowing. Despite the importance of these processes, our understanding of the biochemical properties and regulatory mechanisms of mucociliary
functions are very meager. Several different culture systems
have been developed and used for examining mucociliary
functions in vitro: organ cultures (Sturgess and Reid, 1972;
Suemasu and Mizutu, 1975; Boat and Kleinerman, 1975; Cailleau
et al., 1979), explant outgrowth cultures (Stoner et al.,
1980; Heckman et al., 1978; Lechner et al., 1982, 1983;
Wiesel et al., 1983), and feeder layer cultures (Green, 1980;
Lechner, 1981; Gray et al., 1983). The major drawback to
those systems is the complexity introduced by the presence
of mixed cell types.

A simpler approach to elucidating the nature of mucociliary epithelial cell differentiation is provided by the
dissociated airway epithelial cell cultures which the possible contamination of non-epithelial cell type in culture
can be greatly reduced by the following procedures: selective
digestion, cell separation, and the defined growth environment specific for epithelial cell type. Previous studies

in our laboratory have established the procedures for the isolation and in vitro cultivation of respiratory epithelial cells from various animal tracheas and human tissues (Wu and Smith, 1982; Wu et al., 1982; Nedrud and Wu. 1984; Lee et al., 1984; Wu et al., 1985a, 1985b; Wu, 1985). Our studies demonstrated that dissociated epithelial cell preparation can be serially passaged and clonally cultivated under a serum-free hormone-supplemented medium without the support of the feeder layer or explant tissues.

We have observed that hamster tracheal epithelial (HTE) cells under this defined culture condition can undergo new ciliogenesis and mucus cell differentiation (Lee et al., 1984; Wu et al., 1985b; Wu, 1985). Evidence of cell differentiation are demonstrated at both the morphological and biochemical levels (Wu et al., 1985b). There is a close correlation of results obtained from between the morphological and biochemical studies of mucus cell differentiation. This correlation is important to the purpose of using HTE cell culture as an in vitro model of mucus cell differentiation. In this paper, we use this culture system to study the hormonal and environmental effects on the mucus cell differentiation in vitro. Results of this study should be part of cellular integral physiology of mucus cells.

MATERIALS AND METHODS

Detailed description of this section has been described in previous publications (Lee et al., 1984; Wu, et al., 1985b; Wu, 1985).

RESULTS AND DISCUSSION

Effects of Hormones and Growth Supplements

Previous kinetic studies demonstrated that mucus cell differentiation occurs in culture after the confluency (Wu et al., 1985b). In order to assess the role of various hormones in mucus cell differentiation, the following approaches are needed. The effects of hormones on cell growth were determined in 7-day old primary cultures which are generally in the log phase of cell growth. In case of

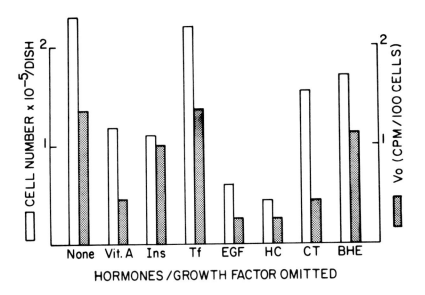

Fig. 1: Effects of omitting 1 hormonal and growth supplement on the growth and the expression of mucus differentiated function of primary HTE cells. Protease-dissociated HTE
cells were plated on collagen gel at a density of 10,000
cells per 35-mm tissue culture dish. The medium was a Ham's
F12 nutrient supplemented with 6 of the following 7 supplements: insulin (Ins), transferrin (Tf), epidermal growth
factor (EGF), hydrocortisone (HC), cholera toxin (CT), bovine hypothalamus extract (BHE) and retinol (Vit. A), i.e.,
one of these factors was omitted. Cell growth (open bars)
was determined 7 days after plating. The activity of mucus
cell differentiation as determined by biochemical method
(see Wu et al., 1985b) was carried out at the 14th day
(filled bars). Results are averages from 2 to 3 dishes. The
variations are generally within 20%.

determing the activity of mucus cell differentiation, the
14-day old cultures were used and carried out as described
previously (Wu et al., 1985b). As shown in Fig. 1, we have
observed that all of these 7 factors are not inhibitors for
the mucus cell differentiation, i.e., they are either

stimulating or no effect. If the inhibition occurs, the omitting this growth supplement should elevate further the activity of mucus cell differentiation. The same result is observed in the growth study. These results indicate that these factors are not only growth supplements but also the supplements for cell differentiation.However, there are differential effects of these factors on cell growth and differentiation. There are factors, like Ins and BHE, which have lesser influence on the activity of mucus cell differentiation than on cell growth. On the other hand, omitting Vit. A or CT is more significantly decrease the biosynthesis of mucin-like than the cell proliferation. This result suggests that both vit. A and CT may play important roles on the regulation of mucin biosynthesis. In case of EGF and HC, their absences severely decrease both the cell growth and differentiation (Fig. 1). It is possible that a severe effect on the survival of cells will damage the ability of cells to differentiate.

Regulation of Mucus Cell Differentiation by Retinoids

Both the in vivo and in vitro (organ culture) studies (Wolbach and Howe, 1925; Sporn et al., 1975; Lotan, 1980) have concluded that vitamin A and its synthetic chemicals (retinoids) are essential for the integrity of mucociliary functions of the respiratory tract epithelium. The studies shown in Fig. 1 not only further support this conclusion but also suggest that the HTE culture can serve as an in vitro model to elucidate the nature of retinoid-mediated cell differentiation.

We have observed that the retinoid treatment has two significant effects on HTE cells. One is an increase of periodic acid-Schiff (PAS) positive cell population in culture, the other is an increase of large molecular weight of glycoprotein synthesis and secretion. In addition to the quantitative change, vitamin A also alters the quality of this large molecular weight of glycoprotein (Fig. 2). In the absence of vitamin A, the void volume (V_o) molecules are sensitive to the hyaluronidase treatment, only 15 to 20% of radioactivity remains in V_o fractions(Fig. 2A and 2B). In contrast, more than 80% of radioactivity is recovered in the V_o fractions (Fig. 2C and 2D) in vitamin A-treated cultures. It is important to point out that the majority of this hyaluronidase-resistant V_o molecules are mucin-like (Wu et al., 1985b). Finally, these quantitative and qualtitative changes in V_o fractions are concentration-dependent on retinoids (data not present). These results suggest the extreme importance of retinoids in the mucus cell differentiation.

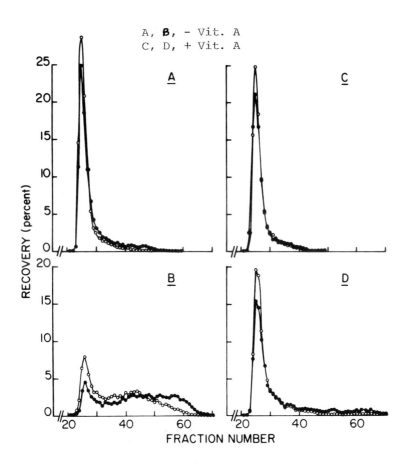

Fig. 2: Sensitivity of V_o fractions to hyaluronidase. HTE cultures were labelled with ^{3}H-glucosamine (o) and ^{35}S-sulfate (●). Radioactive molecules in V_o fractions were prepared and re-chromatography in Sepharose CL-6B column (A,C). B,D; hyaluronidase-treated samples.

Recently, we have carried out kinetic studies in order to determine the level (transcription, translation or others) of retinoid-mediated regulation. Results of this time course study indicated that these quantitative and qualtitative changes described above in V_0 fractions occur 6-18 hours after the treatment of retinoid (data not shown). Furthermore, these changes include also the protein moiety in the V_0 fractions. These results suggest that retinoid may be involved in the regulation of the core protein of mucin.

Effects of Organotypic Culture on Mucus Cell Differentiation

Polarity, or the maintenance of concentration gradients of nutrients and growth regulating factors across basement membranes and cell layers, and the unsymmetrical expression of cellular functions, is a normal in vivo condition for many epithelial cell types. Cells may attach and feed on one side and exhibit specialized differentiated properties from their opposite surface; alternatively, there may be progressively more differentiated cell layers situated further and further from the supporting stromal material.In case of airway epithelia, such an arrangement has its own physiological and functional importance; i.e., conditioning the incoming air. In order to achieve this situation, we have attempted to culture airway cells on floating collagen gel or embedded in collagen gels, as described for mammary (Emerman and Pitelka, 1977; Yang and Nandi, 1983) and other epithelial cells (Chlapowski and Haynes, 1979; Michalopoulos and Pitot, 1975; Leighton et al., 1980; Lille et al., 1980). Thus far, the results have not been encouraging. Airway epithelial cells digest the substrata and hence the cultures cannot be studied long-term.

To provide a system similar to that of a floating gel membrane, a special chamber was developed (Fig. 3). In this chamber a nitrocellulose membrane was glued and cross-linked with gelatin, then a collagen gel substratum was formed on top of the membrane (Whitcutt, 1978). This chamber allows the cells to obtain nutrients from the bottom of the collagen gel. Scanning electron micrographs showed the confluent culture in this chamber differentiated to ciliary beating cells (Fig. 4). The extensive ciliary cell population in these cultures may indicate more active cell differentiation than those immersed in the culture medium. The transmission

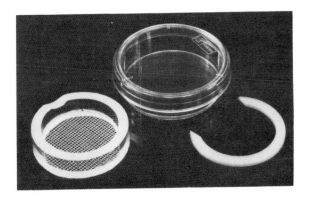

Fig. 3: The organotypic culture system of Jim's chamber.
Left: the Jim's chamber which a polycarbonate or nitrocellulose membrane is glued on. This membrane is further coated
with gelatin, fixed, and used to prepare new collagen gel
substratum for cell culture. Middle: a 35-mm tissue culture
dish to harbor the Jim's chamber. Right: a spacer is used
to raise the Jim's chamber and to allow the feeding of culture from the underneath.

electron micrographs confirm the differentiated features;
i.e., cilia and mucus granules, in the culture (Fig. 5).
Furthermore, as shown in this figure, most of these differentiated features are located in the apical region of the
cell layer (Fig. 5a). Tight junction is also found in this
apical region (Fig. 5b). Most importantly, a columnar epithelial layer resembled that in vivo tracheal epithelium is
observed in some culture area which consists of one-cell
layer (Fig. 5a). These results suggest that the Jim's chamber can be used to culture HTE cells to mimic the in vivo
polarity.

The biochemical studies further support those observed
by morphological technique. We have observed the differential secretion of ^{3}H-glucosamine and ^{35}S-sulfate-labelled
macromolecules (Fig. 6). In the medium, the secretory products were mostly low molecular weight molecules. While, in
the lumen, the products were large molecular weight excluded
from the column and also resistant to hyaluronidase digestion. In case of cell layer, the distribution of molecules

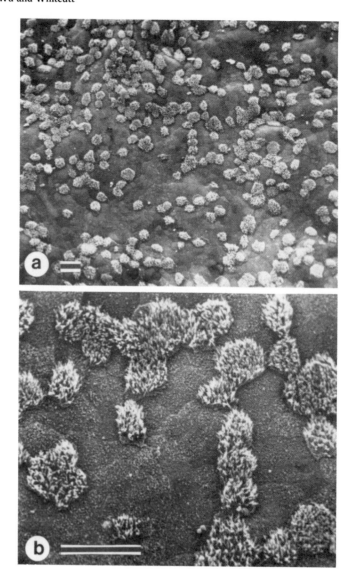

Fig. 4: Scanning electron micrographs of HTE cells maintained
on Jim's chamber for 10 days. HTE cells were initially plated
on the collagen gel substrata in Jim's chamber. Change of
feeding from immerse to feed-up was carried out at day 4.
Bars: 20 um.

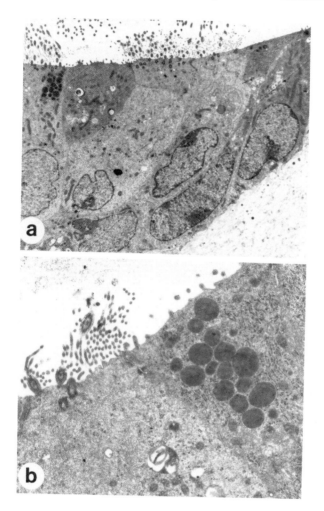

Fig. 5: Transmission electron micrographs of HTE cells cultured in Jim's chamber for 14 days. Experiments were carried
out as described in Fig. 4 except, the cultures were fixed
at day 14. a: a cross-section of HTE culture. (Note: the
columnar appearance of cultured cells on the right, and the
differentiated features, i.e., cilia and mucus granules, in
the apical region.) Original magnification: 4500X. b: enlarged micrographs of a. (Note: tight junction on the left.)
Original magnification: 14,250X.

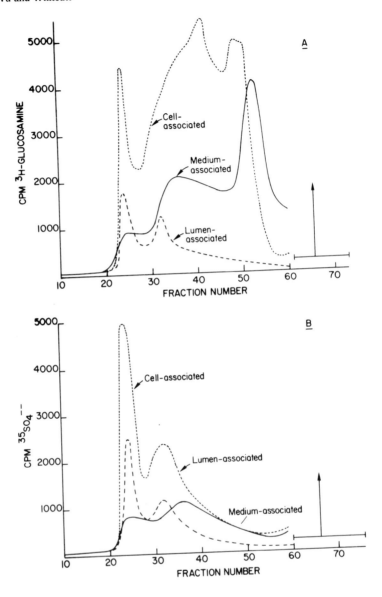

Fig. 6: Differential distribution of ^{3}H-glucosamine (A) and ^{35}S-sulfate (B) labelled macromolecules in HTE cells cultured in Jim's chamber. Media and cell extracts were analyzed in Sepharose CL-6B column with SDS and reducing agent.

was between these two extremes. Large molecular weight of mucin-like molecules were also found in the cell layer. This is consistent with the morphological study (Fig. 5) that mucus granules were formed in these cultures.

Recently, we have compared the activities of mucus cell differentiation between the Jim's chamber culture and the traditional immersed system in order to assess the value of feed-up system. As shown in Table 1, we have not seen significant increase of PAS-positive cell population in Jim's chamber culture system. This result, although is disappointing, suggests that an alteration of feeding method can not further enhance cell differentiation despite some improvement in the cell morphology. It is therefore, in order to understand the nature of mucus cell differentiation, dependent on the interactions between hormonal factors and cells. The collagen gel substrata may provide such an environment for the interactions.

Table 1: Effects of Jim's chamber culture system (or organo-typic culture) on HTE mucus cell differentiation.

	Time#in	Percent PAS-positive population*	
Experiments	culture (days)	Jim's chamber	Immersed system
I	2	0	1
	7	15	12
	10	25	31
	14	21	28
	21	16	20
II	2	3	2
	7	22	26
	11	39	41
	14	31	38
	21	25	35

Change of feeding method in Jim's chamber cultures was carried out at day 4.
* Results were average from two culture dishes, and more than 200 cells from each dish were examined and carried out as described previously (Wu et al., 1985b).

CONCLUSION

Dissociated HTE cell culture system is proved to be an in vitro model for respiratory mucus cell differentiation. We have demonstrated by manipulating the culture condition, that the activity of mucus cell differentiation in culture can be regulated. We have observed that both vitamin A and cholera toxin are important to the induction of mucus cell differentiation in culture. The effects of vitamin A as demonstrated in this study may be related to the synthesis of the core protein of mucin. The effects of cholera toxin in this system are currently under investigated. Although, it is possible to demonstrate the polarity of differentiation in culture through the newly developed organotypic culture in Jim's chamber. However, the quantitation study demonstrated no further enhancement of mucus cell differentiation in culture. These results suggest that either the culture system developed in our laboratory is optimal to the mucus cell differentiation or, the nature of differentiation in most part depends the interactions between hormonal hactors and cells. It is proposed that the use of collagen gel substrata in HTE culture provide the condition of interactions.

ACKNOWLEDGEMENTS

The authors would like to thank Ms. E, Nolan and L. Y. Wang for their excellent techniques for this work. Mr. C. Turner was thanked for performing the ultrastructural analyses of this work. This work was supported in part by a grant from the American Cancer Society (BC-465) to R.W..

REFERENCES

Boat TF, Kleinerman JL (1975). Human respiratory tract secretion. 2. Effects of cholinergic and adrenergic agents on in vitro release of proteins and mucous glycoprotein. Chest 67(Suppl):325-345.
Cailleau R, Crocker TT, Wood A (1979). Attempted long-term culture of human bronchial mucosa and bronchial neoplasmas. J Natl Cancer Inst 62:1027-1037.
Chlapowski FJ, Haynes L (1979). Growth and differentiation of transitional epithelium in vitro. J Cell Biol 83:605-614.

Emerman J, Pitelka DR (1977). Maintenance and induction of morphological differentiation in dissociated mammary epithelium on floating collagen membranes. In Vitro 13: 316-328.

Gray TE, Thomassen DG, Mass MJ, Barrett JC (1983). Quantitation of cell proliferation, colony formation, and carcinogen induced cytotoxicity of rat tracheal epithelial cells grown in culture on 3T3 feeder layer. In Vitro 19: 559-570.

Green H (1980).The keratinocytes as differentiated cell type. Harvey Lecture Series 74:101-138.

Heckman CA, Marchok AC, Nettesheim P (1978). Respiratory tract epithelium in primary culture: Concurrent growth and differentiation during establishment. J Cell Sci 32: 269-291.

Lechner JF, Haugen A, Autrup H, McClendon ZA, Trump BF, Harris CC (1981). Clonal growth of epithelial cells from normal adult human bronchus. Cancer Res 41:2294-2304.

Lechner JF, Haugen A, McClendon ZA, Pettis EW (1982). Clonal growth of adult human bronchial epithelial cells in a serum-free medium. In Vitro 18:633-642.

Lechner JF, McClendon ZA, Laveck MA, Shamsuddin AM, Harris CC (1983). Differential control by platelet factors of squamous differentiation in normal and malignant human bronchial epithelial cells. Cancer Res 43:5915-5921.

Lee TC, Wu R, Brody AR, Barrett JC, Nettesheim P (1984). Growth and differentiation of hamster tracheal epithelial cells in culture. Exp Lung Res 6:27-45.

Leighton J, Tchao R, Stein R, Abaza N (1980). Histophysiologic gradient culture of stratified epithelium. Methods Cell Biol 21:287-307.

Lille JH, MacCallum DK, Jepsen A (1980). Fine structure of subcultivated stratified squamous epithelium growth on collagen rafts. Exp Cell Res 125:153-165.

Lotan R (1980). Effects of vitamin A and its analogs (retinoids) on normal and neoplastic cells. Biochem Biophys Acta 605:33-91.

Michalopoulos G, Pitot HC (1975). Primary cultures of parenchymal liver cells on collagen membranes. Exp Cell Res 94:70-78.

Nedrud JG, Wu R (1984). In vitro mouse megatonegalovirus (MCMV) infection of mouse tracheal epithelial cells require the presence of other cell type. J Gen Virol 65:671-679.

Reid L, Clamp JR (1978). The biochemical and histochemical

nomenclature of mucus. Brit Med Bull 34:5-8.

Sporn MB, Clamon GH, Dunlop MN, Newton DL, Smith JM, Saffio-
tti U (1975). Activity of vitamin A analogues in cell
cultures of mouse epidermis and organ cultures of hamster
trachea. Nature 253:47-49.

Stoner GD, Katoh Y, Fvidart JM, Myers GA, Harris CC (1980).
Identification and culture of human bronchial epithelial
cells. Methods Cell Biol 21A:15-35.

Sturgess J, Reid L (1972). An organ culture study of effects
of drugs on the secretory activity of the human bronchial
submucosal gland. Clin Sci 43:533-542.

Suemasu K, Mizutu T (1975). In vitro culture of human bronchial epithelium. Gann 66:109-110.

Whitcutt MJ (1978). Disposable chamber for co-cultivation
of different cell types. South African J Sci 74:301-303.

Wolbach SB, Howe PR (1925). Tissue changes following deprivation of fat-soluble A vitamin. J Exp Med 42:753-777.

Wu R (1985) In vitro differentiation of airway epithelial
cells. In Schiff LJ (ed.): "In Vitro Models of Respiratory
Epithelium," Boca Raton Florida: CRC Press, Chapter 1.

Wu R, Cheng E, Yankaskas J, Knowles M, Boucher R (1985a).
Growth and differentiation of human nasal epithelial cells
in culture: Serum-free, hormone-supplemented medium and
proteoglycan synthesis. Am Rev Respir Dis 132:311-320.

Wu R, Groelke JW, Chang LY, Porter ME, Smith D, Nettesheim
P (1982). Effects of hormones on the multiplication and
differentiation of tracheal epithelial cells in culture.
In Sirbasku D, Sato GH, Pardee A (eds.): "Growth of Cells
in Hormonally Defined Media", New York: Cold Spring Harbor,
pp 641-656.

Wu R, Nolan E, Turner C (1985b). Expression of tracheal
differentiated functions in serum-free hormone-supplemented
medium. J Cell Physiol in press.

Wu R, Smith D (1982). Continuous multiplication of rabbit
tracheal epithelial cells in a defined hormone-supplemented
medium. In Vitro 18:800-812.

Yang J, Nandi S (1983). Growth of cultured cells using
collagen as substrate. Internat Rev Cytol 81:249-285.

Cellular Endocrinology: Hormonal Control of Embryonic
and Cellular Differentiation, pages 333–360
© 1986 Alan R. Liss, Inc.

Extracellular Matrix Regulation of Cell-Cell Communication
and Tissue-specific Gene Expression in Primary Liver
Cultures

Mishiyasu Fujita, David C. Spray, Haing Choi,
Juan Saez, Douglas M. Jefferson, Elliot Hertz-
berg, Larry C. Rosenberg, and Lola M. Reid
Departments of Molecular Pharmacology, (M.F.,
D.M.J., L.M.R.) Neurosciences, (D.S., J.S.),
Connective Tissue And Orthopedics, (H.C., L.C.R.)
Microbiology and Immunology (L.M.R.) Albert
Einstein College of Medicine, Department of
Biochemistry, Baylor University (E.H.)

ABSTRACT

Epithelial-mesenchymal interactions are effected, in
part, by extracellular matrix components. We have spent
many years analyzing the influence of extracellular matrix,
both as extracts of matrix and as purified matrix components, on the growth and differentiation of normal and neoplastic liver cells. Currently we are focused on analyzing
the influence of the extracellular matrix components, glycosaminoglycans and proteoglycans. We have found that these
factors induce dramatic morphological changes, are potent
inducers of gap junction synthesis and can regulate tissue-
specific gene expression.

With respect to gap junctions: intercellular communication via gap junctions, as measured by dye and electrical
coupling, disappears within 12 hrs in primary rat hepatocytes cultured in serum supplemented media or within 24 hrs
in cells in a serum free, hormonally defined medium designed
for hepatocytes. Glucagon and linoleic acid/BSA were the
primary factors in the HDM responsible for the extended life
span of the electrical coupling. Addition of proteoglycans
or glycosaminoglycans to hormonally defined medium after 24
hrs resulted in reexpression of electrical and dye coupling
when assayed at 96 hrs of culture. The incidence of coupling was less than 5% in hormonally defined medium alone.
Coupling incidence increased to 10-30% with the addition of
10 ug/ml of glycosaminoglycans (i.e., hyaluronic acid,
dermatan sulfate, chondroitin 4- or 6-sulfate, and iota-

or kappa-carrageenan) to hormonally defined medium. By contrast, the same concentrations of chondroitin sulfate proteoglycan, dermatan sulfate proteoglycan, or lambda-carrageenan resulted in dye coupling in more than 70% of the cells, with numerous cells showing dye spread from a single injected cell (in the case of the proteoglycans). The greatest effect of those tested was elicited by the dermatan sulfate proteoglycans, which induced cell-cell communication in 90-100% of the cells. Heparins gave intermediate responses (30-50%). Western blots demonstrated that the amounts of the main intrinsic gap junction polypeptide (27 KDa) extractable from cells correlated with the degree of electrical and dye coupling. Thus, proteoglycans and glycosaminoglycans appear to elicit the formation and function of gap junctions and may thus play a role in the regulation of intercellular communication under normal and pathological conditions.

With respect to gene expression: normal rat hepatocytes maintained in culture on tissue culture plastic and in serum supplemented medium lose their tissue-specific functions within hours to a few days due to loss of synthesis and to rapid degradation of tissue-specific mRNAs. The tissue-specific functions can be maintained by stabilization of the mRNAs (but not by synthesis) if the cells are cultured in a serum-free, hormonally defined medium (HDM). Addition to the serum-free, hormonally defined medium of certain glycosaminoglycans (e.g. heparins), proteoglycans (e.g. dermatan sulfate proteoglycan) or anionic polysaccharides (e.g. carrageenans) resulted in restoration of transcriptional signals for certain tissue-specific mRNAs (albumin, ligandin, alpha-$_1$antitrypsin, and transferrin) accompanied by an equivalent elevation in the cytoplasmic abundance for those same mRNA species. The effects of these factors on the transcriptional signals and on the abundance of these tissue-specific mRNAs was dependent on the dose and the length of exposure to the factors. There was a reduced cytoplasmic abundance in actin and tubulin mRNAs, an effect found to be entirely posttranscriptional.

The biologically active glycosaminoglycans and anionic polysaccharides caused dramatic changes in the morphology of the cells, either contraction or increase in packing density. Some GAGs, such as chondroitin sulfates and dermatan sulfates from cartilage and heparan sulfates from lung or intestine did not show any effects, and others, such as hyaluronic acids, showed weak effects on morphology and gene expression. The biological activity appears to correlate with the degree of sulfation and with the length of the disaccharide polymers. In summary, highly sulfated polyanions, such as GAGs and proteoglycans, proved potentially major regulators in the synthesis and/or the abundance of tissue-specific and common gene mRNAs in normal rat hepatocytes.

I. Chemistry Studies

Purification of Liver-derived Glycosaminoglycans and Proteoglycans

A heparin-like glycosaminoglycan has been isolated from bovine liver. As described in more detail in the next section, it has dramatic effects on cell-cell comminication and gene expression. The procedures used to isolate and characterize the heparin-like species are described below.

Fresh bovine liver was frozen at -20^0C for 2 hours, sliced into 2 mm thick slices with a Cuisinart food processor, then extracted for 3 hours at 4^0C in 4 M GdmCl, 0.05 M EDTA, 0.15 M sodium acetate, pH 7, containing 5 mM PMSF, benzamidine hydrochloride and iodoacetamide as protease inhibitors. The mixture was centrifuged at 8000 RPM for 1 hour. The solution was then subjected to equilibrium density gradient centrifugation in 3 M GdmCl and 2.5 M CsCl at 40,000 rpm for 68 hours to fractionate proteins, nucleic acids and proteoglycans. The gradient was cut into six equal fractions called D1 to D6. Most of the extracted protein was recovered at low buoyant density in fractions D5 and D6. Most of the uronate and glucosamine associated with extracted proteoglycan was recovered in fraction D1.

Fraction D1 was subjected to gel chromatography on Sepharose CL-4B in 4 M GdmCl. Several fractions which contained small amounts of uronate were separated. One called, P (II), showed on toluidine blue stained 4 to 10% gradient slab gels a proteoglycan with a molecular weight that was approximately 400,000. Another, called P (III), was heavily contaminated with nucleic acid based on its high A_{260}, but also contained a glycosaminoglycan (GAG) which appeared as a broad heavily stained band on toluidine blue stained gradient slab gels, whose molecular weight ranged from 7000 to 25,000.

The major uronic acid containing fraction, P (III), obtained by gel chromatography on Sepharose CL-4B in 4 M GdmCl was digested with pancreatic ribonuclease A to remove RNA, then subjected to ion exchange chromatography on DEAE Sephacel in 6 M urea, using a 0 to 1 M NaCl linear gadient. Three main fractions were obtained, two of which had a high A_{260}. However, the third fraction, which eluted at 0.8 M NaCl was high in uronate and showed essentially no absorbance at A_{260} or A_{280} indicating that it was free of nucleic acid and protein. On toluidine blue stained 4 to 20% gradient slab gels, this material appeared as a single, broad heavily stained band whose molecular weight ranged from 7000 to 25,000.

To determine whether the GAG was heparin or heparan sulfate, the susceptibility of the GAG to heparinase and the heparitinase was examined. Optimal conditions for the assay were developed using heparin and heparan sulfate from Miles, and Mathews NIH standards. Maximal degradation was obtained using 2.5 units of enzyme/mg at 35^0C. Time course studies indicated that limit digestion was obtained at 6 hours. The susceptibiilty of the uronic acid-containing fraction from DEAE Sephacel was then examined under these condition. It was based on the A_{232} of the unsaturated disaccharides formed showing the percentage of the GAG degraded by heparinase and heparitinase. No degradation of the GAG occurred with heparitinase, which readily cleaves heparan sulfate. Approximately 25% of the GAG was degraded by heparinase, indicating that the GAG is heparin from liver.

II. Biological Studies

(abbreviations used below: SSM = medium supplemented with 10% serum;
HDM = medium supplemented with a specific mixture of hormones and growth factors and referred to as serum-free, hormonally defined medium; SSM/HDM = medium supplemented with both 10% serum and the specific mixture of hormones and growth factors).

A. Gene Expression in Primary Liver Cultures

The growth and differentiation of normal hepatocytes is regulated by the synergistic effects of hormones, growth factors and components of the extracellular matrix. By using a serum-free, hormonally defined medium designed for normal hepatocytes and by using purified matrix components, we have been able to analyze the effects of each component on gene expression.

Hepatocyte mRNAs divide into two groups by response to culture. The first group includes common genes (alpha-tubulin and beta-actin, etc.) which may be found in all tissues and in any somatic cells (for example epithelial cells, endothelial cells, and mesenchymal cells). The common genes have strong transcriptional signals but are down regulated in vivo such that the cytoplasmic mRNA levels are barely detectable. Dissociation of liver causes the transcription of common genes to increase 100's of fold for 8-16 hours, and then the transcription rates return to normal; thereafter, the cultured liver cells have transcription rates for common genes equivalent to those in vivo. The second group includes liver-specific genes such as albumin, ligandin, P-450, and alpha-antitrypsin. These genes are either not expressed or expressed at very low levels in other tissues and organs. Liver-specific mRNAs are transcribed at high rates in vivo and are expressed as high levels of cytoplasmic mRNAs. When liver is dissociated and cultured (under most conditions), the transcription of liver-specific mRNAs drops within hours to less than 1% of normal in cells in SSM or to 3-10% of normal in cells in HDM. The transcriptional signals do not alter significantly under any hormonal condition (except dexamethasone: see below) and to date, no hormonal condition has been able to restore the normal transcriptional signals for liver-specific mRNAs.

The use of HDM in combination with tissue culture plastic has resulted in culture conditions that permit the cells to survive for approximately one week, that strongly select for the parenchymal cells and that achieve high levels of cytoplasmic mRNAs encoding liver-specific functions. However, the maintenance of normal liver-specific mRNA levels under these conditions has been shown due to increased mRNA stability and not due to sustained liver-specific transcriptional signals.

Dexamethasone is the only hormone, to date, that has a transcriptional component to its influence on primary liver cultures plated onto tissue culture plastic. However, there are only two genes, of those tested, that reproducibly show inductions of mRNA synthesis by dexamethasone: fibronectin and tyrosine aminotransferase (TAT). Albumin could be a third gene, but the data on dexamethasone's influence on albumin synthesis have proven quite variable and inconsistent. Dexamethasone's other effects, for example the well known augmentation in the abundance of tissue-specific mRNAs or the suppression of type I collagen expression, have proven to be via posttranscriptional mechanisms.

B.   The Influence of Anchorage Proteins and Collagens

The use of substrata of purified fibronectin, laminin and collagens (type I and type IV collagen have been tested to date) or extracts enriched in matrix components in combination with the hormonally defined media has resulted in liver cultures that can more readily attach and remain attached to dishes. On the anchorage proteins, laminin and fibronectin, the cultures survived for 10-14 days, whereas on either type I or type IV collagens, they survived for 4-5 weeks. The combination of the HDM plus the anchorage proteins or collagens strongly selected for parenchymal cells. The type of collagen determined whether or not the hepatocytes grew (limited growth on type I collagen or on biomatrices enriched in type III collagen; extensive growth on purified type IV collagen or on EHS biomatrices enriched in type IV collagen). The hepatocytes maintained stably, for the life-span of the culture, high cytoplasmic concentrations of liver-specific mRNAs and yet elevated levels of common gene mRNAs. The maintenance of differentiated functions in liver cultures plated in HDM and on collagens or anchorage proteins was primarily via posttranscriptional regulatory mechanisms (mostly mRNA half-life), although there was a slight increase in transcriptional signals for a few genes in cells cultured on collagens or laminin.

C.   Synergies Between Hormones and Matrix

We have found that use of HDM in conjunction with matrix substrata, either individual matrix components or extracts enriched in matrix, gives cellular responses which strongly implicate synergies in the effects of matrix and hormones. For example, if primary liver cultures are plated onto purified type I collagen and in HDM, the cells show little growth and express normal levels of tissue-specific mRNAs. However, if the cells are plated onto purified type IV collagen and in HDM, the cells show extensive grow and express intermediate levels of tissue-specific functions until the cells become confluent. Such synergies also are evident in hepatomas: the cell line $H_4A_zC_2$, a Reuber rat hepatoma, shows clonal growth on purified collagen and in an HDM but no clonal growth if plated onto tissue culture plastic and in the same HDM. To grow clonally on tissue culture plastic, these cells require several additional hormones and growth factors. Although multiple mechanisms (influence of matrix on hormonal receptors, binding of hormones to matrix components) may explain the synergies, empirically the influence of hormones is dependent, in part, on what substratum is available to the cells.

D. Effects of Glycosaminoglycans and Proteoglycans on Primary Liver Cultures

Glycosaminoglycans (GAGs) and Proteoglycans (PGs) have been found biologically active on cell attachment, on cellular morphology, on cell-cell communication and on gene expression in primary cultures of liver cells. Thus far, several different classes of proteoglycans and types of glycosaminoglycans have been examined. The morphology of the hepatocytes has been analyzed with phase contrast microscopy. Cell-cell communication evaluated by dye coupling among cells. Gene expression has been analyzed by nuclear transcript runons (measuring mRNA synthesis) and by Northern blots which tell the cytoplasmic abundance of particular mRNA species.

1. Morphological Effects

In morphological studies, some of the GAGs and anionic polysaccharides caused the cell layer to contract. The cells contracted, and since the cell-cell contacts remained intact, the entire cell layer contracted as a sheet. If the contraction was sufficiently strong, the cell sheet detached from the dish. Contraction of the cultures occurred by 24-96 hours (depending on which GAG/polysaccharide) with exposure to heparin from both bovine and porcine sources, with high concentrations (100 ug/ml) hyaluronic acid, with lambda-carageenan, and especially with the two forms of dextran sulfate.

Chondroitin sulfate proteoglycan, dermatan sulfate proteoglycan, and liver-derived heparan sulfate proteoglycan (peak II) and heparan sulfate (peak III) did not cause detectable cell layer contraction but did cause an increase in the packing density of the cells. When the cells were packed more tightly, as occurred with the HS III, the cellular membranes became invisible, and individual cells were recognizable primarily by their their nuclei.

Several of the GAGs (e.g. dermatan sulfate, chondroitin-4 and-6 sulfate and the bovine lung-derived heparan sulfate) showed no effect on morphology.

2.   Effects of Glycosaminoglycans and Proteoglycans on Cell-Cell Communication

Gap junctions are specialized regions of intercellular contact containing membrane channels through which cells communicate. Recent progress in the field of gap junction research includes chemical and immunological characterization of the channel-forming protein, identification of the roles that these channels may play in normal and abnormal tissue function and elucidation of controls acting on expression and operation of gap junctions.

There is abundant evidence that gap junctions can be opened or closed by physiological and pharmacological treatment and that in the longer term, formation and loss of gap junctions can be stimulated by various hormones. These latter effects may be to some degree attributable to post-translation processing of the gap junctional protein by functions such as phosphorylation. However, in some cases the hormonal effect is inhibited by the protein and mRNA synthesis inhibitors cycloheximide and camptothecin, suggesting that an earlier step in expression of gap junction protein is responsible.

Our studies establish an association between the presence of certain matrix components and gap junction formation and function assayed as dye coupling, the spread of the intracellularly injected dye Lucifer Yellow CH molecules, and as electrical coupling (junctional conductance-G_j). These studies uniquely demonstrate that cell matrix components can initiate gap junction formation. Physiological processes and pathological conditions are apparently associated with changes in gap junction incidence or strength of electrotonic coupling. Of particular interest is the growing body of evidence associating alterations in gap junction structure and physiology with growth control, tumorigenesis and oncogene expression.

We have studied the physiological and morphological properties of gap junctions connecting pairs of dissociated hepatocytes. In thin section and freeze fracture, gap junctions in tissue examined soon after association are on the free surface, where they are presumably remnants of formerly adjacent cells, and are also found between cells, where they occur as enormous plaques near the intercellular margins, near bile caniculi where they are interspersed among tight junctional lattices, and elsewhere.

We have characterized the effects on conductance of the intercellular gap junctions of two treatments that reduce junctional conductance (g_j) in other tissues: voltage and cytoplasmic acidification. Pairs of hepatocytes were voltage clamped and intracellular pH (pH_i) of one cell of the pair was measured using an intracellular pH sensitive microelectrode. As is the case in other adult mammalian tissues, conductance of hepatocytes gap junctions is insensitive to even large transjunctional or inside-outside potentials of either polarity. As is also the case in other tissues, g_j in hepatocyte pairs is reduced by exposure of the cells to CO_2, which acidifies the cytoplasm. The pK of the relation between g_j and pH_i is about 6.4, which is lower than that of other systems examined and the relation is quite steep (Hill coefficient about 8). Amiloride, a potent inhibitor of Na^+/H^+ exchange, acidifies the hepatocytes by as much as 0.5 pH units. When resting pH is lowered by exposure to CO_2, this pH_i decrement can be sufficient to reduce g_j.

An antibody to rat liver junctions prepared by Dr. E. Hertzberg (Baylor College of Medicine) quickly and irreversibly blocks g_j and dye transfer between hepatocytes when injected into pairs of liver cells. No effects are detected when preimmune serum is injected or when the antibody is applied extracellularly. Based upon the characterization of macroscopic properties of liver gap junctions, we have now demonstrated single channel currents in preparations of isolated liver gap junction membranes.

The membrane-permeable dibutyryl derivative of cAMP

reduces pH_i slightly but quickly increases g_j between hepatocyte pairs (Spray and Bodmer, unpublished). These data suggest that g_j may be regulated by cyclic nucleotides over a time course that is easily studied. Dissociated hepatocytes may thus provide a superior model system in which to study the effects of hormones on gap junction formation and loss. We have also shown that cAMP dependent protein kinase and kinase C phosphorylate gap junctional protein <u>in vitro</u>. In collaboration with Dr. Paul Greengard, we are studying the effects of kinase and its inhibitors injected into cells on junctional conductance.

Pairs of freshly dissociated rat hepatocytes are strongly coupled with respect to ions and the dye Lucifer Yellow CH. When hepatocytes are cultured on tissue culture plastic in serum supplemented medium (SSM), dye coupling disappears within 6-12 hrs. If 1mM dibutyryl cAMP, 8-bromo-cAMP or chlorphenyl-thiol cAMP are added to the cells soon after isolation, they remain dye coupled for at least 24 hours after dissociation. However, if dibutyrl cAMP is added after 12 hours when dye coupling has disappeared, it has no effect. Maintenance of coupling by cAMP derivatives is not affected by the protein and mRNA synthesis inhibitors, cycloheximide and camptothecin. If hepatocytes are cultured on tissue culture plastic and in serum-free medium (no hormones or serum supplements), dye coupling disappears within 18 hours, thus indicating that serum causes a much faster uncoupling process. If plated into the serum-free, hormonally defined medium, dye coupling disappears within 24 hours. The doubling in the survival time of the dye coupling in the HDM as compared to the serum-free medium was found due primarily to the glucagon and linoleic acid/BSA in the HDM.

Using similar techniques we have evaluated the effects of various GAGs and PGs on expression of gap junctions between cells cultured for 3-7 days on tissue culture plastic and in hormonally defined medium supplemented with 10-100 ug/ml of the GAG or PG (See Table 3). Striking effects on induction of dye coupling were produced especially by 10 ug/ml of lambda-carageenan, of P (III) from bovine liver, and of dermatan sulfate proteoglycan and chondroitin sulfate proteoglycan, resulting in 70-100% of the cells tested being capable of communication when assayed at 96 hours of culture. Western blots measuring gap junction protein in the cultures indicated that the level of gap junction protein correlated with the dye coupling and electrical coupling. This is especially noteworthy, since the GAG, PG or polysaccharide (PS) were added either 24, 48, or 72 hours (depending on whether the cells were in SSM, serum-free medium or HDM) after plating the cells, at which time, there is normally little to no dye coupling (and no evidence of gap junction protein in Western blot assays). Thus, these factors are capable of inducing functional gap junctions. At 100 ug/ml, commercial heparin, hyaluronic acid, and i-carageenan were active in inducing dye coupling in 50%-60% of the cells. Weak activity was demonstrated with 100 ug/ml of dermatan sulfate (20% of the cells), chondroitin 4-sulfate (20 % of the cells), chondroitin 6-sulfate (5% of the cells) and k- carageenan (4% of the cells).

3. Gene Expression

In Table 2 are listed the proteoglycans, and glycosaminoglycans that have been tested to date for their influence on gene expression in primary liver cultures. As noted above, primary liver cultures plated onto tissue culture plastic and in a variety of hormonal conditions, regulate their differen- tiation primarily by posttranscriptional mechanisms such as mRNA half-life. GAGs/PGs restore the transcriptional regulation (assayed by nuclear transcript runons assays) in various of the liver-specific mRNAs.

Using nothern blot analysis to measure the cytoplasmic levels of mRNAs in control livers, the liver-specific mRNA species (albumin, ligandin, alpha-$_1$antitrypsin, P450) were expressed at high levels and the common genes at low or barely detectable levels cytoplasmically. In primary liver cultures in SSM, the liver-specific mRNAs disappeared by 5 days and the common gene mRNAs were expressed at high levels throughout. In cultures in HDM, the liver-specific mRNAs remained at high levels (approximately 60-75% of in vivo), and the common gene mRNAs were expressed at high levels that were many times (50X) the levels seen in vivo. Addition of heparin, carageenan or heparan sulfate recently isolated from bovine liver to the culture medium resulted in liver-specific cytoplasmic mRNAs that were at levels equivalent to or above those in vivo. Both commercial heparin and caraggeenan also caused a decrease in the common gene mRNAs (beta-actin, alpha-tubulin). The effect of heparin from bovine lung was equivalent to that from porcine intestinal mucosa (data not shown). Although bovine liver derived heparan sulfate and heparan sulfate proteoglycan), chondroitin sulfate proteoglycan and dermatan sulfate proteoglycan caused an increase in liver-specific mRNA species, they showed no effect on common genes. No effect on gene expression was observed with chondroitin 4-sulfate from whale cartilage, chondroitin 6-sulfate from shark cartilage or dermatan sulfate from porcine skin.

The influence by various forms of carageenan and heparin from several sources on specific mRNA species was dose-dependent (concentrations between 0.1-1000 ug/ml tested). Similar results on Northern blots were obtained with 10 ug/ml of carageenan and 100-1000 ug/ml of heparin indicating that the effect of carrageenan was approximatley 10-100X as potent as heparin. With 48 hours of exposure and at 10 ug/ml, the bovine liver-derived peak 3, P (III), showed similar effects to carageenan (96 hours of exposure at 10 ug/ml) in terms of the augmentation of liver-specific mRNA levels.

Kinetic studies were done with carageenan to ascertain how soon the effects on gene expression occurred and if they were stable. Carageenan was added to hepatocyte cultures for 24, 48, 72, and 96 hours of culture. With respect to liver-specific functions, increasing exposure time resulted in increasing amounts of liver-specific mRNAs and in decreasing amounts of some common genes. Actin was an exception, showing a transient suppressive effect by carageenan on its cytoplasmic mRNA levels. The peak suppressive effect of carageenan on actin mRNA levels was observed between 24-48 hours. By 72 to 96 hours, the actin levels were partially restored to those observed in cultures in HDM (with no carageenan).

The influence of the effect of GAGs/polysaccharides on the common genes also occurred if these factors were added to cells plated onto collagens (type I and IV have been tested). On collagens alone, the cells retained, for several weeks normal levels of tissue-specific mRNA's. However, their common gene mRNA's remained high. However, if cells were plated onto collagens and in HDM with carageenan or with heparan sulfate, the tissue-specific mRNAs remained high and the common genes were suppressed.

The standard responses, i.e. exponential losses of liver-specific mRNAs, of the liver cultures to SSM or HDM/SSM could be counteracted if carageenan was added to the medium. Addition of carageenan (100 ug/ml) to cultures in HDM/SSM resulted in liver-specific functions that were equivalent to those in HDM. Carageenan also caused a suppression of actin and tubulin in cultures in HDM/SSM. By contrast, chondroitin 4-sulfate (100 ug/ml) failed to protect the liver-specific functions and to suppress the common gene mRNAs.

E. Matrix and Neoplastically Transformed Cells

Use of matrix substrata in combination with specific hormonally defined media enabled tumor cells to express morphological, growth and differentiative properties that resembled more their normal counterparts in vivo thus suggesting that some regulatory constraints are extant for neoplastic cells. On collagenous substrata, tumor cells attached and grew more efficiently, with a reduced requirement for serum supplementation for growth. In the development of serum-free, hormonally defined media for hepatoma cells, it was found that collagenous and matrix substrata reduced the hormone requirements for growth both qualitatively and quantitatively.

Whereas normal epithelial cells responded stably to a matrix, tumor cells showed responses that were transient. In studies with rat insulinoma cells and hepatoma cells, the cells were found to respond differently to matrix if cultured in serum supplemented medium (SSM) as opposed to a serum-free, hormonally defined medium (HDM). Growth rates of the hepatomas and of the insulinomas were equivalent if the cells were plated onto tissue culture plastic and in SSM or HDM and if plated onto biomatrix and in SSM. However, if they were plated onto biomatrix and in HDM, the cells underwent growth arrest after one or two divisions. They remained in growth arrest for 10-12 days in the case of the rat and human hepatomas and for 18-20 days in the case of the rat insulinoma. During the growth arrest, tissue-specific functions were augmented 5-50 fold above that observed under any other culture condition. When on matrix and in HDM (but not on tissue culture plastic or on matrix and in SSM) these conditions, the rat insulinoma cells showed a glucose-stimulated insulin secretion. The insulin secretion stimulated by glucose was shown to correlate with an increased mRNA size due to increased adenylation of the mRNA. Thus, matrix combined with HDM can influence differentiation by yet another posttranscriptional mechanism: degree of adenylation of the mRNA, a property thought influential to either mRNA stability or efficiency of translation (Muschel et al, 1986).

The phase of growth arrest accompanied by augmented tissue-specific functions, was transient for all tumor cell lines studied. At the end of growth arrest, regions of the dishes contained cells growing in piles on top of one another. The cells in the piles eventually detached and floated into the medium. If the floating cells or cells in the piles were transferred to dishes with serum- free, hormonally defined medium and biomatrix, they again went into growth arrest. The response of tumor cells to the matrix and defined medium conditions indicate both that tumor cells are capable of responding to regulatory signals and that the cells are able to escape (most probably through the release of degradative enzymes).

Preliminary dye coupling and electrophysiological studies in three human hepatoma cell lines: HepG2, PRL/PRF/5, and SKHep1 have shown differences in the levels of gap junctions that correlate with their degree of differentiation. Thus, the poorly differentiated SKHep1 has never shown gap junctions under any conditions tested; the moderately differentiate PRL/PRF/5 has shown constitutive but regulatable expression of gap junctions; and the minimally deviant HepG2 expresses gap junctions only under conditions similar to those needed for expression in normal hepatocytes. Dye coupling and electrophysiological studies have indicated that 1) SKHep1 cells show no coupling at any cell density in either HDM or SSM; 2) PRL/PRF/5 shows coupling at both subconfluent and confluent densities and in SSM and HDM, but the degree of coupling is much higher in HDM; and 3) HepG2 shows no coupling in SSM at either low or high density, moderate coupling at low densities in HDM, and high degree of coupling at high densities in HDM.

Table 1. Collagens and Anchorage Proteins Tested for Biological Activity on Hepatocytes

Anchorage Protein or Collagen	Cell-Cell Communi-	Gene Expres-

Type	Source/(Dose)	Morphology	cation[1]	sion[2]
None	------	Flat	None	Liver-spc. (P.T.) Common gene (P.T.)
Fibronectin	Human	Flat	not tested	Liver-spc. (P.T.) Common gene (P.T.)
Laminin	Mouse (EHS tumor)	Flat	not tested	Liver-spc. (P.T.) Common gene (P.T.)
Type I Collagen	Rat tail	Cuboidal	100%	Liver-spc. (P.T.)[2] Common gene (P.T.)
Type I	Bovine skin	Cuboidal	100%	Liver-spc. (P.T.)[2] Common gene (P.T.)
Type IV	Human Placenta	Cuboidal	100%	Liver-spc. (P.T.) Common gene (P.T.)

[1]Cell-cell communication was evaluated by spread of Lucifer Yellow Ch molecules injected into cells. The numbers indicate the percentage of cells capable of spreading dye to their neighbors. In each condition, at least 20 cells were injected. When cells were on tissue culture plastic and in serum supplemented medium or in hormonally defined medium, there was little to no spread of dye.

[2]The arrows indicate whether the liver-specific mRNAs or common gene mRNAs have increased or decreased in abundance. The (T.) or (P.T.) or (T./P.T.) indicates whether the increase (or decrease) is due to a change via a transcriptional or posttranscriptional mechanism(s). Thus, if the test condition causes a change in the signals tested by means of the nuclear transcript runons, the regulation is indicated as a transcriptional change. If there is a change in the abundance of the mRNAs (measured by Northern blots) and yet no change in the trancriptional signal, the regulation is posttranscriptional. In some instances, changes in transcriptional signals occurred but were disproportionate to the changes in the Northern blots, thus, there was presumed to be both transcriptional and posttranscriptional regulation.

For cells on tissue culture plastic, the cells regulated almost exclusively posttranscriptionally. On various collagens (and very weakly and transiently with laminin), the cells regulated mostly at a posttranscriptional level; there were a few genes (e.g. P450) in which collagen substrata restored transcriptional controls.

Table 2. Glycosaminoglycans and Proteoglycans Tested for Biological Activity on Hepatocytes

Proteoglycan or Glycosaminoglycan	Source/(Dose)	Morphology	Cell-Cell Communication[1]	Gene Expression[2]
None:				
SSM	-----	Flattened	0	Dedifferentiation
HDM	-----	Flattened	4%	Liver-

			specific (P.T.)	
Dermatan Sulfate (Sigma)	Porcine skin	Slightly Contracted	20% (10 ug/ml) 30% (100 ug/ml)	no effect
Dermatan Sulfate (Sigma)	Porcine intestine	" "	30% (10 ug/ml) 50% (100 ug/ml)	no effect
Dermatan Sulfate	NIH Ref. STD (Matthews)	" "	" "	no effect
Dermatan Sulfate Proteoglycan	Bovine Articular Cartilage (Adult) (10 ug/ml)	Increased Packing Density	90-100%	Liver-specific (T/PT)
Chondroitin 4-Sulfate	Whale Cartilage (Sigma) (1 mg/ml)	Flattened	15-45%	no effect
Chondroitin 6-Sulfate	Shark Cartilage (Sigma) (1 mg/ml)	Flattened	5%	no effect
Chondroitin Sulfate Proteoglycan	Bovine Nasal Cartilage (Adult) (10 ug/ml)	Increased Packing Density	60-80%	Liver-specific (T/PT)
Heparan Sulfate	Bovine Lung, Ref. Std. (Matthew's) (5 mg/ml)	Flattened	0%	no effect
Heparan	Bovine	Flattened	0%	no

Sulfate	Intestine (Linker's; 9% sulfate) (10 ug/ml)			effect
Heparan Sulfate	Bovine Intestine (Linker's; 12% sulfate) (10 ug/ml)	Flattened	0%	no effect
Heparan Sulfate	Bovine Intestine (Linker's; 15% sulfate) (10 ug/ml)	Flattened	0%	no effect
Heparan Sulfate- Proteoglycan, P (II)	Bovine Liver (Rosenberg) (10 ug/ml)	Packing Density	100%	Liver-specific
Heparin	Porcine Intestinal Mucosa (Sigma) (100 ug/ml)	Moderate Contraction	40-70% 40-70%	Liver-specific (T/PT) Common gene (PT)
Heparin	Bovine Lung (Sigma) (100 ug/ml)	" "	" "	" "
Heparin	Bovine Lung, Ref. Std. (Linker's) (100 ug/ml)	" "	" "	" "
Heparin, P (II)	Bovine Liver (Rosenberg) (10 ug/ml)	Packing Density	80-100%	Liver-derived (T/PT) Common gene (PT)
Hyaluronic Acid	Human Umbilical Cord (Sigma) (100 ug/ml)	Flattened 55%	55%	Liver-specific (PT)

Hyaluronic Acid	Ref. Std. (Matthews) (100 ug/ml)	Flattened	30-40%	Liver-specific (PT)

Anionic Polysaccharides

lambda-Carrageenan	Seaweed (Sigma) (10 ug/ml)	Strong Contraction	70%	Liver-specific (T/PT) Common gene (PT)
kappa-Carrageenan	Seaweed (Sigma) (50 ug/ml)	Flattened	14%	Liver-specific (T/PT) Common gene (PT)
iota-Carrageenan	Seaweed (Sigma) (50 ug/ml)	Strong Contraction	30%	Liver-specific (T/PT) Common gene (PT)
Dextran Sulfate	8000 Daltons (Sigma) (10 ug/ml)	Strong Contraction	0%	no effect
Dextran Sulfate	500 K Daltons (Sigma) (2 ug/ml)	Strongest Contraction Observed	10-15%	Liver specific (T/PT) Common gene (PT)

GAG = Glycosaminoglycan; PG = Proteoglycan

[1]Cell-cell communication was evaluated by spread of Lucifer Yellow Ch molecules injected into cells. The numbers

indicate the percentage of cells capable of spreading dye to their neighbors. In each condition, at least 20 cells were injected. When cells were on tissue culture plastic and in serum supplemented medium or in hormonally defined medium, there was little to no spread of dye.

[2]The arrows indicate whether the liver-specific mRNAs or common gene mRNAs have increased or decreased in abundance. The (T.) or (P.T.) or (T./P.T.) indicates whether the increase (or decrease) is due to a change via a transcriptional or posttranscriptional mechanism(s). Thus, if the test condition causes a change in the signals tested by means of the nuclear transcript runons, the regulation is indicated as a transcriptional change. If there is a change in the abundance of the mRNAs (measured by Northern blots) and yet no change in the trancriptional signal, the regulation is posttranscriptional. In some instances, changes in transcriptional signals occurred but were disproportionate to the changes in the Northern blots, thus, there was presumed to be both transcriptional and posttranscriptional regulation.

REFERENCES

Baffet G, Clement B, Glaise D, Guillouzo A, Guguen-Guillouzo C (1982). Hydrocortisone modulates the production of extracellular material and albumin in long-term co-cultures of adult rat hepatocytes with other liver epithelial cells. Biochem and Biophys Res Comm 109:507-512.

Barnes D, Sato G (1984). Methods for Serum-free Culture of Cells "Cell Culture Methods for Molecular and Cellular Biology." New York Vol 1-4 New York: Alan R Liss.

Bennett MVL, Spray DC, eds (1985). "Gap Junctions." New York: Cold Spring Harbor Press (in press)

Ben-Ziev A, Farmer SR, Penman S (1980). Protein-synthesis requires cell-surface contact while nuclear events respond to cell-shape in anchorage-dependent fibroblasts. Cell 21:365-372.

Bernfield M, Banerjee SD, Koda AC, Rapraeger JE (1984). Remodeling of the basement membrane: morphogenesis and maturation. In "Basement Membranes and Cell Movement." Ciba Foundation Symposium #108 pp 1-17.

Berry M, Friend D (1969). J. Cell Biol 43:506-520.

Brock ML, Shapiro DJ (1983). Estrogen stabilizes vitelogenin mRNA against cytoplasmic degradation. Cell 34:207-213.

Caspar DLD, Goodenough DA, Makowski L, Phillips WC (1977). Gap junction structure. I: Correlated electron microscopy and X-ray diffraction. J. Cell Biol 74:605-628.

Choi HU, Tang L-H, Johnson TL, Pal S, Rosenberg LC, Reiner A, Poole AR (1983). Isolation and characterization of a 35,000 molecular weight subunit fetal cartilage matrix protein. J. Biol Chem 258:655-661.

Chung S, Landfear SM, Blumber DD, Cohen NS, Lodish HF (1981). Synthesis and stability of developmentally regulated Dictyostelium mRNA are affected by cell-cell contact and cAMP. Cell 24:785-797.

Clayton DF, Darnell JE (1983). Changes in liver-specific compared to common gene transcription during primary culture of mouse hepatocytes. Mol Cell Biol 3:1552-1561.

Clayton DF, Harrelson AL, Darnell JE Dependence of liver-specific transcription on tissue organization. Mol Cell Biol (in press)

Clement B, Guguen-Guillouzo C, Campion JP, Glaise D, Bourel M, Guillouzo A (1984). Long-term co-cultures of adult human hepatocytes with rat liver epithelial cells: Modulation of albumin secretion and accumulation of extracellular material. Hepatology 4:373-380.

de-Leeuw AM, McCarthy SP, Geerts A, Knook DL 1984. Purified rat liver fat-storing cells in culture divide and contain collagen. Hepatology 4:392-403.

Dermann E, Krauter K, Walling L, Weinberger C, Ray M, Darnell JE, Jr (1981). Transcriptional control in the production of liver-specific mRNAs. Cell 23:731-739.

Diegelmann RF, Guzelian PS, Gay R, Gay S (1983). Collagen formation by the hepatocyte in primary monolayer culture and in vivo. Science 219:1343-1345.

Enat R, Jefferson DM, Ruiz-Opazo N, Gatmaitan Z, Leinwand LA, Reid LM (1984). Hepatocyte proliferation in vitro: its dependence on the use of serum-free, hormonally defined medium and substrata of extracellular matrix. Proc Natl Acad Sci USA 81:1411-1415.

Feramisco JR, Smart JE, Burridge Helfman DM, Thomas GP (1982). Co-existence of vinculin and a vinculin-like protein of higher molecular weight in smooth muscle. J. Biol Chem 257:11024-11031.

Gatmaitan Z, Jefferson DM, Ruiz-Opazo N, Biempica L, Arias I, Dudas G, Leinwand L, Reid LM (1983). Regulation of growth and differentiation of a rat hepatoma cell line by the synergistic interactions of hormones and collagenous substrata. J. Cell Biol 97:1179-1190.

Georgoff I, Secott T, Isom HC (1984). Effect of simian virus

40 infection on albumin production by hepatocytes
cultured in chemically defined medium and plated on
collagen and non-collagen attachment surfaces. J. Biol
Chem 259:9595-9602.

Gomez-Lechon MJ, Garcia MD, Castell JV (1983). Effect of
glucocorticoids on the expression of ¢-
glutamyltransferase and tyrosine aminotransferase in
serum-free-cultured hepatocytes. Hoppe-Seyler's Z.
Physiol Chem 364:501-508.

Grinnell F, Bennett MH (1982). Ultrastructural studies of
cell-collagen interactions. In "Methods in Enzymology."
Structural and Contractile Proteins Part A LW Cunningham
and DW Frederiksen (eds) New York: Academic Press 82:535-
544.

Guguen-Guillouzo C, Guillouzo A (1983). Modulation of
functional activities in cultured rat hepatocytes. Mol
Cell Biochem 53/54:35-56.

Guzelian PS, Lindblad WJ, Diegelmann RF (1984).
Glucocorticoids suppress formation of collagen by the
hepatocyte: Studies in primary monolayer cultures of
parenchymal cells prepared from adult rat liver.
Gastroenterol 86:897-904.

Hasegawa K, Watanabe K, Koga M (1982). Induction of mitosis
in primary cultures of adult rat hepatocytes under serum-
free conditions. Biochem Biophys Res Comm 104:259-267.

Hata R, Ninomiya Y, Nagai Y, Tsukada Y (1980). Biosynthesis
of interstitial types of collagen by albumin-producing
rat liver parenchymal cell (hepatocyte) clones in
culture. Biochem 19:169-176.

Hirsiger H, Giger U, Meyer UA (1984). Stimulation of DNA
synthesis and mitotic activity of chick embryo
hepatocytes in primary culture. In Vitro 20:172-181.

Hixson DC, DeLourdes-Ponce M, Allison JP, Walborg EF, Jr
(1984). Cell surface expression by adult rat hepatocytes
of a non-collagen glycoprotein present in rat liver
biomatrix. Exp Cell Res 152:402-414.

Jefferson DM, Clayton DF, Darnell JE, Jr, Reid LM (1984).
Maintenance of differentiated function in cultured
hepatocytes by mRNA stabilization. Mol & Cell Biol
4:1929-1934.

Jefferson DM, Liverpool C, Reid LM (1984). Hormonal
modulation of steady state levels of specific mRNAs in
primary cultures of adult rat hepatocytes. J. Cell Biol
99:201

Jefferson DM, Reid LM, Giambrone M, Shafritz DA, Zern MA
(1985). Effects of dexamethasone on albumin and collagen

gene expression in primary cultures of adult rat hepatocytes. Hepatology 5:14-20.

Johansson S, Hook M (1984). Substrate adhesion of rat hepatocytes: On the mechanism of attachment to fibronectin. J. Cell Biol 98:810-817.

Kessler JA, Spray DC, Saez JC, Bennett MVL (1984). Modulation of synaptic phenotype: insulin and cAMP independently initiate formation of electronic synapses in cultured sympathetic neurone. Proc Natl Acad Sci USA 81:6235-6239.

Kjellen L, Oldberg A, Hook M (1980). Cell-surface heparan sulfate: Mechanisms of proteoglycan-cell association. J. Biol Chem 255:10407-10413.

Kjellen L, Oldberg A, Hook M (1980). Cell-surface heparan sulfate. J. Biol Chem 255:10407-10413.

Kjellen L, Pettersson I, Hook M (1981). Cell-surface heparan sulfate: An intercalated membrane proteoglycan. Proc Natl Acad Sci USA 78:5371-5375.

Kleinman HK, Klebe RJ, Martin GR (1981). Role of collagenous matrices in the adhesion and growth of cells. J. Cell Biol 88:473-485.

Kleinman HK, McGarvey ML, Hassell JR, Martin GR (1984). Formation of a supramolecular complex is involved in the reconstitution of basment membane components. Biochem 22:4969-4974.

Kleinman HK, McGarvey ML, Hassell JR, Star VL, Cannon FB, Laurie GW, Martin GR (1984). Basement membrane matrisome. a defined supramolecular complex with biological activity.

Koda JE, Bernfield M (1982). Heparan sulfate proteoglycan binding to collagen involves the native fibril. J. Cell Biol 95:126a.

Kraemer PM (1971). Heparan sulfates of cultured cells. I. Membrane-associated and cell-sap species in Chinese hamster cells. Biochemistry 10:1437-1445.

Kraemer PM (1971). Heparan sulfates of cultured cells. II. Acid-soluble and acid-precipitable species of different cell lines. Biochemistry 10:1445-1451.

Leivo I (1983). Basement membrane-like matrix of teratocarcinoma-derived endodermal cells: Presence of laminin and heparan sulfate in the matrix at points of attachment to cells. J. Histochem and Cytochem 31:35-45.

Liotta LA, Tryggvason K, Garbisa S, Hart I, Foltz CM, Shafie M (1980). Metastastic potential correlates with enzymatic degradation of basement membrane collagen. Nature 284:67-68.

Marceau N, Goyette R, Valet JP, Deschenes J (1980). The
effect of dexamethasone on formation of a fibronectin
extracellular matrix by rat hepatocytes in vitro. Exp
Cell Res 125:497-502.
Marceau N, Goyette R, Guidoin R, Antakly T (1982).
Hormonally-induced formation of extracellular biomatrix
in cultured normal and neoplastic liver cells: Effect of
dexamethasone. Scan Electron Microsc Pt. 2 815-823.
Marceau N, Goyette R, Pelletier G, Antakly T (1983).
Hormonally-induced changes in the cytoskeleton
organization of adult and newborn rat hepatocytes
cultured on fibronectin precoated substratum: Effect of
dexamethasone and insulin. Cell Mol Biol 29:421-435.
Martinez-Hernandez A (1984). The hepatic extracellular
matrix. I: Electron immunohistochemical studies in normal
rat liver. Lab Inv 51:57-74.
Mather J (ed) (1984). Mammalian cell culture: The use of
serum-free hormone supplemented media. New York: Plenum
Press Inc.
Michalopoulos G, Cianciulli HD, Novotry AR, Kligerman AD,
Strom SC, Jirtle RL (1982). Liver regeneration on studies
with rat hepatocytes in primary culture. Cancer Res
42:4673-4682.
Miller EJ, Gay S (1982). Collagen: An overview. "Methods
Enzymology." Structural and Contractile Proteins Part A
LW Cunningham and DW Frederiksen (eds) New York: Academic
Press 82:3-32.
Miller EJ, Rhodes RK (1982). Preparation and
characterization of the different types of collagen. In
"Structural and Contractile Proteins." Part A
Extracellular Matrix Methods in Enzymology LW Cunningham
and DW Frederiksen (eds) New York: Academic Press 82:33-
64.
Miyanaga O, Evans C, Cottam GL (1983). The effect of
dexamethasone on pyruvate kinase activity in primary
cultures of hepatocytes. Biochimica et Biophyssica Acta
758:42-48.
Muschel R, Khoury G, Reid LM (1986). Regulation of insulin
expression a rat insulinoma cell line by hormones and
matrix. Mol and Cell Biol 6:337-341.
Nakamura T, Nakayama Y, Ichihara A (1984). Reciprocal
modulation of growth and liver functions of mature rat
hepatocytes in primary culture by an extract of hepatic
plasma membranes. J. Biol Chem 259:8056-8058.
Narita M, Jefferson DM, Fujita M, Miller EJ, Clayton DF,
Rosenberg LC, Reid LM (1985). Hormonal and Matrix

Regulation of differentiation in primary liver cultures.
Internat. Symposium on Growth and Differentiaion of Cells
in Defined Environments. New York: Springer Verlag
pp. .
Ocklind C, Odin P, Obrink B (1984). Two different cell
adhesion molecules-cell-CAM 105 and a calcium-dependent
protein-occur on the surface of rat hepatocytes. Exp Cell
Res 151:29-45.
Oldberg A, Hook M (1977). Structure and metabolism of rat
liver heparan sulphate. J. Cell Biol 164:75-81.
Oldberg A, Kjellen L, Hook M (1979). Cell-surface heparan
sulfate: Isolation and characterization of a proteoglycan
from rat liver membranes. J. Biol Chem 254:8505-8510.
Oldberg A, Ruoslahti E (1982). Interactions between
chondroitin sulfate proteoglycans, fibronectin, and
collagen. J. Biol Chem 257:4859-4863.
Orkin RW, Gehron P, McGoodwin EB, Martin GR, Valentine T,
Swarm R (1977). A murine tumor producing a matirx of
basement membrane. J. Exp Med 145:204-220.
Prinz R, Klein U, Sudhakaran PR, Sinn W, Ullrich K, von
Figura K (1980). Metabolism of sulfated
glycosaminoglycans in rat hepatocytes. Synthesis of
heparan sulfate and distribution into cellular and
extracellular pools. Biochimica et Biophysica Acta
630:402-413.
Rajan TV, Halay ED, Potter TA, Evans GA, Seidman JG,
Margulies DH (1983). H-2 hemizygous mutants from a
heterozygous cell line: role of mitotic recombination.
EMBO 2:1537-1542.
Rapraeger AC, Bernfield M (1983). Heparan sulfate
proteoglycans from mouse mammary epithelial cells. A
putative membrane proteoglycan associates quantitatively
with lipid vesicles. J. Biol Chem 258:3632-3636.
Reid LM, Fujita M, Saez JC, Hertzberg E, Spray D (1985).
Glycosaminoglycans and proteoglycans induce gap junction
expression and function in primary liver cell cultures.
J. Cell Biol (in press)
Reid LM, Jefferson DM (1984). Cell culture studies using
extracts of extracellular matrix to study growth and
differentiation in mammalian cells. In "Mammalian Cell
Culture." Mather J.P. (ed) pp. 239-280.
Reid LM, Jefferson DM (1984). Culturing hepatocytes and
other differentiated cells. Hepatology 4:548-559.
Reid LM, Narita M, Fujita M, Murray Z, Liverpool C,
Rosenberg L (1985). Matrix and Hormonal Regulation of
Differentiation in Liver Cultures. In "Isolated and

Cultured Hepatocytes." A and C Guillouzo (eds) INSERM Inc. Paris. pp. .

Rich MA, Pearlstein E, Weissmann G, Hoffstein ST (1981). Cartilage proteoglycans inhibit fibronectin-mediated adhesion. Nature 293:224-226.

Rigby PW, Kieckmann M, Rhodes C, Berg P (1977). Labelling of deoxyribonulceic acid to high specific activity in vitro by nick translation of with DNA polymerase. J. Mol Biol 113:237-251.

Robinson J, Viti M, Hook M (1984). Structure and properties of an under-sulfated heparan sulfate proteoglycan synthesized by a rat hepatoma cell line. J. Cell Biol 98:946-953.

Rosenberg L, Wolfenstein-Todel C, Margolis R, Pal S, Strider W (1976). Proteoglycans from bovine proximal humeral articular cartilage: Structural basis for the polydispersity of proteoglycan subunit. J. Biol Chem 251:6439-6444.

Rosenberg L, Tang L, Choi H, Pal S, Johnson T, Poole AR, Roughley P, Reiner A, Pidoux I (1983). Isolation, characterization and immunohistochemical localization of a dermatan sulfate-containing proteoglycan from bovine fetal epiphyseal cartilage. In "Limb Development and Regeneration." Part B New York: Alan R. Liss Inc. pp. 67-84.

Rosenberg L, Varma R (1982). An overview of proteoglycans in physiology and pathology. In "Glycosaminoglycans and Proteoglycans in Physiological and Pathological Processes of Body Systems.: Varma R. and Varma R. (ed) S Karger AG Basel Switzerland pp. 1-5.

Rubin J, Hook M, Obrink B, Timpl R (1981). Substrate adhesion of rat hepatocytes: Mechanism of attachment to collagen substrate. Cell 24:463-470.

Ruoslahti E, Hayman EG, Engvall E (1980). Molecular interactions of fibronectin. Prog Clin Biol Res 41:821-828.

Saber MA, Zern MA, Shafritz DA (1983). Use of in situ hybridization to identify collagen and albumin mRNA in isolated mouse hepatocytes. Proc Natl Acad Sci USA 80:4017-4020.

Saez JC, Nairn AC Hertzberg E, Greengard P, Bennett MVL, Spray DC (1985). cAMP increases junctional conductance and induces phosphorylation of the principal gap junctional polypeptide. Proc Natl Acad Sci USA (submitted).

Spray DC, Harris AL, Bennett MVL (1981). Equilibrium

properties of a voltage dependent junctional conductance. J. Gen Physiol 77:75-94.

Spray DC, White RL, Mazet F, Bennett MVL (1985). Regulation of gap junctional conductance. Amer J. Physiol 248:H753-764.

Spray DC, Bennett MVL (1985). Physiology and pharmacology of gap junctions. Ann Rev Physiol 47:281-202.

Spray DC, Ginzberg RD, Morales EA, Bennett MVL, Babayatsky M, Gatmaitan Z, Arias I (1984). Physiological and morphological properties of gap junctions between dissociated pairs of rat hepatocytes. J. Cell Biol 99:344a.

Spray DC, Saez JC, Gregory WA, Hertzberg EL (1985). Gap junctions between cultured hepatocytes are maintained by cAMP derivatives, agents that disrupt or stabilize the cytoskeleton and reduce intracellular pH. J. Cell Biol (in press).

Strom SC, Michalopoulos G (1982). Collagen as a substrata for cell growth and differentiation. "Methods in Enzymology." Structural and Contractile Proteins Part A LW Cunningham and DW Frederiksen (ed) New York: Academic Presss 82:544-555.

Williams GM, Bermudez E, San RHC, Goldblatt PJ, Laspia MF (1978). Rat hepatocyte primary cultures: IV. Maintenance in defined medium and the role of production of plasminogen activator and other proteases. In Vitro 14:824-837.

Wilson EJ, McMurray WC (1983). Effects of hormones on the maintenance and mitochondrial functions of rat hepatocytes cultured in serum-free medium. Can J. Biochem Cell Biol 61:636-643.

Winterbourne DJ, Mora PT (1981). Cells selected for high tumorigenicity or transformed by simian virus 40 synthesize heparan sulfate with reduced degree of sulfation. J. Biol Chem 256:4310-4320.

Woods A, Hook M, Kjellen L, Smith CG, Rees DA (19). Relationship of heparan sulfate proteoglycans to the cytoskeleton and extracellular matrix of cultured fibroblasts. J. Cell Biol

Yamada K, Akiyama S (1984). Cell interactions with extracellular matrix. pp 77-148.

This research was supported by a grant from the American Cancer Society (BC-439D) and by NIH grants (P30CA1330, CA30117, AM17702, NS19830, NS16524, AM34614, AMHD21498, GM30667, NS07512). This research was also supported by a grant in aid from the American Heart Association (to DCS). Lola Reid and Elliot Hertzberg receive salary support through Career Development Awards (NIH CA00783 and HD00713, respectively).

Cellular Endocrinology: Hormonal Control of Embryonic
and Cellular Differentiation, pages 361–369
© 1986 Alan R. Liss, Inc.

ENDOTHELIAL CELL GROWTH FACTOR

Thomas Maciag and Wilson H. Burgess

Department of Cell Biology
Biotechnology Research Center
4 Research Court
Rockville, Maryland 20850

Introduction: The endothelium constitutes a quiescent monolayer of cells which form the inner-lining of blood vessels in vivo (1). The endothelial cell is responsible for a variety of unique physiological functions that include (i) the formation of a selective barrier for the translocation of blood constituents and macromolecules to underlying tissues, (ii) the maintenance of a non-thrombogenic interface between blood and tissue and (iii) the maintenance of function as a metabolic organ responsible for the control of hemostasis (1,2,3). In addition, endothelial cells are an important component for the development of new capillaries and blood vessels (1,2,3,4). Although the endothelial cell possesses a relatively low mitotic index in vivo (5), this quality is modulated in a dynamic manner during the process of angiogenesis (1,2,3,4,5) which involves the organized migration and proliferation of the endothelial cell at an accelerated rate. The process of neovascularization which occurs during the development of the vasculature in the embryo (3,4), also occurs post-developmentally during the pathophysiology of a variety of disease states which include psoriasis, arthritis, diabetic retinopathy, chronic inflammatory conditions and tumor development (1,2,3,4). Thus, the identification and characterization of factors, that modulate the migration and proliferation of the endothelial cell, is fundamental to the elucidation of biochemical mechanisms which modulate the neovascular response.

It is the central role of the endothelial cell as a modulator of a variety of physiological and pathological states which has lead this laboratory to focus our attention on the cell biology of the human endothelial cell. Techniques introduced by Jaffe, et al., (7) have provided reliable methodologies (5) for the establishment of primary, non-proliferative in vitro populations of human endothelial cells. Although these methods are valuable for obtaining enriched populations of human endothelial cells, these cells possess limited utility due to their low mitotic index in vitro (5,6). Thus, the state of human endothelial cell quiescence in vitro presented an opportunity to identify factors that influence the proliferative potential of the human endothelial cell.

The discovery of a polypeptide mitogen for human endothelial cells was influenced by the contributions of G.H. Sato and his colleagues (7). Serum, a potent mitogen for the proliferation of many mammalian cells in vitro, is a poorly defined biological fluid. The concept that serum contributes hormones and growth factors for the stimulation of cell proliferation, stimulated our interest since the human endothelial cell is refractory to the mitogenic influence of plasma and serum (8,9). It therefore appeared reasonable that a biological assay for endothelial cell polypeptide mitogens could be established since a putative endothelial cell growth factor would synergize with serum-derived mitogens and promote human endothelial cell division. This argument was accurate since it was possible to identify a polypeptide present in bovine neural tissue that enhanced the proliferation of human endothelial cells in vitro (10). The bovine polypeptide mitogen was named endothelial cell growth factor (ECGF) since it was possible to demonstrate that the biological activity of the polypeptide was chemically and physically unique (10).

The Biological Properties of ECGF: A number of biological attributes are associated with the mitogen and are listed in Table 1. The ability of ECGF to stimulate human endothelial proliferation in vitro was highlighted by the delay of the premature senescence of the human endothelial cell in vitro (11,12). It is possible to achieve between 40 to 60 cumulative population doublings (CPD) by the addition of ECGF to the cell culture medium. The delay of premature in vitro senescence by mitogens has been documented for other human cell types, most notably with serumstimulated fibroblast (13) and epidermal growth factor-induced keratinocyte proliferation (14). Although, ECGF has found wide utility as a general mitogen for the serial propagation of human endothelial cells derived from artery (15), vein (12) and capillary (16), a correlation between in vivo age and advanced CPL has not been established.

TABLE I: Biological Attributes of ECGF In Vitro:

1. Potent endothelial cell and fibroblast mitogen (10,11,18,20).

2. Reduces the serum requirement for endothelial cell proliferation (12).

3. Delays the premature senescence of the human endothelial cell (3,11,12).

4. Potent chemotactic signal for human endothelial cells (17).

5. Biological activity is modulated by heparin (11,18,24).

6. Permits the attainment of stable human endothelial cell clones (11).

Thornton and her colleagues (11) have contributed significantly to the biology of the human endothelial cell by the introduction of heparin into the ECGF-supplemented cell culture medium. Although heparin itself, possess no mitogenic activity, the glycosaminoglycan induces a phenotypic change in the confluent human endothelial cell monolayer and potentiates the biological activity of ECGF. The heparin-induced phenotype is characterized by an ECGF-dependent increase in human endothelial cell monolayer density observed at confluence. Although the mechanism of the heparin-induced, ECGF-dependent phenotype is not known, it is reasonable to suggest it involves a structural interaction between the glycosaminoglycan and the polypeptide mitogen.

In addition to the mitogenic attributes associated with ECGF, the polypeptide is also a potent stimulator of human endothelial cell chemotaxis in vitro (17). The chemotactic activity of ECGF is also potentiated by heparin, an observation consistent with the enhanced mitogenic activity of the polypeptide in the presence of heparin (11,12). Platelet-derived growth factor (PDGF), a potent polypeptide mitogen for mesenchymal cells, is also a chemotactic signal. Although the chemotactic and mitogenic activities of PDGF have been separated (19), similar studies have not been performed with ECGF.

Although ECGF was discovered as an endothelial cell mitogen, recent data demonstrate that other cell types are responsive to the mitogenic attributes associated with ECGF. Human diploid fibroblasts and Balb/c 3T3 cells are responsive to ECGF as a mitogen (10,18), however, it is not known whether these cells can respond to ECGF as a chemotactic signal. It will be of interest to determine whether other cell types which are responsive to ECGF, especially those cells derived from the neural crest.

The Chemical Properties of ECGF: A rapid and efficient purification protocol for ECGF has recently been established (20). This procedure generates 100-200 micrograms of ECGF per Kg of bovine brain and requires approximately two days to complete. The success of this purification procedure is attributed to the extraction of bovine neural tissue at neutral pH to minimize proteolytic digestion (10), the presence of EDTA to inactivate Ca^{2+}-dependent brain-derived proteases, the conversion of the high molecular weight (Mr) form of ECGF to a low Mr ECGF species (21) and the ability of heparin to bind ECGF (22). The purification procedure has been described in detail and has resulted in the identification of multiple forms of ECGF (20). Although these forms share similar isoelectric points and biological activities, the polypeptide mitogens can be separated by gradient elution from heparin-Sepharose, reversed-phase HPLC and SDS-PAGE (20). These polypeptides have been named alpha- and beta-ECGF and are defined on the basis of apparent Mr and retention time off reversed-phase supports (20). Thus, alpha-ECGF with an apparent Mr= 17,000 elutes prior to beta-ECGF which possesses an apparent Mr= 20,000 (20). Although the amino acid composition of the two forms of ECGF are similar, alpha- and beta-ECGF are different when the polypeptides are examined by digestion with CNBr and trypsin (20). Beta-ECGF contains two tryptic peptide fragments which are unique and these fragments reside in the smaller of the two polypeptide chains resolved by reduced SDS-PAGE of the CNBr digestion (20). These data demonstrate that both alpha- and beta-ECGF are single chain polypeptides containing a single methionine residue central to a disulfide bond(s).

Automated Edman degradation of intact alpha-ECGF reveals an amino-terminal sequence identical to the sequence reported for the amino-terminal region (starting at residue 7) of acidic-fibroblast growth factor (FGF) (27). In contrast, sequential release of amino acids from intact beta-ECGF was not observed (20). However, Edman degradation of CNBrmodified beta-ECGF revealed a sequence similar to the sequence reported for the COOH-terminal CNBr fragment of acidic-FGF (23). Likewise, the COOH-terminal fragment derived from alpha- and beta-ECGF generate a sequence identical to the COOH-terminus of acidic-FGF (23). These data demonstrate that the amino-terminus of beta-ECGF is blocked and suggest that the beta-ECGF contains an amino-terminal extension of alpha-ECGF.

The Family of Endothelial Cell Polypeptide Mitogens: Polypeptide growth factors for endothelial cell proliferation have been described by other laboratories. These factors have been named either on the basis of the source of the polypeptide or the target cell for the growth factor. Table 2 represent a list of these endothelial cell polypeptide mitogens and the chemical and physical properties established for each polypeptide. The

TABLE II: Putative Representatives of the Endothelial Cell Polypeptide Mitogen Family: The following polypeptide mitogen are potential members of the family of endothelial cell polypeptide mitogen. Heparin elution refers to the molarity of NaCl which elutes the polypeptide from immobilized heparin. Immuno and receptor competant refers to the ability of the polypeptide to bind anti-ECGF antibodies and the ECGF receptor.

POLYPEPTIDE	TISSUE SOURCE	Mr	pI	IMMUNO COMPETENT	RECEPTOR COMPETENT	HEPARIN ELUTION
Alpha-ECGF	Brain, Hypothalamus	17,000(20)	5-6 (21,32)	+	+	1.0(20)
Beta-ECGF	Brain, Hypothalamus	20,000(20)	5-6 (21,32)	+	+	1.0(20)
Acidic-FGF	Brain	17,000(33)	5-6 (33)	+	+	1.0(34)
EDGF-II	Eye, Retina	17,000(35)	5-6 (35)	+	+	0.9(35)
Alpha-HGF	Brain, Hypothalamus	16,000(36)	N.D	N.D.	N.D.	1.0(36)
AGF-I	Brain	17,500(37)	5.5 (37)	N.D.	N.D.	1.0(37)
Acidic-HDGF	Hypothalamus	N.D.	5.0 (38)	N.D.	N.D.	1.0(38)
RDGF	Retina	16,000(39)	5.0 (40)	N.D.	N.D.	1.0(40)
ECGF	Human Brain	18,500(41)	5.2 (41)	N.D.	N.D.	1.2(41)

* N.D. = not determined

relationship between these polypeptides has been extended to include immunological and receptor binding criteria for three of the endothelial cell polypeptide mitogens (24). It has been demonstrated that acidic-FGF and eye-derived growth factor-II (EDGF-II) compete for (^{125}I)-ECGF binding to the ECGF receptor and are recognized by monoclonal antibodies prepared against ECGF. These data argue that a new family of polypeptide growth factors exist which presently comprises acidic-FGF, ECGF and EDGF-II. It is reasonable to suggest that alpha-heparin-binding growth factor (25), retina-derived growth factor (26) and alpha-hypothalamus-derived growth factor (27,38) are also members of the endothelial cell polypeptide mitogen family although membership must be verified by sequence analysis.

The ECGF Receptor: Binding studies performed with (^{125}I.)-ECGF on a variety of mammalian cells suggest that endothelial cells and fibroblasts possess a high affinity receptor for the poly-peptide mitogen (18). The number of receptors and the Kd for ECGF does not appear to vary significantly among the cell types examined (Table 3). It is also apparent that the ECGF receptor is conserved among verterbrate species since bovine, human, rabbit and murine cells possess the high affinity binding domain (18). A comparison of the half-maximum activity of ECGF to stimulate (^{3}H)-thymidine incorporation with the Kd for receptor binding on a variety of cell types suggests that only a small number of the receptors for ECGF need to be occupied to generate a mitogenic signal. The receptor for ECGF apprears to be specific for this polypeptide mitogen since known hormones and growth factors (EGF, NGF, insulin, etc) do not compete for receptor binding (18).

Although the mechanism of ECGF-induced signal transduction is not known, binding data performed at 4°C and 37°C suggest that the ECGF:ECGF receptor complex is rapidly internalized

TABLE III: Mitogenic and Receptor Binding Properties of ECGF.

CELL TYPE	HALF-MAXIMUM MITOGENIC ACTIVITY (M X 10^{10})	K_d (M X 10^{10})	RECEPTOR NUMBER PER CELL (X 10^4)
Human Umbilical Vein Endothelial Cell	0.7+0.2	2+1	4.0
Murine Lung Capillary Endothelial Cell	0.6+0.3	4+2	4.0
Rabbit Aortic Endothelial Cell	1.9+0.5	8+3	2.0
Bovine Pulmunary Vein Endothelial Cell	0.6+0.3	2+1	4.0
Bovine Aorta Endothelial Cell	1.5+0.7	6+3	2.0
Balb/c 3T3 Cells	1.4+0.2	4+2	3.0
Human Foreskin Fibroblasts	2.0+0.6	7+3	2.0

(18). These data are consistent with the behavior of other polypeptide ligand:receptor systems (28). Thus, it is reasonable to suggest that the receptor for ECGF is a membrane protein and preliminary evidence obtained from covalent affinity cross-linking studies with (^{125}I)-ECGF are consistent with this suggestion (Friesel, R., Burgess, W.H. and Maciag, T., unpublished observation).

Murine monoclonal antibodies specific for ECGF have been synthesized (22). These antibodies have been characterized by their ability to bind ECGF and inhibit the biological activity of the polypeptide mitogen (18,22,24). In this manner, antibodies that bind ECGF and inhibit biological activity and antibodies that bind ECGF and inhibit mitogenic activity have been characterized (18). Those antibodies which inhibit ECGF-induced biological activity have been further characterized by their ability to inhibit (^{125}I)-ECGF receptor binding. Indeed, those antibodies which inhibit the biological activity of ECGF also prevent the polypeptide from occupying the ECGF receptor (18). This correlation was not observed with the antibodies which bind ECGF but do not inhibit ECGF-induced biological activity (18,22). These data demonstrate that the binding of ECGF to a receptor present on the surface of the endothelial cell is requisite for induction of the mitogenic signal and there exist epitopes present within the structure of ECGF that do not participate in receptor binding. Since ECGF-induced endothelial cell chemotaxis is also inhibited by anti-ECGF antibodies (17), the chemotactic properties attributed to ECGF also involve receptor occupancy.

Is Heparin A Cofactor for ECGF Function?: Clinical preparations of heparin potentiate the mitogenic activity of crude (11) and pure (18,24) preparations of ECGF. In addition, the chemotactic activity of the ECGF polypeptide is also potentiated by heparin (17). The ability of ECGF to bind to heparin and augment the biological activities of the polypeptide suggests that the structural interaction which occurs between the growth factor and the glyco-saminoglycan may involve stabilization of the structure of the polypeptide mitogen by heparin. This hypothesis was examined by studying the interaction of ECGF with two biological affinity systems, the ECGF receptor and anti-ECGF antibodies. Scatchard analysis of (^{125}I)-ECGF binding on endothelial cells in the presence and absence of heparin demonstrate that heparin enhances the binding of ECGF to its receptor. A decrease in the dissociation constant (K_d) for ECGF from 5×10^{-10}M to 2×10^{-10}M was observed with no alteration in the total number of ECGF receptors present on the endothelial cell surface (18). This change in K_d in the presence of heparin is consistent with the potentiation of ECGF-induced mitogenic activity by heparin. Indeed, the half-maximum activity for ECGF was altered from 5×10^{-11}M in the absence of heparin to 1×10^{-11}M in the presence of heparin (18). Furthermore, the potentiation of ECGF-induced mitogenic activity by heparin was observed to be dependent upon the concentration of heparin with the half-maximum activity of heparin equal to approximately 10ug per ml (18). These data suggest that heparin interacts structurally with ECGF and perhaps induces a conformation change within the structure of the polypeptide which favors the presentation of the mitogen to its receptor. Alternatively, heparin may also interact with the ECGF receptor in a manner which augments the binding of ECGF.

Heparin also potentiates the binding of anti-ECGF antibodies to ECGF. An alteration in the K_d for antibody:antigen dissociation from 10^{-7} to 5×10^{-8} was independently observed for two anti-ECGF monoclonal antibodies (18). These data demonstrate that heparin is able to alter immunological epitopes present within the structure of ECGF. Heparin is also able to restore biological activity to purified preparations of ECGF that have lost biological potency upon storage (18). The biological activity of ECGF is labile to extremes of temperature and pH and after extended periods of time in storage losses a majority of its biological potency (10,18). Adsorption of "denatured" ECGF by heparin-Sepharose and elution with 1M NaCl restores biological potency to the ECGF polypeptide. The specific activity of the ECGF preparation increases 100-fold (2×10^{-8}M to 1×10^{-10}M) as a result of heparin adsorption. These data are consistent with the alteration of K_d for ECGF by immunological and receptor criteria and further suggest that heparin induces conformational changes in the structure of the polypeptide mitogen. Thus, we suggest that heparin is indeed a cofactor for ECGF. Although the precise mechanism is not clear, the structural interaction between the polypeptide may involve the induction of a favored conformation in the tertiary structure of ECGF which results in the formation of a more suitable polypeptide comformation for receptor binding. This hypothesis needs to be confirmed with spectroscopic methods.

The Significance of the Endothelial Cell Growth Factor and Future Directions: Further characterization of the members of the endothelial cell family of polypeptide mitogens must be performed at the structural level. Indeed the complete primary structure of acidic- and basic-FGF are major contributions to our understanding the role of this family in mesenchymal cell proliferation (23,29) but must be extended to include other putative members of this family (Table 2). We anticipate that this information will result in further characterization of this polypeptide family at the genetic level and ultimately provide cDNA and genomic clones. This information promises to rigourously define the relationship between the basic and the acidic polypeptide mitogen families on the basis of intron-exon structures and chromosomal localizations.

The site(s) and mechanism(s) of ECGF synthesis and delivery are not known. Although ECGF is present in neural tissue, it is unclear how the polypeptide is delivered to the endothelial cell in vivo, if at all. Since, we have not been able to detect the presence of ECGF in either serum or plasma with ECGF antibodies, it is possible that the polypeptide is delivered by a paracrine mechanism which may involve synthesis by fibroblasts or other mesenchymal cells or perhaps be carried by circulating cells. The recent observation that the macrophage contains basic-FGF (30) and c-sis (31) argues in favor of the latter hypothesis. Likewise, the spectrum of biological targets for ECGF must also be addressed. We anticipate that those cells responsive to ECGF either as a mitogen or modulator of cellular homeostasis, will include mammalian cell types other than the endothelial cell since fibroblasts contain receptors for, and respond to, ECGF (18).

The mechanism of ECGF-induced signal transduction also requires further characterization. Although it is known that a down-regulatable receptor for ECGF exists on the cell surface of the endothelial cell, the biochemical character of this poly-peptide must be established. Likewise, the activation of intra-cellular modulators concomitantly expressed as a result of ECGF receptor occupancy will provide further definition for the endo-thelial cell polypeptide family of mitogens and aid in the eluci-dation of the mechanism by which ECGF modulates endothelial cell proliferation.

REFERENCES:

(1) Folkman, J., Ann. Intern. Med., 82,96 (1975)
(2) Gimbrone, M.A. Jr., Prog. Hemostasis Thromb., 3,1 (1976)
(3) Maciag, T., Prog. Hemostasis Thromb., 7,167 (1984)
(4) Folkman, J. and Haudenschild, C., Nature, 288,551 (1980)
(5) Gimbrone, M.A. Jr., Cotran, R.S., and Folkman, J., J. Cell Biol., 60,673 (1974)
(6) Jaffe, E.A., Nachman, R.J., Becker, C.G., and Minick, C.R., J. Clin. Invest., 52,2745 (1973)
(7) Bottenstein, J., Hayashi, I., Hutchings, S., Masui, H., Mather, J., McCluse, D., Ohasa, S., Rizzino, A., Sato, G.H., Serrero, G., Wolfe, R., and Wer, R., Methods in Enzy., 58,94 (1978)
(8) Thorgiersson, G. and Robertson, A.L. Jr., Atherosclerosis, 31,231 (1978)
(9) Wall, R.L., Harker, L.A., Quadracci, L.J., and Stricker, G.E., J. Cell. Physiol., 96,203 (1978)
(10) Maciag, T., Cerundolo, J., Ilsley, S., Kelley, P.R., and Forand, R., Proc. Natl. Acad. Sci. U.S.A., 76,5674 (1979)
(11) Thorton, S.C., Mueller, S.N., and Levine, E.M., Science, 222,623 (1983)
(12) Maciag, T., Hoover, G.A., Stimerman, M.B., and Weinstein, R., J. Cell Biol., 91,420 (1981)
(13) Cristofalo, V.J. and Sharf, B.B., Exp. Cell Res., 76,419 (1973)
(14) Reinwald, J.G. and Green, H., Nature, 265,421 (1977)
(15) Glassberg, M.K., Bern, M.M., Coughlin, S.R., Haudenschild, C.C., Hoyer,L.W., Antoniades, H.N., and Zetter, B.R., In Vitro, 18,859 (1982)
(16) Folkman, J., Haudenschild, C.C., and Zetter, B.R., Proc.-Natl. Acad. Sci.U.S.A., 76,5217 (1979)
(17) Terranova, V.P., DiFlorio, R., Lyall, R.M., Hic, S., Friesel, R., and Maciag, T., J. Cell Biol., 101,2330 (1985)
(18) Schreiber, A.B., Kenney, J., Kowalski, W.J., Friesel, R., Mehlman, T., and Maciag, T., Proc. Natl. Acad. Sci.-U.S.A., 82,6138 (1985)
(19) Senior, R.M., Huang, J.S., Griffin, G.L., and Deuel, T.F., J. Cell Biol., 100,351 (1985)
(20) Burgess, W.H., Mehlman, T., Friesel, R., Johnson, W., and Maciag, T., J. Biol. Chem., 260,11389 (1985)
(21) Maciag, T., Hoover, G.A., and Weinstein, R., J. Biol.-

Chem., 257,5333 (1982)

(22) Maciag, T., Mehlman, T., Friesel, R., and Schreiber, A.B., Science, 225,932 (1984)

(23) Gimenez-Gallego, G., Rodkey, J., Bennett, C., Rios-Candelor, M., DiSalvo, J., and Thomas, K.A., Science, 230,1385 (1985)

(24) Schreiber, A.B., Kenney, J., Kowalski, J., Thomas, K.A., Gimenez-Gallego, G., Loret, C., Burgess, W.H., Mehlman, T., Friesel, R., Johnson, W., and Maciag, T., J. Cell Biol., 101,1623 (1985)

(25) Lobb, R.R. and Fett, J.W., Biochemistry, 23,6925 (1984)

(26) D'Amore, P.A., Glaser, B.M., Brunson, S.K., and Fenselau, A.H., Proc. Natl. Acad. Sci. U.S.A., 78,3068 (1981)

(27) Lobb, R.R., Harper, J.W., and Fett, S.W., Analytical Biochem., In Press

(28) James, R. and Bradshaw, R.A., Ann. Rev. Biochem., 53,259 (1984)

(29) Esch, F., Baird, A., Ling, N., Ueno, N., H.U.F., Denoroy, L., Klepper, R., Gospodarowicz, D., Bohlen, P., and Guillemin, R., Proc. Natl. Acad. Sci. U.S.A., 82,6507 (1985)

(30) Esch, F., Ueno, N., Baird, A., Hill, F., Denoroy, L., Ling, N., Gospodarowicz, D., and Guillemin, R., Biochem. Biophys. Res. Commun., 131,554 (1985)

(31) Jaye, M., McConathy, E., Drohan, W., Tong, B., Denel, T.F., and Maciag, T., Science, 228,882 (1985)

(32) Burgess, W.H., Mehlman, T., and Maciag, T., unpublished observation

(33) Thomas, K.A., Rios-Candelor, M., and Fitzpatrick, S., Proc. Natl. Acad. Sci. U.S.A., 81,357 (1984)

(34) Thomas, K.A., Rios-Candelor, M., Gimenez-Gallego, G., DiSalvo, J., Bennett, C., Rodkey, J., and Fitzpatrick, S., Proc. Natl. Acad. Sci. U.S.A., 82,6409 (1985)

(35) Courty, J., Loret, C., Moenner, M., Chevallier, B., Lagente, O., Courtois, Y., and Barritault, D., Biochemie, 67,265 (1985)

(36) Lobb, R.R., Strydom, D., and Fett, J.W., Biochem. Biophys. Res. Commun., 131,586 (1985)

(37) Pettman, B., Weibel, M., Sensenbrenner, M., and Labourdette, G., FEBS Letters, 189,102 (1985)

(38) Klagsbrun, M. and Shing, Y., Proc. Natl. Acad. Sci. U.S.A., 82,805 (1985)

(39) Lobb, R., Sasse, J., Shing, Y., D'Amore, P.A., Sullivan, R., Jacobs, J., and Klagsbrun, M., J. Biol. Chem., 261,1924 (1986)

(40) D'Amore, P.A. and Klagsbrun, M., J. Cell Biol., 99,1545 (1984)

(41) Conn, G. and Hatcher, V.B., Biochem. Biophys. Res. Commun., 124,262 (1984)

Cellular Endocrinology: Hormonal Control of Embryonic
and Cellular Differentiation, pages 371–388
© 1986 Alan R. Liss, Inc.

REFLECTIONS ON THE EVOLUTION OF THE REGULATION OF
SPERMATOGENESIS

Irving B. Fritz
Banting and Best Department of Medical Research
University of Toronto
112 College Street
Toronto, Ontario, M5G 1L6 CANADA

A) INTRODUCTION AND STATEMENT OF THE HYPOTHESIS

The overall pattern of spermatogenesis has been
remarkably well conserved during evolution (Figure 1).
Gametogenesis is essentially the same in sponges (Fell,
1974) as in mammals (Clermont, 1972). In contrast, complex
patterns of regulation of spermatogenesis differ radically
among organisms in various phyla (Roosen-Runge, 1977).

In mammals, and indeed in most if not all vertebrates,
the development of germ cells depends upon a functioning
neuroendocrine system. Regulatory hormones, primarily androgens and pituitary gonadotropins, act directly on somatic
cells of the gonad, and not on germinal cells. From data
reviewed elsewhere (Fritz, 1978 and 1984), the conclusion
emerges that in the sexually mature normal testis, gonadal
somatic cells permit expression of the phenotypic programs
inherent in germ cells by providing an appropriate microenvironment. When optimally functioning, gonadal somatic
cells create a unique cytoarchitectural and physical-
chemical microenvironment within the mammalian seminiferous
tubule required to maintain necessary levels of nutrients,
cofactors and modulating components; and also to allow
immunologic privilege for germinal cells during their
successive stages of development (for reviews, see Fritz,
1978; Fritz and Tung, 1985) (Figure 2).

In this communication, we shall advance the concept
that fundamental characteristics of cell interactions of
the sort described in the seminiferous tubules of mammals

have much in common with those of cell interactions in gonad-like structures of less complex animals, including sponges. In these cases, gonadal somatic cells are also

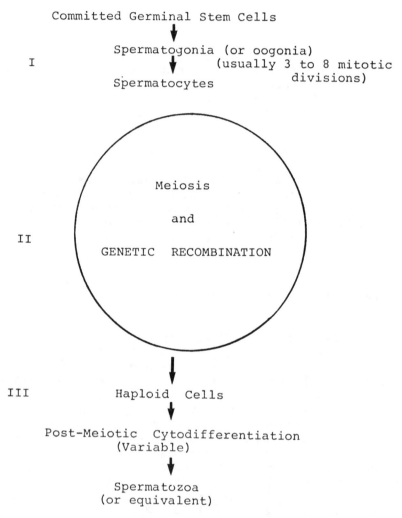

Figure 1. <u>Typical Animal Spermatogenesis, From Eukaryotic Microbes to Mammals</u>
(For reviews, see Clermont, 1972; Roosen-Runge, 1977; Bell, 1982).

postulated to provide an environment which either permits, or fails to permit, implementation of expression of the programs for spermatogenesis. The regulation of gonadal somatic cell functions thereby serves as part of a cascade in the control of spermatogenesis. Simply stated, the

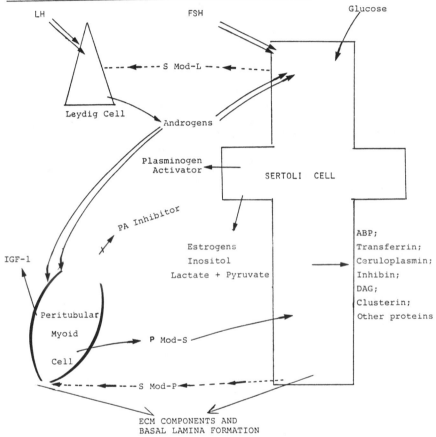

Figure 2. Regulation of Activities of Mammalian Gonadal Somatic Cells
For reviews, see the text. Abbreviations are "LH" for luteinizing hormone; "FSH" for follicle stimulating hormone; "PA" for plasminogen activator; "ABP" for androgen binding protein; "DAG" for dimeric acidic sulfated glycoprotein; "ECM" for extracellular matrix; "IGF-1" for insulin-like growth factor 1 (somatomedin C); "P" for peritubular myoid cell; "S" for Sertoli cell; "L" for Leydig cell; and "Mod" for modulates.

regulation of spermatogenesis in general is postulated to be mediated effectively by modulation of gonadal somatic cell functions, and by control of the milieu in which germinal cells develop.

In this view, increasingly complex levels of regulators of germinal cell development have evolved which have the capacity to respond to changes in the external environment by turning on or turning off gonadal somatic cell functions. The hypothesis to be presented by no means excludes concomitant changes during evolution of other mechanisms by which gonadal somatic cells may influence germinal cell development; nor does it exclude special cases in which spermatogenesis might proceed in a unique environment provided by alternative cytoarchitectural arrangements. We shall examine the possibility that the complex neuroendocrine control of mammalian spermatogenesis is superimposed upon ancient modulating mechanisms whose prototypes exist in gonads of more primitive animals, such as sponges, and even in eukaryotic microbes. We wish to explore how the evolution of the neuroendocrine regulation of gonadal somatic cell functions may be related to the concomitant evolution of mechanisms which control spermatogenesis in response to environmental stimuli.

B) THE ADVANTAGES OF SEX

It is evident, even by casual inspection of the processes of "typical spermatogenesis" (Figure 1), that meiosis and genetic recombination occupy center stage. The advantages thus offered for generating genetic diversity are unique (Smith, 1978; Bell, 1982). It has been conjectured that "the 'invention' of sexuality must have occurred very early in the history of organisms and was an essential step in evolution - perhaps second only to the origin of life itself" (Metz and Monroy, 1985). Still, Nature was extraordinarily inventive in making countless variations on the theme of asexual reproduction (for review see Giese and Pearse, 1974), concomitant with the initiation of an apparently infinite number of approaches to sexual reproduction. Even after 'inventing' sexuality, Nature hedged its bets, and conserved techniques whereby life cycles of many organisms continue to have both sexual and asexual forms of reproduction (Campbell, 1974; Bell, 1982).

A theme common to the control of sexual reproduction in many species relates to changes in gametogenesis in response to changes in the environment. In most animals who reproduce sexually, it becomes necessary to have mechanisms for gametes from male and female members of the species, respectively, to come into contact at roughly the same time and place, in a setting compatible with mating. More complex mechanisms may have evolved from simpler ones associated with the responses of gonads from sponges and jellyfish to changes in the environment (Figure 3). For example, increased crowding of Hydra results in a switch from asexual to sexual forms of reproduction, mediated perhaps by an increase in pCO_2 (Campbell, 1974). Whatever the effective environmental stimulus is, it appears likely that somatic precursor cells in sponges or jellyfish can give rise to germinal cells and to nurse cells, resulting in the formation of a "spermary follicle" (homologous to the seminiferous tubule), in which both cell types remain closely associated (Figure 3) (Willmer, 1970; Fell, 1974). What factors modulate the unequal division of precursor cells to generate germinal stem cells and nurse cells as daughter cells? The effective environmental signal is postulated to trigger an increase in the ratio of modulating factors to mitogenic factors, or to trigger changes in the responsiveness of precursor cells to the factor (Figure 3). The primitive somatic cell-germ cell interactions depicted in sponges may represent a prototype for more complex somatic cell-germ cell relations which subsequently evolved. Increased information clearly is required concerning levels of specific growth or mitogenic factors, and specific modulating factors, in cells of sponges and jellyfish during sexual and asexual states. As discussed below, it is not unlikely that some of the modulating and mitogenic factors discovered in mammalian tissues may also be present in less complex organisms (Nial, 1982).

C) THE CONTROL OF GONADAL SOMATIC CELL FUNCTIONS

In organisms in which fate maps are rigidly followed, such as in nematodes like Caenorhabditis elegans, the genetic program determines the development of gonadal somatic cells and germinal cells, apparently independent of neural or systemic hormonal influences (Kratochwil, 1982; Ward, 1985). Ablation of the gonadal somatic cells with a

laser beam has been shown to alter germinal cell development (Kimble, 1985). Under usual circumstances, however,
spermatogenesis proceeds according to an inflexible genetic
program, dependent only on an environment compatible with
the support of the whole nematode.

In contrast, in organisms in which spermatogenesis is
less strictly predetermined, and in which environmental
factors such as seasonal variations may play an important
regulatory role, the functions of gonadal somatic cells are
greatly altered during different states. As indicated

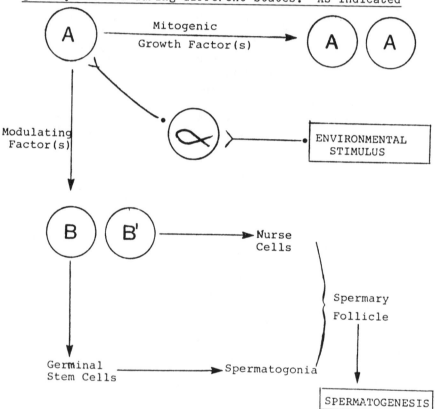

Figure 3. Differentiation of Sponge Cells to Form Spermary
Follicle: Potential Importance of Ratio of Modulation
Factors to Growth Factors
For details, see the text, and reviews by Willmer (1970)
and Fell (1974). A, α, and B represent different cell
types.

earlier, gonadal somatic cells in mammals turn on spermatogenesis by providing the correct milieu for germ cell
development (Figure 2). Steady state spermatogenesis
normally occurs in many mammals, such as mice and men, from
the time of adolescence until old age. However, there are
interesting variants among mammals, including species like
deer, mink, rams and cattle, which produce spermatozoa
during only one season of the year (Lodge and Salisbury,
1970; Sadleir, 1972). Seasonal variation in reproduction
is of course the rule in most arthropods, fishes, amphibia,
reptiles and birds.

Spermatogensis in normal adult non-cycling mammals can
be arrested by interrupting the pathways between the central nervous system and the gonads at any of a number of
sites (Setchell, 1978; 1982). The important role of the
neuroendocrine system in the regulation of reproduction has
long been appreciated (Harris, 1955). It is well recognized that spermatogenesis ceases following removal of the
gonadotrophic hormones by hypophysectomy, or by lowering
levels of gonadotropin releasing hormone (GnRH) produced by
hypothalamic nuclei. It appears likely that in seasonally-
breeding animals, the low levels of GnRH are responsible
for the diminution in spermatogenesis during the non-
breeding periods. In the case of the golden hamster, the
neural control of levels of gonadotrophin hormones can
clearly be shown to be associated with responses to light,
since optic enucleation elicits a failure of gametogenesis
comparable to that observed after hypophysectomy (Gravis,
1978).

The neuroendocrine system has also been shown to be
crucial to the regulation of spermatogenesis in insects
(Scharrer, 1959), and in several other classes of non-
vertebrates. In starfish, a "gonad stimulating substance"
can be extracted from radial nerves which functions in a
manner comparable to that of pituitary gonadotrophins in
chordates (Kanatani, 1985) (Figure 4). The homologies can
be carried further: in all known cases, the systemic
messenger is a peptide, under neural regulation, which acts
on gonadal somatic cells to elicit the formation of one or
more products (local messengers) which influence germinal
cell development. In the case of starfish, 1-methyladenine
is produced by ovarian follicular cells (or by testicular A
cells), under the control of "gonadal stimulating substance". The 1-methyladenine then acts to allow oocytes

arrested in the diplotene stage to resume meiosis
(Figure 4). The resumption of meiosis elicited in starfish
oocytes by 1-methyladenine is completely homologous to that
observed in amphibian oocytes subjected to progesterone.
Progesterone is produced by <u>Xenopus</u> ovarian granulosa cells
when stimulated by gonadotrophic hormones. In both cases,
the local messenger stimulates the synthesis by oocytes of
a "maturation-promoting factor" (MPF). Intracellular injection of MPF elicits resumption of meiosis in isolated
<u>Xenopus</u> oocytes, independent of the presence of
progesterone or other systemic or local messengers (Masui,
1985).

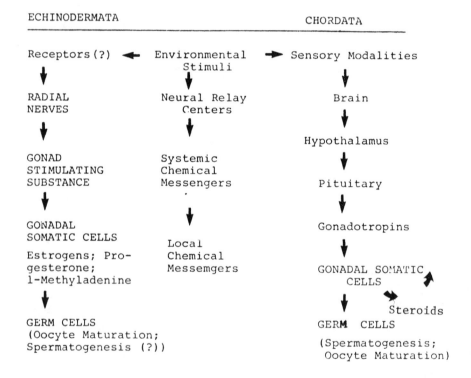

ECHINODERMATA   CHORDATA

Receptors(?) ◄── Environmental ──► Sensory Modalities
    ↓   Stimuli   ↓
                      ↓
RADIAL   Neural Relay   Brain
NERVES   Centers   ↓
    ↓   ↓
                                        Hypothalamus
GONAD   Systemic   ↓
STIMULATING   Chemical
SUBSTANCE   Messengers   Pituitary
    ↓   ↓   ↓
GONADAL   Gonadotropins
SOMATIC CELLS   ↓   ↓
                   Local
Estrogens; Pro-   Chemical
gesterone;   Messemgers   GONADAL SOMATIC
1-Methyladenine   CELLS
    ↓   ↓   ↓
                                                 Steroids
GERM CELLS   GERM CELLS
(Oocyte Maturation;
Spermatogenesis (?))   (Spermatogenesis;
                                       Oocyte Maturation)

Figure 4. <u>Regulation of Germ Cell Development: Homologies
Between Starfish and Man</u>
For details, see the text, and reviews by Harris (1955);
Kanatani (1985).

The generalization emerges that the functions of somatic gonadal cells in sponges, starfishes and men are regulated by reactions to changes in the environment, mediated by a variety of mechanisms, and that gonadal somatic cell products influence the development of neighboring germinal cells (Figures 2-4).

D) EVOLUTION OF PARACRINE FACTORS CONTROLLING GONADAL FUNCTIONS

In a review of "The Evolution of Peptide Hormones", Nial (1982) develops the argument that the evolution of hormones may well have begun in unicellular organisms. For example, chorionic gonadotropin-like material (hCG) is present in bacteria (Maruo et al., 1979). Since hCG shares a common subunit with mammalian follicle stimulating hormone (FSH), luteinizing hormone (LH) and thyrotropin (TSH), it seems likely that all of these hormones could be present in unicellular organisms.

More remarkably, the eukaryotic microbe Achlya (a fungus) reproduces sexually only when there are cooperating partners of appropriate mating type. Two specific sterols, secreted by the female and male, respectively, are required to elicit sexual reproduction (for review, see Horgen, 1981). Pheromones synthesized by the interacting partners are sterols which are homologous to some of the paracrine factors produced by gonadal somatic cells of more complex organisms. Thus antheridiol, secreted constitutively by female Achlya strains, elicits the formation of sex organs in males and also induces the male to synthesize a different sterol, oogoniol (Horgen, 1981). These sterols are homologous to the paracrine steroid testosterone, which is secreted by mammalian testicular interstitial cells in response to LH or to hCG (Setchell, 1978, 1982). Achlya represents the first eukaryotic microbe in which characterized steroid-like compounds have been shown to exert complex physiological and biochemical effects. The entire male organism responds to antheridiol, a pregnenolone derivative, and the entire female organism responds to oogonial, a sterol structurally similar to mammalian steroids. In this sense Achlya itself is the target tissue to the sterol, resulting in differentiation of gonadal-like structures, the generation of haploid gametes, and the ultimate formation of zygotes (Horgen, 1981).

We have previously referred to the presence of steroids (estrogen and progesterone) in starfish gonadal follicles (Kanatani, 1985). Thus, early in evolution both gametogenesis and steroidogenesis take place in the gonad. Although it is not yet clear how far back this set of dual functions extends, it is not inconceivable that the first gamete-producing gonad also contains nurse cells which synthesize steroids . The effects of steroids on Achyla referred to above certainly support such a possibility.

Paracrine agents other than steroids are produced by mammalian gonadal somatic cells. These include mitogenic factors and modulating proteins secreted by peritubular cells, and a variety of peptides and other components synthesized by Sertoli cells (Feig et al., 1983; Skinner and Fritz, 1985a; Fritz, 1978; 1984; Mather, 1984; Fritz et al., 1985). Recently, the presence of many mammalian peptide hormones (including insulin) in molluscs, insects and Tetrahymena has been demonstrated (for reviews, see Nial, 1982; Roth et al., 1982). It is therefore possible that paracrine agents identified as products of mammalian gonadal somatic cells are also synthesized by somatic cells in gonads of less complex organisms, and that comparable regulatory roles may exist. It remains to be determined which, if any, of the platelet derived growth factor, the epidermal growth factor or the insulin-like growth factor families (Heldin and Westermark, 1984) play crucial roles in the regulation of gametogenesis in organisms of most ancient origin. Similarly, the phylogeny of specific receptors to these agents, as well as to other hormones, paracrine factors, and autocrine factors (Csaba, 1980) remains to be delineated.

E) THE ROLE OF GONADAL SOMATIC CELLS IN THE CONTROL OF MAMMALIAN SPERMATOGENESIS

The major somatic cells in seminiferous tubules of mammalian testes are peritubular myoid cells and Sertoli cells. The anatomy and functions of these cells have been reviewed extensively (Dym and Fawcett, 1970; Fawcett, 1975; Fritz, 1978; 1984; Russell, 1980; Waites and Gladwell, 1982; Stefanini et al., 1985). The nature of the interactions between these two cell types has also been recently considered (Fritz et al., 1985; Fritz and Tung, 1985). Consequently, it is necessary only to summarize information which seems most relevant to our current topic.

The control of functions of mammalian gonadal somatic cells is mediated by systemic hormones (FSH on Sertoli cells, and androgens on both Sertoli and peritubular cells); and by paracrine factors elaborated by each cell type (Figure 2). Sertoli cells and peritubular cells interact at many levels: 1) They function cooperatively to synthesize extracellular matrix components, deposit them in an organized matrix, form basal laminae, and generate a complex tubule-like structure containing a basement membrane (Tung and Fritz, 1980; Skinner et al., 1985; Fritz and Tung, 1985). 2) They support the survival of each other in culture in a serum-free medium under conditions in which neither would survive in monoculture (Tung and Fritz, 1980). 3) Peritubular cells under androgen regulation synthesize P Mod-S, a protein having an Mr of approximately 70 kDa, which stimulates Sertoli cells to produce specific products (e.g. androgen binding protein and transferrin) (Skinner and Fritz, 1985a and b). In addition, peritubular cells synthesize a protein which is mitogenic, and which is reactive with an antibody against IGF-1 (in preparation).

The modulation by systemic hormones and paracrine factors of functions of Sertoli cells and peritubular cells (Figure 2) is thought to be required for germinal cell developmental programs to be expressed. When gonadal somatic cells are not functioning optimally (as in off-seasons for seasonal breeders, or prior to adolescence), spermatogenesis cannot proceed to completion. The neuroendocrine control of germinal cell development in mammals therefore appears to be mediated exclusively via hormonal actions on gonadal somatic cells, without direct effects on germinal cells. The properties of Sertoli cells and peritubular cells, and the regulation of their functions, are rapidly becoming better understood. Although exact mechanisms by which these gonadal somatic cells influence germinal cell development remain to be delineated, it is likely that multiple interactions are required, ranging from the provision of suitable cytoarchitectural arrangements for compartmentation, to the supply of specific nutrients and cofactors.

Complex pathways described for the regulation of the functions of gonadal somatic cells in mammals presumably evolved in response to the pressure for increased reproductive success. Animals possessing steady state spermatogenesis probably have better chances of fathering offspring and propagating the species than animals without such a capacity. However, this increased capability imposes a need for additional levels of regulation, super-imposed upon pre-existing strategies for modulation of spermatogenesis in response to environmental stimuli (Lofts, 1968; Bell, 1982). At different levels of complexity, the courtship rituals of man, birds, fish, horseshoe crabs and snails may be regarded as extensions, with apparently infinite variations, superimposed upon the mating patterns of more ancient organisms (Herbert, 1972).

On the other hand, there are interesting exceptions to the requirement for gonadal somatic cell regulation of spermatogenesis. For example, relatively large adult Urechis caupa females (sea worms) (about one meter in length) acquire very small husbands (about one mm in length) who live in their coelomic cavities. The males of the species donate spermatogonia, and these germ cells undergo "typical spermatogenesis" while swimming or floating in the coelomic fluid of the female, (Gould-Somero, 1975). Unless maternal somatic cells become attached to the floating syncytia of germinal cells in ways not yet detected, it appears that spermatogenesis in this species can proceed perfectly well in the absence of nurse-like cells such as Sertoli cells, perhaps because the coelomic fluid provides precisely the correct milieu. Other organisms also have been reported to support sperm-atogenesis without benefit of intimate contact with gonadal somatic cells, such as certain annelids (Roosen-Runge, 1977; Pilsworth and Setchell, 1981). Culture conditions have been found which support much but not all of amphibian spermatogenesis in the absence of somatic cells (Risley, 1983). These observations provide very important clues which should prove helpful in determining the significance of the dependency of germinal cell development upon neigh-boring somatic cells in most species, and in offering an understanding of mechanisms involved.

F) SUMMARY AND CONCLUSIONS

We have developed the concept that mechanisms evolved very early for the modulation of spermatogenesis in response to changes in the external environment, and that these ancient control mechanisms were retained during subsequent evolution. In nearly all animals, the regulation of germinal cell development is postulated to be mediated through the control of gonadal somatic cell functions, associated with the creation and maintenance of an optimal milieu within the spermary or seminiferous tubule in which gametogenesis takes place. In primitive organisms, a small number of stages intervenes between environmental stimuli and subsequent alteration of gonadal somatic cell functions (Figure 5). In contrast, in more complex organisms, the number of intervening stages is greatly amplified and modulated via neuroendocrine mechanisms involving receptors, transducers, and various sorts of relays and messengers (Figure 5).

The evolution of these neural and endocrine controls appears to have occurred in lock-step with the evolution of increasing layers of complexity of regulators of spermatogenesis. This is not unduly surprising, since the requirement to have functionally fertile male and female partners of the same species together at the same time and place would require considerable integration of behavioral and recognition mechanisms during courtship and mating. The

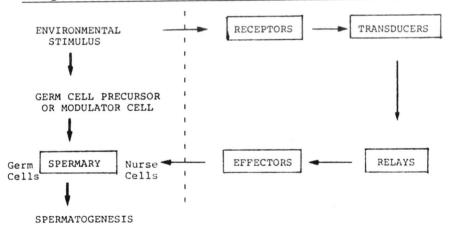

Figure 5. Comparison of Influences of Environmental Stimuli on Spermatogenesis in Simple and Complex Metazaon Organisms
For primitive organisms (left dotted line), see Figure 3; for complex organisms (right of dotted line) see Figure 4. For details, see the text.

nature of these neural mechanisms is likely to prove no less complex than that of mechanisms in the gonad required for successful gamatogenesis.

The neuroendocrine regulation of spermatogenesis in starfish and in chordates is postulated to act in a manner completely homologous to the ways in which external environmental stimuli influence spermatogenesis in more primitive organisms (Figures 3-6). In both sets of cases, the gonadal somatic cells (nurse cells) are the ultimate targets which mediate the effective turning on or turning off of spermatogenesis. The hormone-responsive nurse cells are postulated to achieve this simply by creating a microenvironment in the vicinity of germinal cells which permits the expression of program required for development, or by failing to do so (Figure 6). In mammals, Sertoli cells and peritubular cells, only when optimally stimulated by hormones and paracine factors, are thought to form a functional unit which provides this necessary microenvironment (Figure 2). In less complex organisms, other nurse cell arrangements exist to nourish the syncytia of developing germ cells with the mixture of nutrients, salts, etc. required for a gametogenesis to take place in a protected milieu (Figures 5 and 6).

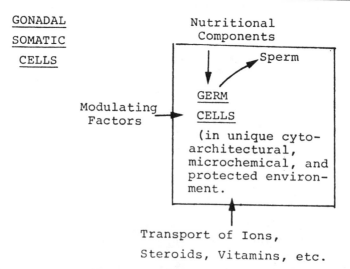

Figure 6. Control of Implementation of Program for Germinal Cell Development

ACKNOWLEDGMENT

It is a pleasure to thank my colleagues especially
Pierre Tung, for many stimulating discussions of topics
related to this article. Work reported from this
laboratory was supported by a grant from the Canadian MRC.
I am grateful to Donna McCabe and Fern Teodoro for their
excellent help in assembling and typing the manuscript.

REFERENCES

Bell G (1982). The Masterpiece of Nature: The Evolution
    and Genetics of Sexuality. London: Croom Helm pp 1-392.
Campbell RD (1974). Cnidaria. In: Reproduction of Marine
    Invertebrates. Vol I (AC Giese and JS Pearse, eds). NY:
    Academic Press pp 133-183.
Clermont Y (1972). Kinetics of spermatogenesis in mammals:
    seminiferous epithelial cycle and spermatogonial renewal.
    Physiol Rev 52:198-236.
Csaba G (1980). Phylogeny and ontogeny of hormone
    receptors: the selection theory of receptor formation and
    hormonal imprinting. Biol Rev 55:47-63.
Dym M, Fawcett DW (1970). The blood-testis barrier in the
    rat and the physiological compartmentation of the
    seminiferous epithelium. Biol Reprod 3:500-532.
Fawcett DW (1975). The ultrastructure and functions of the
    Sertoli cell. In: Handbook of Physiology. Vol V of
    Section 7 (RO Greep and DW Hamilton, eds). Washington:
    Amer Physiol Soc pp 21-55.
Feig LA, Klagsbrun M, Bellve AR (1983). Mitogenic
    polypeptide of the mammalian seminiferous epithelium:
    biochemical characterization and partial purification. J
    Cell Biol 97:1435-1443.
Fell PE (1974). Porifera. In: Reproduction of Marine
    Invertebrates. Vol I (AC Giese and JS Pearse, eds). NY:
    Academic Press pp 51-132.
Fritz IB (1978). Sites of action of androgens and follicle
    stimulating hormone on cells of the seminiferous tubule.
    In: Biochemical Actions of Hormones, Vol V (G Litwack,
    ed). NY: Academic Press pp 249-281.
Fritz IB (1984). Past, present and future of molecular and
    cellular endocrinology of the testis. In: Recent
    Progress in Cellular Endocrinology of the Testis (JM
    Saez, MG Forest, A Dazard, J Bertrand, eds). Paris:
    Editions INSERM 123:15-54.

Fritz IB, Skinner MK, Tung PS (1985). The nature of somatic cell interactions in the seminiferous tubule. In: Development and Functions of the Reproductive Organs (A Eshkol and A Tsafriri, eds). NY: Raven Press in press.

Fritz IB, Tung PS (1985). The role of interactions between peritubular cells and Sertoli cells in mammalian testicular functions. In: Gametogenesis and the Early Embryo (JG Gall, ed). 44th Symposium Society Develop Biol. NY: Alan R Liss Inc in press.

Giese AC, Pearse JS (1974). Introduction, general principles. In: Reproduction of Marine Invertebrates, Vol I (AC Giese and JS Pearse, eds). NY: Academic Press pp 1-49.

Gould-Somero M (1975). Echiura. In: Reproduction of Marine Invertebrates, Vol III (AC Giese and JS Pearse, eds). NY: Academic Press pp 227-311.

Gravis CJ (1978). Testicular involution after optic enucleation: ultrastructure and alkaline phosphatase cytochemistry of the peritubular tissue. Am J Anat 151:213-226.

Harris GW (1955). Neural Control of the Pituitary Gland. London: Edward Arnold Ltd pp 1-285.

Heldin CH, Westermark B (1984). Growth factors: mechanisms of action and relation to oncogenes. Cell 37:9-20.

Herbert J (1972). Behavioral patterns. In: Reproduction in Mammals, Vol IV: Reproductive Patterns (CR Austin and RV Short, eds) Cambridge: University Press pp 34-68.

Horgen PA (1981). The role of the steroid sex pheromone antheridiol in controlling the development of male sex organs in the water mold Achlya. In: Sexual Interactions in Eukaryotic Microbes (DH O'Day and PA Horgen, eds). NY: Academic Press pp 155-178.

Kanatani H (1985). Oocyte growth and maturation in starfish. In: Biology of Fertilization. Vol I: Model Systems and Oogenesis (CB Metz and A Monroy, eds) NY: Acadmemic Press pp 119-140.

Kimble J (1985). Control of post-embryonic germ cell line development in Caenorhabditis. In: Gametogenesis and the Early Embryo (JG Gall, ed). 44th Symposium, Society Develop Biol. NY: Alan R Liss, Inc in press.

Kratochwil K (1982). Embryonic induction. In: Cell Interactions and Development. Molecular Mechanisms (KM Yamada, ed). NY: Wiley pp 100-122.

Lodge JR, Salisbury GW (1970). Seasonal variation and male reproductive efficiency. In: The Testis Vol III (AD Johnson, WR Gomes, NL Vandemark, eds). NY: Academic Press pp 139-165.

Lofts B (1968). Patterns of testicular activity. In: Perspectives in Endocrinology. Hormones in the Lives of Lower Vertebrates (EJW Barrington, CB Jorgensen, eds) NY: Academic Press pp 239-304.

Maruo T, Cohen J, Segal SJ, Kiode SS (1979). Production of choriogonadotropin-like factor by a microorganism. Proc Natl Acad Sci USA 76:6622-6626.

Masui Y (1985). Meiotic arrest in animal oocytes. In: Biology of Fertilization. Vol I, Model Systems and Oogenesis (CB Metz, A Monroy, eds). NY: Academic Press pp 189-220.

Mather JP (1984). Intratesticular regulation: evidence for autocrine and paracrine control of testicular function. In: Mammalian Cell Culture (MP Mather, ed). NY: Plenum Press pp 167-193.

Metz CB, Monroy A (1985). Preface. In: Biology of Fertilization, Vol 1 (CB Metz and A Monroy, eds). NY: Academic Press.

Nial HD (1982). The evolution of peptide hormones. Ann Rev Physiol 44:615-624.

Pilsworth LM, Setchell BP (1981). Spermatogenic and endocrine functions of the testes of invertebrate and vertebrate animals. In: The Testis (H Burger, D de Kretser, eds). NY: Raven Press pp 9-38.

Risley MS (1983). Spermatogenic cell differentiation in vitro. Gamete Res 4:331-346.

Roosen-Runge EC (1977). The Process of Spermatogenesis in Animals. Cambridge: Cambridge University Press pp 1-200.

Roth J, LeRoith D, Shiloach J, Rosenzweig JL, Lesniak MA, Havrankova J (1982). The evolutionary origins of hormones, neurotransmittors, and other intracellular chemical messengers. New England J Med 306:523-527.

Russel LD (1980). Sertoli-germ cell interrelations: a review. Gamete Res 3:179-202.

Sadleir RMFS (1972). Environmental effects. In: Reproduction in Mammals, Vol IV: Reproductive Patterns (CR Austin and RV Short, eds). Cambridge: University Press pp 69-93.

Setchell BP (1978). The Mammalian Testis. London: Elek pp 1-432.

Setchell BP (1982). Spermatogenesis and spermatozoa. In: Reproduction in Mammals Vol I: Germ Cells and Fertilization (CR Austin and RV Short, eds). Cambridge: Cambridge University Press, 2nd edition pp 63-101.

Scharrer E (1959). General and phylogenetic interpretations of neuroendocrine interrelations. In: Comparative Endocrinology (A Gorbman, ed). NY: Hohn Wiley pp 233-249.

Skinner MK, Fritz IB (1985a). Testicular peritubular cells secrete a protein under androgen control that modulates Sertoli cell functions. Proc Nat Acad Sci (USA) 82:114-118.

Skinner MK, Fritz IB (1985b). Androgen stimulation of Sertoli cell functions is enhanced by peritubular cells. Molec Cell Endocrinol 40:115-122.

Skinner MK, Tung PS, Fritz IB (1985). Cooperativity between Sertoli cells and testicular peritubular cells in the production and deposition of extracellular matrix components. J Cell Biol 100:1941-1947.

Smith JM (1978). The Evolution of Sex. Cambridge: Cambridge University Press pp 1-194.

Stefanini M, Conti M, Geremia R, Ziparo E (1985). Regulatory mechanisms of mammalian spermatogenesis. In: Biology of Fertilization Vol 2: Biology of the Sperm (CB Metz and A Monroy, eds). NY: Academic press pp 59-102.

Tung PS, Fritz IB (1980). Interactions of Sertoli cells with myoid cells in vitro. Biol Reprod 23:207-217.

Waites GMH, Gladwell RT (1982). Physiological significance of fluid secretion in the testis and blood-testis barrier. Physiol Rev 62:624-671.

Ward S (1985). The asymmetric localization of gene products during development of Caenorhabditis spermatozoa. In: Gametogenesis and the Early Embryo (JG Gall, ed). 44th Symposium, Society Develop Biol. NY: Alan R Liss, Inc in press.

Willmer EN (1970). Cytology and Evolution. NY: Academic Press, 2nd ed. pp 121-154.

Section 5. MECHANISM OF HORMONE ACTION ON CELLULAR DIFFERENTIATION

Cellular Endocrinology: Hormonal Control of Embryonic
and Cellular Differentiation, pages 391–399
© 1986 Alan R. Liss, Inc.

DNA METHYLATION AND DRUG RESISTANCE IN VARIANTS OF
C3H10T1/2 Cl 8 CELLS

Lesley A. Michalowsky and Peter A. Jones
USC Comprehensive Cancer Center
2025 Zonal Avenue, Los Angeles, CA   90033.

One of the mechanisms by which eukaryotic cells regulate gene expression and differentiation is by the methylation of specific cytosine residues within DNA (Riggs and Jones, 1983). About 3% of the cytosines in mammalian DNA are enzymatically modified to 5-methylcytosine shortly after replication.   5-Methylcytosine is the only modified base in mammalian DNA and is found predominantly in the sequence 5'CpG3'. Significantly, this doublet is statistically underrepresented in eukaryotic DNA (Josse et al., 1961).

The extent and pattern of genomic DNA methylation varies with cell type, and is species and tissue-specific (Gama-Sosa et al., 1983; Ehrlich et al., 1983; Razin and Szyf, 1984).   The generation of tissue-specific patterns during development may occur by sequential changes in the methylation patterns of cells (Razin and Riggs, 1980; Razin, 1984).   Once established, the methylation patterns may be faithfully inherited for many generations, thus ensuring the fidelity of the information code (Stein et al., 1982).   Patterns of DNA methylation are maintained by DNA methyltransferase enzymes (Simon et al., 1978) that recognize hemimethylated DNA as their specific substrate (Gruenbaum et al., 1982).   In addition, de novo DNA methyltransferases function to impose sequence specific patterns of DNA methylation at sites previously not methylated (Groudine and Conklin, 1985).   These methylase enzymes mediate the site-specific changes in cytosine modification patterns.   Such changes within genes may represent regulatory signals vital, but not necessarily sufficient, for the induction of transcription within that gene.

Highly specific DNA-protein interactions most probably regulate gene expression in eukaryotes. 5-Methylcytosine has been shown to affect protein-DNA interactions (Razin and Riggs, 1980) and in this way may modulate the activity of certain genes. It is not known whether DNA methylation at specific sites exerts its biological effects directly or via conformational changes in chromatin.

Studies on the differential states of DNA methylation in various tissues at different stages of development have shown correlations between DNA methylation and gene activity (McGhee and Felsenfeld, 1980). Active genes are hypomethylated in expressing cells whereas they are methylated in cells in which they are not being transcribed (Doerfler, 1983). The question of DNA methylation being a cause or consequence of gene inactivation has been addressed by the in vitro methylation of genes before their introduction into eukaryotic cells (Busslinger et al., 1983; Langer et al., 1984). These experiments have suggested that transcriptional inactivity is a result of methylation. Furthermore, the methylation status of the 5' region of the gene is more important in modulating gene expression than methylation at other regions (Keshet et al., 1985).

However, not all eukaryotic genes are regulated by DNA methylation (Bird, 1984) and alterations in methylation patterns do not always occur during changes in gene expression (McKeon, 1982). Ribosomal RNA genes and vitellogenin genes are expressed even when heavily methylated (Macleod and Bird, 1983; Gerber-Huber et al., 1983). DNA methylation may therefore represent a topographical coding constraint which constitutes part of the multilevel control system of eukaryotic gene expression. Undermethylation of specific cytosine residues may be a necessary, but not sufficient, condition for the expression of some but not all genes.

Experiments using 5-azacytidine (5-aza-CR) or 5-azadeoxycytidine (5-aza-CdR) have provided further evidence for a causative role for hypomethylation in gene expression. These nucleotide analogs are powerful inducers of gene expression and cell differentiation in many experimental systems (Jones, 1985). 5-Aza-CR can be incorporated into DNA, but cannot be methylated (Jones and Taylor, 1980) and inhibits DNA methylation probably by forming a tight complex with the DNA methyl transferase, thus preventing the progression of the enzyme along the DNA duplex (Taylor and Jones, 1982; Christman et al., 1985).

Biologically active doses of 5-aza-CR are potent inhibitors of DNA methylation, and are strong inducers of gene expression. Thus, the dramatic phenotypic alterations induced by these analogs are thought to be due to changes in the methylation patterns of treated cells (Riggs and Jones, 1983).

5-Aza-CR can alter the differentiated state of certain eukaryotic cells. For example, 5-aza-CR treatment of the non-muscle mouse embryo cell line (10T1/2) results in the formation of twitching muscle cells (Constantinides et al., 1977). This phenotypic change presumably reflects the concerted switching of many genes, or the activation of some "master switch" that then invokes the simultaneous expression of muscle-specific genes. The analog does, in addition, have marked effects on the transcription of individual, selectable gene products. The expression of thymidine kinase, for example, is increased 10^5-10^6 fold following exposure to the drug (Harris, 1983). The activation frequencies of certain housekeeping genes are many orders of magnitude greater than those expected for the activity of mutagenic agents. Indeed, 5-aza-CR is not significantly mutagenic in eukaryotic cells (Landolph and Jones, 1982; Delers et al., 1984; Kerbel et al., 1984) and yet it induces somatically heritable changes in genetic programming.

Another example of the dramatic effects of 5-aza-CR is the reactivation of genes located on the inactivated X-chromosome in female mammals. Treatment with the analog induces the expression of such genes as HGPRTase, (Mohandas et al., 1981) and glucose-6-phosphate dehydrogenase (Wolf et al., 1984). Since 5-aza-CR treatment leads to hypomethylation, it is likely that DNA methylation is somehow responsible for X chromosome inactivation (Wolf and Migeon, 1982).

Although much of the recent interest in azanucleosides has been directed to their powerful effects on gene expression, the analogs were originally developed as cancer chemotherapeutic agents (Vesely and Cihak, 1978). The chemotherapeutic potency of 5-aza-CdR is hindered by the development of resistance to the antineoplastic drug (Vesely et al., 1967). This resistance represents a serious problem in the treatment of cancer, and may be caused by decreased drug transport, decreased activity of activating enzymes, or increased levels of drug detoxification (Vesely et al., 1970). For some drugs, the molecular basis of drug resistance has also been associated with gene amplification (Mariani and Schimke, 1984). The precise mechanism of 5-aza-

CdR resistance remains unknown, although this would be of special interest in view of the dramatic effects of the drug on cellular differentiation.

We have therefore derived a series of 10T1/2 mouse cell lines that are resistant to 5-aza-CdR and will be useful for studying drug resistance, DNA methylation and gene expression. The cell line T17 was derived from C3H10T1/2 C18 cells after multiple treatments with increasing concentrations of 5-aza-CdR (Flatau et al., 1984). Drug treatment lasted for 24 hr. before the medium was changed and the cells allowed to recover. Treated cells were passaged every 7 to 10 days, and the treatment cycle with increasing 5-aza-CdR concentrations was repeated. T17 cells were exposed 17 times to 5-aza-CdR concentrations ranging from 1 µM to 100 µM.

Successive 5-aza-CdR treatments resulted in progressively decreased levels of overall DNA methylation (Table 1). Clones isolated from mass cultures exposed to 5-aza-CdR for a specific number of times showed similar amounts of cytosine modification as did the respective mass culture. This demonstrated that the cultures were homogeneous with regard to overall 5-methylcytosine content, and that the treatments were not selecting for cells with low methylation levels. Cells were isolated with 5 methylcytosine contents as low as 0.6%, which represented an 80% decrease from the level of 3.22% in the parental C3H10T1/2 cells. Clones with methylation levels lower than 0.45% were not obtained even after further drug treatments. Our failure to derive cell lines with less than 0.45% 5-methylcytosine may be due to the fact that methylation levels below this limit result in abnormal patterns of gene expression and cell death.

Significantly, the decreased DNA modification levels of the 10T1/2 derivatives were not stable. The genomic content of 5-methylcytosine increased as the cells were passaged in the absence of further drug treatment. Clones isolated from the mass cell culture also underwent de novo methylation suggesting that the increased methylation levels were not due to a selection of preexisting cells with high methylation levels within the population. The remethylation phenomenon has previously been observed with the passage of 5-aza-CR-treated clones of T lymphoid cells (Gasson et al., 1983). This suggests that de novo methylation can occur in cultured cells, and thus provides an excellent system for studying the role of de novo methylation in gene silencing.

Table 1.   Effects of multiple 5-aza-CdR treatments on the overall DNA methylation levels of 10T1/2 derivatives.

$$\% \ 5mCyt = \frac{[\ 5mCyt\ ]}{[\ 5mCyt\ ] + [\ Cyt\ ]} \ x \ 100$$

Number of 5-Aza-CdR Treatments	Mass Culture	Clones from Mass Culture		
0	3.22	3.27	3.28	3.31
7	1.30	1.11	1.29	1.65
12	1.04	1.04	1.34	1.38
16	0.64	0.73	0.73	0.89
20	0.45	0.62	0.63	0.75

We are currently studying the remethylation of house-keeping genes, non-expressed genes and mouse satellite sequences in order to plot the development of new methylation patterns. The clones may exhibit a hierarchy of remethylation of certain classes of genes, thus initiating gene switching and phenotypic changes in the cell lineage.

Cytotoxicity assays revealed that the 5-aza-CdR-treated cell lines were 30 times more resistant to the toxic effects of 5-aza-CdR than the parental 10T1/2 cells (Table 2). Furthermore, the resistant phenotype was stable when the cells were passaged at least 30 times in the absence of 5-aza-CdR. Slight cross-resistance to 5-aza-CR was evident.

Table 2:   Drug resistance of 10T1/2 and Aza-CdR-treated 10T1/2 derivatives.

	50% Lethal Dose, µM	
	10T1/2	T17
Aza-CdR	0.1	3.0
Aza-CR	3.5	25.0
Ara-C	0.3	0.7

Resistance to pyrimidine analogs may be due to altered activities of the enzymes responsible for transporting, activating, or detoxifying the nucleosides. Incorporation studies showed that the resistant cells incorporated the same amount of 5-aza-CdR as did 10T1/2 cells, thus suggesting that the emergence of resistance was not due to inefficiencies of drug transport and utilization. Moreover, the 10T1/2 derivatives were not significantly more resistant to ara-C (Table 2) which is a nucleoside analog whose detoxification involves the same deaminase enzymes utilized in azanucleoside metabolism. The development of drug resistance in these 10T1/2 variants was therefore not due merely to decreased drug transport or to increased drug inactivation. The cell lines may consequently be important for the characterization of the mechanism of 5-aza-CdR resistance. Furthermore, the results of these studies may be valuable in elucidating mechanisms common to other types of drug resistance, as well as being significant in molecular analysis of gene regulation.

ACKNOWLEDGEMENTS

This work was supported by grant CA 39913 from the National Cancer Institute, Bethesda, Maryland.

REFERENCES

Bird AP (1984). DNA methylation-how important in gene control? Nature 308:503-504.
Busslinger M, Hurst J, Flavell RA (1983). DNA methylation and the regulation of globin gene expression. Cell 34:197-206.
Christman JK, Schneiderman N, Acs G (1985). Formation of highly stable complexes between 5-azacytosine-substituted DNA and specific non-histone nuclear proteins. Implications for 5-azacytidine-mediated effects on DNA methylation and gene expression. J Biol Chem 260:4059-4068.
Constantinides PG, Jones PA, Gevers W (1977). Functional striated muscle cells from non-myoblast precursors following 5-azacytidine treatment. Nature 267:364-366.
Delers A, Szpirer J, Szpirer C, Saggioro D (1984). Spontaneous and 5-azacytidine-induced re-expression of ornithine carbamoyl transferase in hepatoma cells. Mol Cell Biol 4:809-812.
Doerfler W (1983). DNA methylation and gene activity. Ann Rev Biochem 52:93-124.

Ehrlich M, Gama-Sosa MA, Huang L-H, Midgett RM, Kuo KC, McCune RA, Gehrke C (1983). Amount and distribution of 5-methylcytosine in human DNA from different types of tissues or cells. Nuc Acids Res 10:2709-2721.

Flatau E, Gonzales FA, Michalowsky LA, Jones PA (1984). DNA methylation in 5-aza-2'-deoxycytidine resistant variants of C3H10T1/2 Cl 8 cells. Mol Cell Biol 4:2098-2102.

Gama-Sosa MA, Midgett R, Slagel VA, Githens S, Kuo KC, Gehrke CW, Ehrlich M (1983). Tissue specific differences in DNA methylation in various mammals. Biochim Biophys Acta 740:212-219.

Gasson JC, Ryden T, Bourgeois S (1983). Role of de novo DNA methylation in the glucocorticoid resistance of a T-lymphoid cell line. Nature 302:621-623.

Gerber-Huber S, May FEB, Westley BR, Felber BK, Hosbach HA, Andres A-C, Ryffel, GU (1983). In contrast to other Xenopus genes the estrogen-inducible vitellogenin genes are expressed when totally methylated. Cell 33:43-51.

Groudine M, Conklin KF (1985). Chromatin structure and de novo methylation of sperm DNA: implication for activation of paternal genome. Science 228:1061-1068.

Gruenbaum Y, Cedar H, Razin A (1982). Substrate and sequence specificity of a eukaryotic DNA methylase. Nature 295:620-622.

Harris M (1982). Induction of thymidine kinase in enzyme-deficient Chinese hamster cells. Cell 29:483-492.

Jones PA (1985). Altering gene expression with 5-azacytidine. Cell 40:485-486.

Jones PA, Taylor SM (1980). Cellular differentiation, cytidine analogs and DNA methylation. Cell 20:85-93.

Josse J, Kaiser AA, Kornberg A (1961). Enzymatic synthesis of deoxyribonucleic acid. VII Frequencies of nearest neighbor base sequences in deoxyribonucleic acid. J Biol Chem 236:864-875.

Kerbel RS. Frost P, Liteplo R, Carlow D, Elliot BE (1984). Possible epigenetic mechanisms of tumor progression: induction of high frequency heritable but phenotypically unstable changes in the tumorigenic and metastatic properties of tumor cell populations by 5-azacytidine treatment. J Cell Physiol Suppl 3:87-97.

Keshet I, Yisraeli J, Cedar H (1985). Effect of regional DNA methylation on gene expression. Proc Natl Acad Sci (USA) 82:2560-2564.

Landolph JR, Jones PA (1982). Mutagenicity of 5-azacytidine and related nucleosides in C3H10T1/2 Cl 8 and V79 cells. Cancer Res 42:817-823.

Langer K-D, Vardimon L, Renz D, Doerfler W (1984). DNA methylation of three 5'-CCGG-3' sites in the promoter and 5' region inactivate the E2a gene of adenovirus type 2. Proc Natl Acad Sci (USA) 81:2950-2954.

Macleod D, Bird AP (1983). Transcription in oocytes of highly methylated rDNA from Xenopus laevis sperm. Nature 306:200-203.

McGhee JD, Felsenfeld G (1980). Nucleosome structure. Ann Rev Biochem 49:1115-1156.

McKeon C, Ohkubo H, Pastan I, deCrombuggle B (1982). Unusual methylation pattern of the α2(1) collagen gene. Cell 29:203-210.

Mariani BD, Schimke RT (1984). Gene amplication in a single cell cycle in Chinese hamster ovary cells. J Biol Chem 259:1901-1910.

Mohandas T, Sparkes RS, Shapiro LJ (1981). Reactivation of an inactive human X chromosome: Evidence for X inactivation by DNA methylation. Science 211:393-396.

Razin A (1984). DNA methylation patterns: Formation and Biological functions. In Razin A, Cedar H, Riggs AD (eds): "DNA methylation. Biochemistry and Biological Significance" Springer-Verlag p. 127-146.

Razin A, Riggs AD (1980). DNA methylation and gene function. Science 210:604-610.

Razin A, Szyf M (1984). DNA methylation patterns. Formation and function. Biochim et Biophys Acta 782:331-342.

Riggs AD, Jones PA (1983). 5-Methylcytosine, gene regulation and cancer. Adv in Cancer Res 40:1-30.

Simon D, Grunert F, v. Acken U, Doring HP, Kroger H (1978). DNA-methylase from regenerating rat liver: purification and characterization. Nuc Acids Res 5:2153-2167.

Stein R, Gruenbaum Y, Pollack Y, Razin A, Cedar H (1982). Clonal inheritance of the pattern of DNA methylation in mouse cells. Proc Natl Acad Sci (USA) 79:61-65.

Taylor SM, Jones PA (1982). Mechanism of action of eukaryotic DNA methyltransferase. Use of azacytosine-containing DNA. J Mol Biol 162:679-692.

Vesely J, Cihak A (1978). 5-Azacytidine: mechanism of action and biological effects in mammalian cells. Pharm Ther 2:813-840.

Vesely J, Cihak A, Sorm F (1967). Biochemical mechanisms of drug resistance. Development of resistance to 5-azacytidine and simultaneous depression of pyrimidine metabolism in leukemic mice. J Cancer 2:639-646.

Vesely J, Cihak A, Sorm F (1970). Association of decreased uridine and deoxycytidine kinase with enhanced RNA and DNA polymerase in mouse leukemic cells resistant to 5-azacytidine and 5-aza-2'-deoxycytidine. Cancer Res 30:2180-2186.

Wolf SF, Dintzis S, Toniolo D, Presico G, Lunnen KD, Axelman J, Migeon BR (1984). Complete concordance between glucose-6-phosphate dehydrogenase activity and hypomethylation of CpG clusters: implications for X-chromosome dosage compensation. Nucl Acids Res 12:9333-9348.

Wolf SF, Migeon BR (1982). Studies of X-chromosome DNA methylation in normal human cells. Nature 295:667-671.

Cellular Endocrinology: Hormonal Control of Embryonic and Cellular Differentiation, pages 401-415
© 1986 Alan R. Liss, Inc.

ROLE OF CYTODIFFERENTIATION AND CELL-CELL COMMUNICATION IN THE ANDROGEN DEPENDENT EXPRESSION OF α_{2u} GLOBULIN GENE IN RAT LIVER

A.K. Roy, F.H. Sarkar, A.C. Nag and M.A. Mancini

Department of Biological Sciences, Oakland University, Rochester, Michigan 48063

INTRODUCTION

The discovery of the bacterial operon for the regulation of gene expression through specific DNA binding proteins during early sixties led to an intense search for a similar mechanism in the eukaryotic system. Since hormones were known to be involved in the regulation of specific gene expression, the intermediate events between hormone uptake and target gene expression naturally became the subject of immediate scrutiny. Such studies resulted in the development of several well-characterized model systems and many conceptual advances were made. These include: (a) appreciation of the critical role of specific receptor proteins in hormone action (Jensen et al., 1962; Gorski et al., 1968); (b) mediation of certain types of hormone action through activation of adenyl cyclase (Robison et al, 1981); (c) sequence-specific binding of steroid hormone receptors to target genes (Payvar et al., 1981); and (d) close relationship between the mode of action of several peptide hormones and the growth factors such as the products of so called "oncogenes", (Hunter, 1984). All of these advances took place despite the enormous structural complexity and cellular heterogeneity of eukaryotic tissues. Because of their physiological abnormalities, the established animal cell lines were of limited use for the study of hormone action. Thus, many investigators were attracted to physiologically relevant models which are simple enough for critical biochemical analysis (reviewed by Goldberger & Deeley, 1980).

Such a reductionist approach with simple models has played an important role in elucidation of the biochemical basis of hormone action. However, this approach has underestimated many important control mechanisms, especially cell-cell interactions which may greatly influence the overall coordination of hormonal control of gene expression under a complex architectural network as encountered in the multicellular organism. As we know today, Goldberger's most simplified transcriptionally regulated system (i.e. chicken liver) looks considerably more complex than initially perceived. These complications appear to be an integral part of the eukaryotic gene regulation which may have been overlooked in simple model systems. Some of these issues have received considerable attention in this symposium and have been addressed in other chapters.

α_{2u} Globulin in the Rat Liver and its Hormonal Regulation

Earlier studies in our laboratory, aimed at the identification and characterization of various proteins in the rat urine, led to the discovery of an 18 kilodalton major male rat urinary protein called α_{2u} globulin (Roy, Neuhaus and Harmison, 1966; Roy et al., 1983). This protein was found to be synthesized and secreted by the hepatic parenchymal cells. Primarily because of its low molecular weight, it is rapidly filtered through the kidneys and appears as the principal urinary protein. It is normally present only in the liver of mature male rats where it appears at puberty (approx. 40 days) and reaches a peak level at about 75-85 days of age. A gradual age-dependent decline begins around 150 days and ultimately around 800 days there is a total cessation of α_{2u} globulin synthesis (Fig. 1). α_{2u} globulin can be induced in the female rat after ovariectomy followed by androgen treatment. Besides androgen, several other hormones including pituitary growth hormone, insulin, glucocorticoid and thyroxine synergistically influence the multihormonal regulation of α_{2u} globulin (Roy, 1973, Roy et al., 1980). In the mature male rat, normal hepatic synthesis of α_{2u} globulin can be totally inhibited by daily treatment of estrogenic hormones (Roy, McMinn and Biswas, 1975).

α_{2u} globulin is coded by a multigene family comprising of about 30 gene copies per haploid genome (Kurtz, 1981). Both the cDNA and the natural gene have been cloned and

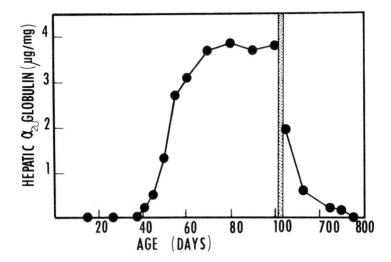

Figure 1. Age-dependent changes in hepatic α_{2u} globulin in the male rat. Hepatic content of α_{2u} globulin is presented as radioimunoassayable α_{2u} globulin per mg of hepatic protein within the liver cytosol. A change in the scale from a unit of 20 days to 100 days is represented at the dotted bar. (From Roy et al., J. Biol. Chem. 258, 10123, 1983)

sequenced (Dolan et al., 1982; Roy & Chatterjee, 1985). Studies on the hormonal regulation of this protein so far have shown that except thyroxine all other hormonal modulators seem to primarily influence the synthesis of α_{2u} globulin mRNA.

Studies in our laboratory have identified a 3.5S cytoplasmic androgen binding protein (CAB) which does not translocate into the nucleus (Roy, 1979). A close correlation between the presence of this cytoplasmic androgen binding protein and the ability of the liver to respond to androgenic induction has been established. For example, both prepubertal and senescent rats, which lack the cytoplasmic androgen binding protein, also do not synthesize

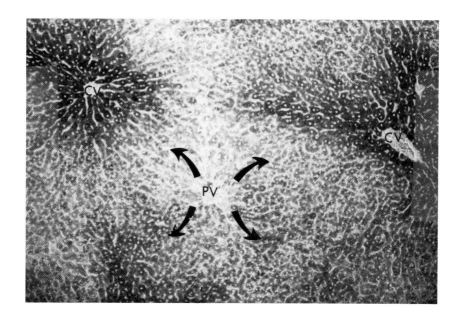

Figure 2. Perivenous concentration of α_{2u} globulin producing hepatocytes. Paraffin section of the adult male rat
liver was immunostained with monospecific antibody to α_{2u}
globulin. The arrows show the direction of blood flow.
PV, portal vein; CV, central vein.

α_{2u} globulin under androgenic stimulation. Because of its
cytoplasmic localization, CAB may have a cytoplasmic regulatory role in mRNA stabilization as proposed for a similar
cytoplasmic estrogen binding protein of the frog liver
(Brock and Shapiro, 1983).

Cellular Architecture of the Rat Liver and Histological
Distribution of α_{2u} Globulin Producing Hepatocytes

    The functional unit of the mammalian liver is organized
as lobules where the peripheral area of this lobular struc-

ture receives the incoming blood supply from branches of both the hepatic artery and the portal vein and the outgoing blood drains into a central vein. Each hepatic lobule is a polygonal prism and in a cross section it is seen as a hexagonal unit where the portal vessels (along with the hepatic artery) form the vertices and surround a central hepatic vein. Cords or plates of hepatocytes radiate from the periphery of the central vein as spokes of a wheel. Thus from a biochemical standpoint the hepatocytes located around the portal vessels (periportal hepatocytes) are in an advantageous position with respect to nutrition and oxygen-rich environment as compared to those located near the central vein (perivenous hepatocytes). Both histological and cytofluorometric analysis of the adult male rat hepatocytes show two distinct cell populations, one of which is much more active in the synthesis of α_{2u} globulin than the other (Antakly et al., 1982; Motwani et al., 1984). Despite their positional disadvantage, in the normal male rat, the perivenous hepatocytes are distinctly more active in the synthesis of α_{2u} globulin than their periportal counterparts (Fig. 2).

Both during androgenic induction of α_{2u} globulin in the ovariectomized female rat, and during puberty in the male rat, the first immunoreactive hepatocytes begin to appear around the perivenous area (Fig. 3, frame A). The relative proportion of α_{2u} globulin positive hepatocytes in the perivenous area of the maturing male and androgen-treated female rats show a general correlation with the amount of α_{2u} globulin mRNA within the total poly(A) containing hepatic RNA. This observation may give an impression that cytodifferentiation alone and not differential regulation of gene expression by sex hormones is the reason for increased synthesis of α_{2u} globulin in the male rat. However, results from other studies show that sex hormones are involved in exerting a differential regulatory influence on the synthesis of α_{2u} globulin by the competent hepatocytes. For example, immunocytochemical staining of age-matched control and estrogen-treated male rats shows a dramatic decrease in the cellular level of α_{2u} globulin. Likewise in the in vitro liver perfusion system a single bolus of androgen within a short period (90 min) causes about tenfold increase in the hepatic synthesis of α_{2u} globulin (Murty, Rao and Roy, 1985). These results indicate that both hormone-mediated increase in competent hepatocytes and the rate of synthesis of α_{2u} globulin within these com-

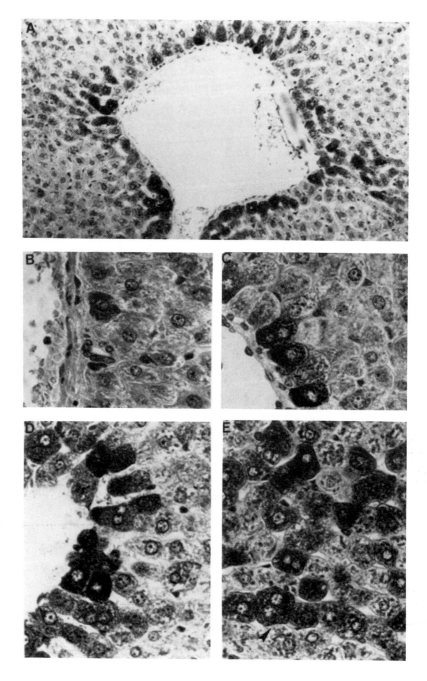

petent cells are responsible for modulating the rate of production of this protein by the liver.

Role of Cytodifferentiation and Cell Recruitment in the Androgenic Induction

Examination of the early stages of the inductive events both during the normal pubertal maturation in the male and during the androgenic induction of ovariectomized females revealed that competent α_{2u} globulin producing cells first appear as a single layer of hepatocytes attached to the central vein. Figure 3 shows the appearance of α_{2u} globulin producing hepatocytes during sexual maturation of the male rat. A similar pattern is also observed in the ovariectomized female rat after androgen treatment. Examination of the early stages of α_{2u} globulin synthesis during puberty in the male shows at least three temporal phases in the attainment and propagation of cellular competency. In the first phase a few cells attached to the wall of the central vein become competent to produce α_{2u} globulin (Figure 3, frame B). In the second phase this inductive process along the venous wall proceeds until a monolayer of hepatocytes attached to the vascular matrix (wall of the central vein) gain competency to synthesize α_{2u} globulin (Figure 3,

Figure 3. Initial induction of α_{2u} globulin in the hepatocytes situated around the central vein and propagation of the induction process during maturation in the male. A, liver from a 40 day-old rat showing a layer of α_{2u} globulin producing (competent) cells attached to the wall of the central vein. B-D, show progressive conversion of cells from non-competent to competent type during maturation (38, 40 & 42 days). In frame B only a solitary competent cell attached to the central vein is seen (circled). Frame C shows the progression of the induction process along the central vein. Frame D shows propagation of the competency within the cells belonging to the same cord. Frame E presents further evidence for the vertical propagation of competency. Adjacent cells in a non-competent cord even with membrane contact (arrow) fail to confer competency (liver from a 45 day-old rat).

frame C). In phase three hepatocytes belonging to the same cord and situated vertically on the competent cells begin to synthesize α_{2u} globulin (Figure 3, frame D). Cords of hepatocytes synthesizing α_{2u} globulin are generally separated from an adjacent non-competent cord by bile canaliculi. These observations indicate that cell to cell contact plays a critical role in the conversion of non-competent to competent hepatocytes for the expression of α_{2u} globulin gene.

The observations described above raise several interesting questions and possibilities. (1) Are the stromal cells of the venous wall the primary target of the inducing hormone which subsequently causes cytodifferentiation of the adjacent hepatocytes through secondary mediators? (2) What is the possible mechanism of the vertical propagation of the inductive influence? and, (3) Do α_{2u} globulin producing cells differ from the non-competent variety with respect to other gene expression?

Cunha and his associates have extensively studied prostatic development in tissue recombinants composed of urinary bladder epithelium and urogenital sinus mesenchyme (Cunha et al., 1983). These studies clearly indicate that androgen mediated cytodifferentiation and differential gene expression in epithelial cells are indirect events. Using Tfm and wild-type tissue recombinants they have shown that the presence of androgen receptors in the supporting stromal cells and not in the overlying bladder epithelium dictates the androgen mediated cytodifferentiation and prostate specific gene expression in the epithelial layer. Since hepatic blood vessels are derived from the mesenchymal tissue a similar mechanism for androgen action on the hepatocytes around the central vein is a distinct possibility.

The next question concerns the mechanism for the vertical propagation of the inductive influence. Certain morphological observation presented in figure 3 may provide important clues to the process. (a) the process of propagation absolutely requires cell-to-cell contact, (b) effective propagation is limited only to adjacent cells on the same cellular cord. A non-producing cell belonging to a different cord fails to gain competency. Thus, it seems that not only cell-to-cell contact but also a specific type of contact is essential to confer competency from one cell to another.

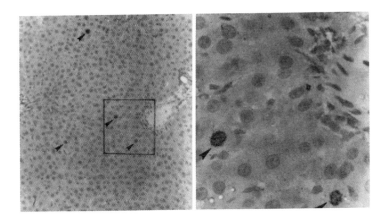

Figure 4. Tritiated thymidine incorporation into the hepatocyte nuclei of an ovariectomized female rat after 4 days of androgen treatment. The labeled nuclei are marked with arrowheads. The right frame shows a magnified picture of the periportal zone (boxed area in the left frame).

(c) In most cases, vertical transmission of competency is an all or none process, i.e. the process proceeds from one cell to the next and does not proceed to the third cell until the newly competent cell has attained a certain degree of competency. This indicates that saturation kinetics of the effector-receptor interaction may be operational in the transfer of competency. This concept will be elaborated further under the "epilogue".

A recent publication by Spolski, Schneider and Wangh (1985) showing massive (40% to 70%) cell proliferation in the frog liver after 4-6 days of estrogen treatment may indicate a totally different means for propagation of the competency process. A large increase in mitotic activity after estrogenic stimulation may suggest that initial cytodifferentiation is followed by progressive proliferation of the competent cells. We have considered such a possibility for α_{2u} globulin. Figure 4 shows the autoradiographic picture of a liver section from an ovariectomized female rat treated for 4 days with androgen followed by pulse-labelling of the mitotically active nuclei with ^{3}H-thymidine. The picture shows only a small number (less than 1%) of the hepatocytes are active in DNA synthesis, and more importantly, these cells are localized in the vicinity of the portal area rather than around the central vein. These results suggest that cell proliferation is not the mechanism for the propagation of the competency process.

We have addressed the question concerning the extent of cytodifferentiation needed to convert a non-competent hepatocyte to a competent hepatocyte by simply separating the producing and non-producing cells through fluorescence activated cell sorting and analyzing the protein patterns by SDS-polyacrylamide gel electrophoresis. Results which are presented in Fig. 5 show that besides α_{2u} globulin these cells mainly differ only in two other gene products one of which may represent another androgen inducible protein. Irrespective of the identity of these two proteins the important point is that cytodifferentiation which confers competency for the synthesis of α_{2u} globulin does not involve extensive changes in specific gene expression.

EPILOGUE

Although relatively novel to endocrinologists, the critical role of cell-cell communication in cytodifferentiation and organogenesis is a well-established concept among developmental biologists. The biochemical nature of such communicative signals, however, has not been clearly established. In recent years, studies from several laboratories especially those of Cunha, Sirbasku and Moscona (Cunha et al., 1983; Sirbasku, 1981; Linser and Moscona, 1982) have indicated that stimulation of specific gene expression and proliferation of the epithelial cells by androgens, estrogens and glucocorticoid may be indirectly mediated through secondary mediators. These secondary mediators are produced after the primary interaction of the steroid hormone on the underlying non-epithelial cells. Our results are consistent with such a concept. However, it should also be emphasized that although androgens may indirectly influence the perivenous hepatocytes to cause cytodifferentiation and confer competency to produce α_{2u} globulin, modulation of α_{2u} globulin synthesis in the competent cells is also directly influenced by the sex-hormones. This conclusion is supported

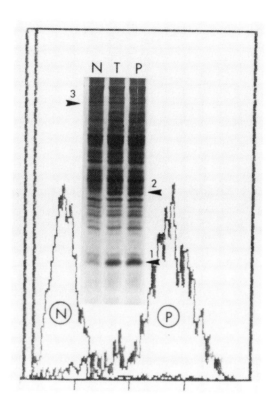

Figure 5. Protein patterns of α_{2u} globulin positive and negative hepatocytes separated by fluorescence activated cell sorting. Hepatocytes were isolated from a 50-day-old male rat and separated into positive (P) and negative (N) cell populations. SDS-polyacrylamide gel electrophoretic patterns of total cellular proteins are shown in the inset. N, negative, T, total and P, positive cells. Arrow heads mark the protein bands that show marked difference between negative and positive populations. Band 1, α_{2u} globulin; Band 2, a 33 kilodalton protein; Band 3, a 90 kilodalton protein. Unlike bands 1 & 2, band 3 is present in a higher concentration in the negative cells.

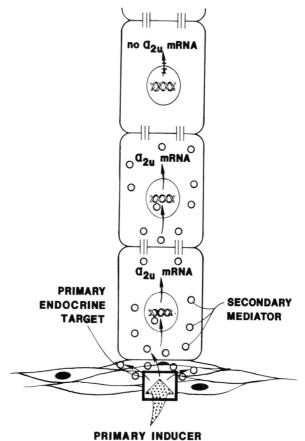

PRIMARY INDUCER

Figure 6. Model for the hormonal induction of α_{2u} globulin in the perivenous hepatocytes and the vertical propagation of the inductive influence through a secondary mediator. Cells in the venous wall are depicted as the primary target for the inducing hormone. This primary action produces a secondary mediator which can be channeled within the cells of the same hepatic cord. The secondary mediator is considered to be essential for the conversion of non-competent cells to competent cells. In addition to the cardinal influence of the secondary mediator, the model also proposes a direct role of androgen on the α_{2u} globulin producing cells.

by the results of the in vitro perfusion experiments and the immunocytochemical demonstration of the inhibition of α_{2u} globulin synthesis in the competent cells after estrogen treatment. The cytoplasmic androgen binding protein may play an important role in this regulatory process.

Despite membrane contact both in the lateral and vertical directions, the propagation of competency only proceeds within the component cells of a cord in a venous to portal direction. This may suggest the role of specific junctional complexes rather than simple membrane contact as a prerequisite for the transmission of the inductive signal. If the signalling process is mediated via a small molecule (1000 daltons or less), gap junctions may provide a channel for such a mediator. Vertical transmission of competency in all or none fashion may indicate a well known endocrinological phenomenon, i.e. presence of vast excess of "spare receptors" for the inductive signal. In every case examined, the target tissue contains an amount of receptor which is greater than the number required for evoking the maximum cellular response. If the same mechanism is operative in the transfer of competency, spare receptors in the newly recruited competent cell will continue to sequester the effector molecules and prevent their flow into the adjacent cell even after it has become totally competent to express α_{2u} globulin gene. The effector molecules can only overflow into the next cell after the spare receptors are saturated. A model based on these considerations is presented in Figure 6. The basic tenets of this model can be subjected to experimental verification.

ACKNOWLEDGMENTS

This work was supported by NIH grant AM-14744. The authors wish to thank Drs. B. Chatterjee and B. Winkler for valuable comments.

REFERENCES

Antalky T, Lynch KR, Nakhasi HL, Feigelson P (1982). Cellular dynamics of the hormonal and developmental induction of α_{2u} globulin as demonstrated by immunocytochemistry and specific mRNA monitoring. Am J Anat 165:211-224.

Brock ML, Shapiro DJ (1983). Estrogen stabilizes vitellogenin mRNA against cytoplasmic degradation. Cell 34:207-
214.

Cunha GR, Chung LWK, Shannon JM, Taguchi O, Fujii H (1983)
Hormone-induced morphogenesis and growth: Role of mesenchymal-epithelial interactions. Rec Prog Horm Res 39:559-
598.

Dolan KP, Unterman R, McLaughlin M, Nakhasi HL, Lynch KR,
Feigelson P (1982). The structure and expression of very
closely related members of the α_{2u} globulin gene family.
J Biol Chem 256:3634-3636.

Goldberger RF, Deeley RG (1980). The effect of estrogen on
gene expression in avian liver. In Roy AK, Clark JH (eds):
"Gene Regulation by Steroid Hormones I," New York:
Springer-Verlag, pp 32-57.

Gorski J, Toft D, Shyamala G, Smith D, Notides A (1968).
Hormone receptors: Studies on the interaction of estrogen
with the uterus. Recent Prog Horm Res 24:45-80.

Hunter T (1984). The proteins of oncogenes. Scientific
American 70-79.

Jensen EV, Jacobsen HJ (1962). Basic guides to the mechanism
of estrogen action. Rec Prog Horm Res 18:387-414.

Kurtz DT (1981). Rat α_{2u} globulin is coded by a multigene
family. J.Mol Appl Gen 1:29-38.

Linser P, Moscona AA (1982). Developmental and experimental
changes in retinal glia cells: Cell interactions and control of phenotype expression and stability. In Moscona
AA, Monroy A (eds) : "Current Topics in Developmental
Biology, Vol. 18," New York: Academic Press, pp 155-188.

Motwani NM, Caron D, Demyan WF, Chatterjee B, Poulik D,
Hunter S, Roy AK (1984). Monoclonal antibody to α_{2u} globulin and immunocytofluorometric analysis of α_{2u} globulin
synthesizing hepatocytes after androgenic induction on
aging. J Biol Chem 259:3653-3657.

Murty CVR, Rao KVS, Roy AK (1985). Independent regulatory
influence of androgen and growth hormone on the hepatic
synthesis of α_{2u} globulin. Endocrinology 116:109.

Payvar F, Wrange Ö, Carlsedt-Duke J, Okret S, Gustafson J,
Yamamoto K (1981). Purified glucocorticoid receptors bind
selectively in vitro to a cloned DNA fragment whose transcription is regulated by glucocorticoids in vivo. Proc
Natl Acad Sci USA 78:6628-32.

Robison GA, Butcher RW, Sutherland EW (1981). Cyclic AMP,
New York, Academic Press.

Roy AK, Chatterjee B, Demyan WF, Milin BS, Motwani NM, Nath
TS, Schiop MJ (1983). Hormone and age-dependent regulation

of α_{2u} globulin gene expression. Recent Prog Horm Res 39: 425-461.

Roy AK, Chatterjee B (1985). Gene regulation by androgens. In Handbook on Receptor Research: Sex Steroid Receptors. Auricchio, F (ed), Field Educational Italia, Rome, pp 157-177.

Roy AK, Chatterjee B, Demyan WF, Nath TS, Motwani NM (1982). Pretranslational regulation of α_{2u} globulin in the rat liver by the growth hormone. J Biol Chem 257:7834-7838

Roy AK, Chatterjee B, Prasad MSK, Unakar NJ (1980). Role of insulin in the regulation of the hepatic mRNA for α_{2u} globulin in diabetic rats. J Biol Chem 255:11614-18.

Roy AK (1973). Androgen dependent synthesis of α_{2u} globulin in the rat: Role of the pituitary gland. J Endocrinol 56: 295-301.

Roy AK, Neuhaus OW, Harmison CR (1966). Preparation and characterization of a sex-dependent rat urinary protein. Biochim Biophys Acta 127:72-81.

Roy AK (1979). Hormonal regulation by α_{2u} globulin synthesis in rat liver. Biochemical Actions Horm 6:481-517.

Roy AK, McMinn D, Biswas NM (1975). Estrogenic inhibition of the hepatic synthesis of α_{2u} globulin in the rat. Endocrinology 97:1501-1508.

Sirbasku DA (1981). New concepts in the control of estrogen responsive tumor growth. Branbury Report 8:425-443.

Spolski RJ, Schneider W, Wangh LJ (1985). Estrogen-dependent DNA synthesis and parenchymal cell proliferation in the liver of adult male Xenopus frogs. Dev Biol 108:332-340.

Cellular Endocrinology: Hormonal Control of Embryonic
and Cellular Differentiation, pages 417–431
© 1986 Alan R. Liss, Inc.

CYTOPLASMIC FACTORS REGULATING CELLULAR DIFFERENTIATION

Jerry W. Shay

University of Texas Southwestern Medical School,
Department of Cell Biology, Dallas, Texas 75235

Introduction

Cell enucleation and fusion provide a technology to
determine if the cell cytoplasm contains stable regulatory substances that might modulate nuclear gene expression. Enucleation separates cells into nuclear and
cytoplasmic components termed karyoplasts and cytoplasts,
respectively. A cytoplasmic hybrid or cybrid is defined
as the viable, proliferating fusion product of a cytoplast and a whole cell. It has been reported that added
cytoplasm can have either a permanent (Gopalakrishan and
Anderson, 1979; Lipsich et al., 1979; Gopalakrishan et
al., 1977; Ber and Wiener, 1978), long-lived (2-8 weeks)
(Linder, 1980; Kahn et al., 1981), short-lived (1-2 days)
(Lipsich et al., 1979; Clark and Shay, 1982), or no
effect on the phenotype of the whole cell recipient. In
the present experiments cytoplasts derived from a non-
tumorigenic cell line (AMT) were fused to either Y-1
adrenal tumor cells or T984-15 a non-differentiating
mesenchymal tumor cell line cloned from a myoblast line
(Shay et al., 1981). The resulting cybrids were compared
to the parental cells as to differentiation phenotype and
tumorigenicity. In the Y-1 experiments, cytoplasmic
factors inhibited steroidogenesis for 2-3 weeks but had
no effect on tumorigenicity. Additional experiments
indicated that this cytoplasmic inhibition was not due to
trauma of the enucleation and fusion procedures, time
required to resynthesize the steroidogenic machinery, or
to mitochondria (Clark and Shay, 1982). In the T984-15
experiments, AMT cytoplasmic factors induced myogenesis
and suppressed tumorigenicity (Shay et al, 1981).

Although 20 of 20 of the parental T984-15 subclones produced tumors and none differentiated into muscle, only 2 of 27 cybrids were tumorigenic while 17 of 27 produced differentiated muscle. This series of experiments supports the notion that factor(s) in the non-tumorigenic cytoplasm are able, in some but not all cell types, to induce long-term, heritable suppression of tumorigenicity and that this phenomenon is not necessarily related to the ability of the cells to differentiate in culture. Since a DNA hypomethylating agent, 5-azacytidine, also results in both suppression of tumorigenicity of T984-15 cells and activation of myogenesis (Walker et al., 1984; Walker and Shay, 1984), one possible mechanism to explain cytoplasmic modification of nuclear gene expression may involve alterations in DNA methylation (Shay, 1983).

Materials and Methods
    Enucleation and Fusion
        Cytochalasin B is a fungal metabolite that causes rapid and dramatic change in the morphology of cells growing in monolayer culture (Carter, 1967). Cell enucleation can occur in virtually all cells by combining treatment of cells with cytochalasin B and exposure to a centrifugal field (Prescott et al., 1972; Wright and Hayflick, 1972). As can be seen in Figure 1, (phase contrast light micrographs of CHO cells), within 20 minutes after beginning centrifugation in medium containing 10 µg/ml cytochalasin B, 37°C, the nuclei of most cells bulge out from the main body of the cells (1a).

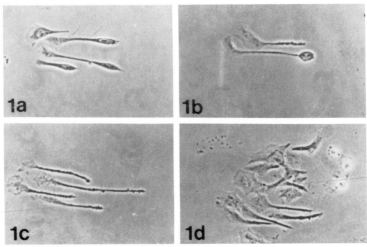

1a   1b

1c   1d

By 40 min (1b, 1c) most cells have lost their nuclei and the anucleate cytoplasms are greatly distorted (frequently reaching over 100 μm in length). If the distorted cytoplasms are placed in medium not containing cytochalasin B, they quickly recover and regain a morphology (1d) similar to the original whole cells (Shay et al., 1975). The precise techniques vary slightly, depending on the cell line in use, but in general it is now possible to easily separate populations of mammalian cells into nuclear (karyoplast) and cytoplasmic (cytoplast) parts. Both karyoplasts and cytoplasts degenerate within 48 hr after enucleation (Shay et al., 1974). The observation that karyoplasts which contain 5-10% of the cell cytoplasm and an intact plasma membrane cannot survive and/or regenerate their lost parts is interesting. It is possible, however, to fuse cells and cell components using inactivated virus or polyethylene glycol to produce viable proliferating hybrids, cybrids, and reconstituted cells (Fig. 2).

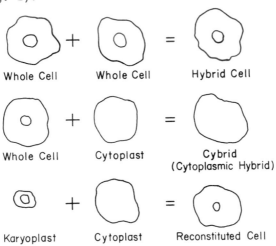

Whole Cell + Whole Cell = Hybrid Cell

Whole Cell + Cytoplast = Cybrid (Cytoplasmic Hybrid)

Karyoplast + Cytoplast = Reconstituted Cell

FIGURE 2

A cybrid is the viable proliferating fusion product of a cytoplast with a whole cell (Bunn, 1982; Bunn et al., 1974) while a reconstitued cell is the viable proliferating fusion product of a cytoplast with a karyoplast (Bunn, 1982, Veomett et al., 1974). The main difference between reconstituted cells and cybrids is that the former does not involve as much dilution of the donor cytoplasm by the recipient cytoplasm.

Using these techniques, it is possible to investigate nuclear cytoplasmic interactions and to determine if cytoplasmic regulatory substances might act to modify nuclear gene expression (for a more thorough review of this subject see Shay, 1983; for reviews of techniques to enucleate and fuse cells, as well as methods to select cybrids and reconstitued cells from a mixed population of parental cells and fusion products, see Shay, 1982).

Cells Lines

The tumorigenic Y-1 line was originally derived from a murine adrenal tumor (Buonassisi et al., 1962) and was obtained from the American Type Culture Collection, Rockville, MD, and Dr. Bernard Schimmer. The T984-15 tumorigenic murine cell line was clonally isolated from C17-S1-D-T984 (Jacob et al., 1978) on the basis of the morphologic criterion of the absence of terminal differentiation into myotubes (Shay et al., 1981). The nontumorigenic A-MT-BU-A1 (hereafter designated AMT) was originally derived from MT-29240 in Dr. Hayden Coon's laboratory and was obtained from Drs. Malech and Wivel, NIH. The AMT cell line is contact-inhibited, contains intracisternal A virus particles, but is non-tumorigenic as tested by lack of growth in soft agar and nude mice. In addition, the AMT cell line is chloramphenicol- and BrdU-resistant allowing for genetic selection of various cybrids and reconstituted cells. All cells were grown in DMEM (low glucose) supplemented with 10% fetal bovine serum in a humidified atmosphere containing 95% air and 5% CO_2. All cells utilized in these experiments, as well as hybrids, cybrids, and reconstituted cells, were found to be free of Mycoplasma contamination.

Tumorigenicity Testing

Logarithmically growing cultures were detached from the substrate using 0.5% trypsin, washed with medium containing serum, and resuspended in DMEM without serum. Using a 20 or 21g needle, 0.2 ml of the cell suspension was injected into the subcutaneous tissue on the back of 4-8 week old congenital athymic nude Balb/c male and female mice to give a total innoculum ranging from $5x10^5$ to $5x10^6$ cells/animal. Animals were kept a minimum of 6 months or sacrificed when 1-2 cm diameter tumors were observed, which ever occurred first.

Differentiation Testing

As can be seen in Figure 3a, Y-1 cells are flat and epitheloid in shape prior to ACTH treatment. Upon the addition of 100 milliunits/ml ACTH Y-1 cells round up (Fig. 3b) and increase steroid secretion greater than 10-fold. Y-1 cells and enucleated Y-1 cells (Fig. 3c) secrete a basal level of 0.032 - 0.036 µg of steroid per mg of cell protein per 30 min as determined by fluorimetric analysis. Surprisingly, enucleated Y-1 cells treated with ACTH also round up (Fig. 3d) and secrete steroids similarily to whole cells (0.440 - 0.560 µg of steroid per mg of cell protein per 30 mins) (Clark and Shay, 1982).

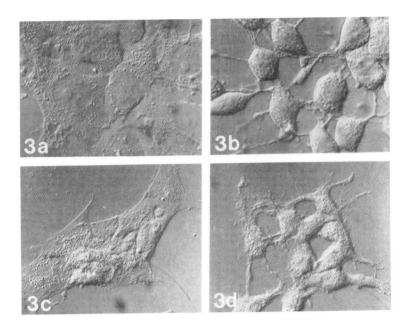

Differentiation of T984-15 cells was determined by placing subclones in culture and observing if myotube formation occurred. Muscle specific myosin was identified by immunoperoxidase staining with the use of a monoclonal antibody (CCM-52) which was raised against chick myosin but which cross-reacts with mouse myosin. (The antibody was obtained from Dr. Radovan Zak, U. of Chicago) (Walker et al., 1984.)

Results and Discussion

As illustrated in Figure 4, somatic cell hybrids were isolated by fusing AMT and Y-1 cells in the presence of medium containing HAT (hypoxanthine, aminopterin, and thymidine) and CAP (chloramphenicol) as previously described (Shay and Clark, 1979). Resistance to the antibiotic chloramphenicol was due to a mitochondrial mutation and thus served as a cytoplasmic genetic marker. Under these selection conditions only the hybrid cells survived. The unfused AMT cells did not grow because of the HAT while the unfused Y-1 cells did not grow because of the CAP.

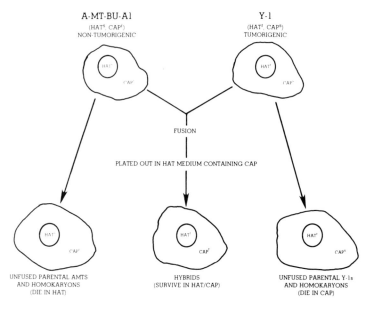

FIGURE 4

Although 6 of 6 control Y-1 clones produced tumors in nude mice and 6 of 6 AMT clones were nontumorigenic using the identical conditions, only 1 of 3 hybrid clones were tumorigenic. This indicated that either nuclear or cytoplasmic AMT factors were capable of suppressing the Y-1 cell tumorigenic potential. Various reconstituted cells were then produced. When Y-1 cytoplasts were fused to Y-1 karyoplasts, all clones examined were tumorigenic whereas none of 6 clones of Y-1 cytoplasts fused to AMT karyoplasts were tumorigenic. However, when AMT cyto-

plasts were fused to Y-1 karyoplasts (Figure 5) 6/6
clones were tumorigenic.

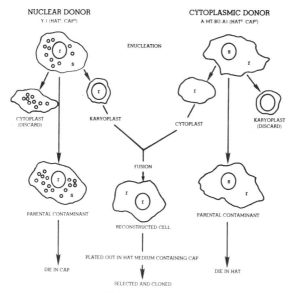

NUCLEAR DONOR
Y-1 (HAT', CAP³)

CYTOPLASMIC DONOR
A·MT·BU·AI (HATˢ CAPᴿ)

ENUCLEATION

CYTOPLAST
(DISCARD)

KARYOPLAST

CYTOPLAST

KARYOPLAST
(DISCARD)

FUSION

PARENTAL CONTAMINANT

RECONSTRUCTED CELL

PARENTAL CONTAMINANT

PLATED OUT IN HAT MEDIUM CONTAINING CAP

DIE IN CAP

SELECTED AND CLONED

DIE IN HAT

FIGURE 5

These experiments indicated that AMT cytoplasmic factors
were not capable of suppressing the Y-1 tumorigenic
potential nor were Y-1 cytoplasts capable of making AMT
tumorigenic. However, when the reconstituted cells were
fluorimetrically quantitated for steroid production, an
interesting result was observed, AMT cytoplasm was able
to suppress steroidogenesis in Y-1 karyoplasts. Upon
ACTH treatment, Y-1 cells rounded up and produced
elevated levels of steroids, whereas AMT control cells
and Y-1(k) x AMT(c) did not round up or produce steroids.
After 3 weeks in culture the Y-1(k) x AMT(c) clones again
became responsive to ACTH induced rounding and steroid
production. In order to determine if this inhibition of
steroidogenesis was due to the trauma of enucleation and
fusion, Y-1(k) x Y-1(c) were similarly produced as a
control. In all instances these reconstituted cells were
capable of rounding up and producing steroids.

Another possibility was that the delay in steroidogenesis was due to a lack of adrenal cytoplasmic components in the Y-1(k) x AMT(c) clones. In order to test
this possibility, cybrids were produced by fusing Y-1
whole cells to AMT(c). Similarly to the reconstituted

cells, the cybrids were also inhibited in steroidogenesis. Thus, resynthesis of adrenal cell cytoplasmic components was an unlikely explanation for the inhibition since the cybrids contained the steroidogenic machinery. In addition to genetic isolation of cybrids, physical isolation of cybrids was accomplished using a fluorescence activated cell sorter and a procedure as illustrated in Figure 6.

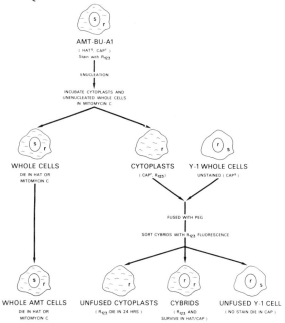

FIGURE 6

Using Rhodamine-123, a non toxic mitochondrial specific stain, populations of cybrids could be isolated and tested for steroidogenesis immediately after fusion. Using either the genetic or physical isolation techniques Y-1 whole cells fused to AMT(c) were non-responsive to ACTH induced rounding and steroidogenesis. The result was thus not a consequence of the specific selection technique employed.

Another possibility was that the AMT cytoplasts contained long-lived cytoplasmic factors capable of suppressing steroidogenesis. Because mitochondria are important in the biogenesis of steroids, experiments were conducted to determine if the AMT mitochondria were responsible for the inhibition of steroidogenesis in the

Y-1(k) x AMT(c) reconstituted cells. Two approaches were used, the first of which involved transferring isolated mitochondria from AMT cells to Y-1 cells as previously described (Clark and Shay, 1982). The mitochondrial transformants were produced by taking CAP-resistant mitochondria from AMT cells, mixing with Y-1 cells, and selecting for growth in the presence of CAP. Such transformants were isolated and in all instances were responsive to ACTH, thus indicating that mitochondria were not likely candidates for the AMT cytoplasmic factor that inhibited Y-1 steroidogenesis. The second approach was to treat AMT cells with the mitochondrial poison Rhodamine 6G, enucleating the AMT cells, fusing to Y-1 cells, and finally isolating cybrids using the fluorescence activated cell sorter. Such cybrids did not round or produce steroids for approximately 3 weeks. These experiments indicated that nonmitochondrial cytoplasmic factors were responsible for the inhibition of response to ACTH.

As a final series of experiments, isolated microcytospheres (Maul and Weibel, 1982) were fused to Y-1 cells. Microcytospheres are small cytoplasmic fragments predominantly containing ribosomes which are isolated from cytochalasin B treated cells as described in Fig. 7.

PRODUCTION OF MICROCYTOSPHERES

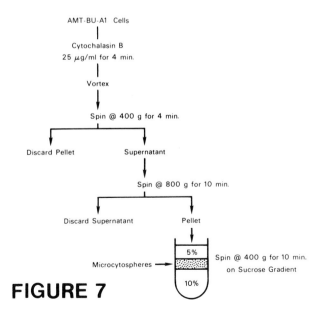

AMT-BU-A1 Cells
|
Cytochalasin B
25 μg/ml for 4 min.
|
Vortex

Spin @ 400 g for 4 min.

Discard Pellet   Supernatant

Spin @ 800 g for 10 min.

Discard Supernatant   Pellet

Microcytospheres → 5% Spin @ 400 g for 10 min.
                    10% on Sucrose Gradient

FIGURE 7

As is illustrated in Figure 8, microcytospheres isolated from AMT cells [previously stained with a non-toxic long chain fatty acid conjugated to fluorescein (F-18)], were fused to Y-1 cells and sorted on the fluorescence activated cell sorter. Individual cells were then tested for ACTH induced rounding.

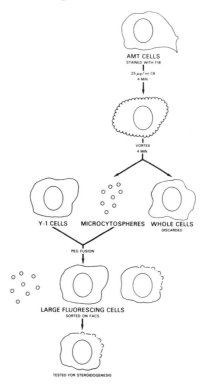

AMT CELLS
STAINED WITH F18

25 µg/ml CB
4 MIN

VORTEX
4 MIN

Y-1 CELLS   MICROCYTOSPHERES   WHOLE CELLS
DISCARDED

PEG FUSION

LARGE FLUORESCING CELLS
SORTED ON FACS

TESTED FOR STEROIDOGENESIS

FIGURE 8

Of 270 cells isolated that had been fused to microcytospheres, 84 or 31% were unable to round upon ACTH treatment. F-18 stained Y-1 control cells sorted and tested were able to round (297/300), and steroidogenesis was not inhibited. It is not clear why only 31% of the Y-1 cells fused to AMT microcytospheres were inhibited, but it is possible that there is a dose-dependent effect (e.g., more than one AMT microcytosphere might be required to inhibit Y-1 steroidogenesis).

In the experiments in which Y-1 cells were fused to AMT cytoplasts or cytoplasmic fragments, there was long-term suppression of differentiated function (e.g., steroidogenesis inhibition) but no suppression of tumorigenicity using the AMT cytoplasts. In a second series of experiments AMT cytoplasts were fused to another tumorigenic cell line T984-15. Figure 9 illustrates the procedure for isolating cybrids produced by fusing AMT(c) and T984-15 cells.

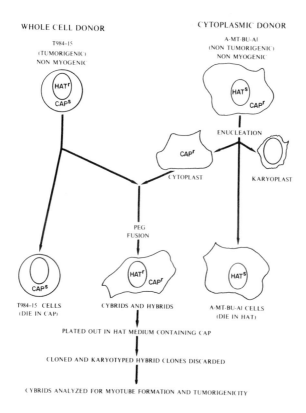

WHOLE CELL DONOR

CYTOPLASMIC DONOR

T984-15
(TUMORIGENIC)
NON MYOGENIC

A-MT-BU-AI
(NON TUMORIGENIC)
NON MYOGENIC

HAT^r
CAP^s

HAT^s
CAP^r

ENUCLEATION

CAP^r

CYTOPLAST

KARYOPLAST

PEG
FUSION

CAP^s

HAT^r
CAP^r

HAT^s

T984-15 CELLS
(DIE IN CAP)

CYBRIDS AND HYBRIDS

A-MT-BU-AI CELLS
(DIE IN HAT)

PLATED OUT IN HAT MEDIUM CONTAINING CAP

CLONED AND KARYOTYPED HYBRID CLONES DISCARDED

CYBRIDS ANALYZED FOR MYOTUBE FORMATION AND TUMORIGENICITY

FIGURE 9

The results of these experiments were dramatic. Of 27 cybrids clones isolated, only two were found to be tumorigenic. As one control the parental T984-15 cell line was subcloned and 20/20 subclones produced tumors in nude mice. In another control experiment (Fig. 10) cytoplasts from the tumorigenic Y-1 cells were fused to T984-15 and 10/10 isolated clones were tumorigenic.

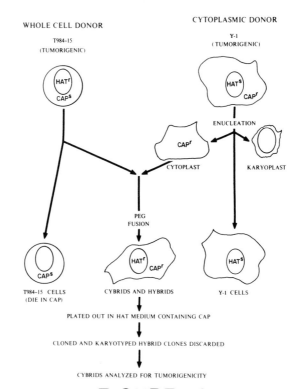

WHOLE CELL DONOR

T984-15
(TUMORIGENIC)

CYTOPLASMIC DONOR

Y-1
(TUMORIGENIC)

ENUCLEATION

CYTOPLAST

KARYOPLAST

PEG
FUSION

T984-15 CELLS
(DIE IN CAP)

CYBRIDS AND HYBRIDS

Y-1 CELLS

PLATED OUT IN HAT MEDIUM CONTAINING CAP

CLONED AND KARYOTYPED HYBRID CLONES DISCARDED

CYBRIDS ANALYZED FOR TUMORIGENICITY

FIGURE 10

The results of these experiments indicate that cytoplasmic factors from the nontumorigenic AMT cells can suppress tumorigenicity of T984-15 cells, but cytoplasmic factors from a tumorigenic cell (Y-1) cannot. Since in the earlier series of experiments cytoplasmic factors from AMT cells did not suppress the tumorigenic potential of Y-1 cells, it suggests there may be something about T984-15 cells that make them more permissive for modification.

When the AMT(c) x T984-15 cybrid clones were examined for their differentiation phenotype, it was observed that 17/27 clones differentiated into myotubes in cell culture. Since all subclones of the parental T984-15 were found to be non-differentiating (0/20) and 17/27 cybrids were capable of myogenesis, it appeared as if there was a general correlation between induction of differentiation and suppression of tumorigenic potential. This correlation was not a stringent one since, of the two cybrids clones which continued to make tumors, one was myogenic while the other one was not.

Using the DNA hypomethylating agent 5-azacytidine to treat T984-15 cells, essentially the same results were observed as with cybridization with AMT cytoplasts (Walker et al., 1984). While 20 of 20 untreated subclones of T984-15 produced tumors when injected into nude mice, 14 of 15 T984-15 subclones which were treated for 24 hours with 5 µg/ml 5-azacytidine displayed suppressed tumorigenesis under identical conditions. Thus, two separate epigenetic mechanisms appear to uncouple differentiation and tumorigenicity in the T984-15 cell line. However, since 5-azacytidine generally resulted in both a suppression of tumorigenicity and activation of myogenesis, one possible mechanism to explain the cybrid modification of gene expression may involve alterations in DNA methylation. Because DNA hypomethylation generally correlates with gene expression it is possible that 5-azacytidine treatment and the cybridization procedures activated a suppressor gene(s) which in turn decreased the potential of treated T984-15 cells to produce tumors. Since hypomethylation is necessary but not sufficient to induce gene expression, this may help explain why Y-1 cells were not suppressed by identical cybridization procedures.

In conclusion, cytoplasmic factors from AMT cells are able to have long-lived effects on the phenotypes of Y-1 and T984-15 cells. While the examples presented in this article are consistent with cytoplasmic-mediated changes in DNA methylation patterns, additional mechanisms equally consistent could be proposed. The isolation and purification of specific cytoplasmic substances, their introduction via microinjection into cells and their effects on purified genes, may help elucidate the mechanism of cytoplasmic modification of nuclear gene expression.

Acknowledgements

The contributions of two of my former graduate students, Dr. Mike A. Clark and Dr. Cheryl Walker, are gratefully acknowledged. Supported in part by grants from N.S.F. and the Meadow's Foundation.

References

Ber, R. and Wiener, F. (1978) Phenotypic trait transferred by cybridization. Cytogenics and Cell Genetics 21:304-308.

Buonassisi, V., Sato, G. and Cohen, A.I. (1962) Hormone producing cultures of adrenal origin. Proc Natl Acad Sci (USA) 48: 1184-1190

Bunn, C.L., Wallace, D.C., and Eisenstadt, J.M. (1974) Cytoplasmic inheritance of chloramphenicol resistance. Proc Natl Acad Sci (USA) 71: 1681-1685

Bunn, C.L. (1982) The influence of cytoplast-to-cell ratio on cybrid formation. In: Techniques in Somatic Cell Genetics (ed. J.W. Shay) Plenum Pub. Co., New York pp 189-199

Carter, S.B. (1967) Effects of cytochalasins on mammalian cells. Nature 213: 261-264

Clark, M.A. and Shay, J.W. (1982) Long-lived cytoplasmic factors that suppress adrenal steriodogenesis. Proc Natl Acad Sci (USA) 79: 1144-1148

Darmon, M., Serrero, G., Rizzino, A. and Sato, G. (1981) Isolation of myoblastic, fibro-adipogenic and fibroblastic clonal cell lines from a common precursor and study of their requirements for growth and differentiation. Exp. Cell Res. 132: 313-327

Gopalakrishnan, T.V., Thompson, E.B., and Anderson, W.F. (1977) Extinction of hemoglobin inducibility in Friend erythroleukemia cells by fusion with cytoplasm of enucleated mouse neuroblastoma or fibroblast cells. Proc Natl Acad Sci (USA) 74: 1642-1646

Gopalakrishnan, T.V. and Anderson, W.F. (1979) Epigenetic activation of phenylalanine hydroxylase in mouse erythroleukemia cells by the cytoplast of rat hepatoma cells. Proc Natl Acad Sci (USA) 76: 3932-3936

Jacob, H., Buckingham, M.E, cohen, A., Dupont, L., Fiszman, M. and Jacob, F. (1978) A skeletal muscle cell line isolated from a mouse teratocarcinoma undergoes apparently normal differentiation in vitro. Exp. Cell Res 114: 403-408

Kahn, C.R., Gopalakrishnan, T.V., and Weiss, M.C.(1981) Transfer of heritable properties by cell cybridization: Specificity and the role of selective pressure. Somatic Cell Genetics 7:L 547-565

Linder, S. (1980) Teratoma cybrids: An analysis of the post-fusion effects of myoblast cytoplasms on embryonal carcinoma cells. Exp Cell Res 130: 159-167

Lipsich, L.A., Kates, J.R. and Lucas, J.J. (1979) Expression of a liver-specific function by mouse fibroblast nuclei transplanted into rat hepatoma cytoplasts. Nature 281: 74-76

Maul, G.G. and Weibel, J. (1982) Production of micro-cytospheres. In: Techniques in Somatic Cell Genetics. (ed. J.W. Shay) Plenum Pub. Co., New York, pp. 237-242

Prescott, D.M., Myerson, D. and Wallace J. (1972) Enucleation of mammalian cells with cytochalasin B. Exp Cell Res 71: 480-485

Shay, J.W. and Clark, M.A. (1979) Nuclear control of tumorigenicity in cells reconstructed by PEG induced fusion of cell fragments. J. Supramol Struct Cellular Biochem 11: 33-49

Shay, J.W., Porter, K.R. and Prescott, D.M. (1975) The surface morphology and fine structure of CHO cells following enucleation. Proc Natl Acad Sci (USA) 71: 3059-3063

Shay, J.W., Lorkowski, G. and Clark, M.A. (1981) Suppression of tumorigenicity in cybrids. J Supramol Struct Cellular Biochem 16: 75-82

Shay, J.W. (1982) Techniques in Somatic Cell Genetics. (ed, J.W. Shay) Plenum Pub. Co., New York

Shay, J.W. (1983) Cytoplasmic modification of nuclear gene expression. Mol and Cellular Biochem 57: 17-26

Veomett, G., Prescott, D.M., Shay, J.W. and Porter, K.R. (1975) Reconstruction of mammalian cells from nuclear and cytoplasmic components. Proc Natl Acad Sci (USA) 71: 1999-2002

Walker, C., Ranney, D.F. and Shay, J.W. (1984) 5-azacytidine-induced uncoupling of differentiation and tumorigenicity in a murine cell line. JNCI 73: 877-885

Walker, C. and Shay, J.W. (1984) 5-azacytidine-induced myogenesis in a differentiation defective cell line. Differentiation 25: 259-263

Wright, W.E. and Hayflick, I. (1972) Formation of anucleate and multinucleate cells in normal and SV40 transformed WI-38 cells by cytochalasin. B Exp Cell Res 74: 187-194

Cellular Endocrinology: Hormonal Control of Embryonic
and Cellular Differentiation, pages 433-443
© 1986 Alan R. Liss, Inc.

HORMONAL   CONTROL   OF   DEVELOPMENTALLY   REGULATED   ADIPOSE
GENES

D. M. Knight, A. B. Chapman, F. M. Torti, and
G. M. Ringold

Department of Pharmacology, Stanford University
School of Medicine, Stanford, California 94305

INTRODUCTION

The differentiation of multipotent cells involves
widespread changes in gene expression as they progress
along a defined lineage towards their final specialized
phenotypes. A particular cell type must not only possess
the regulatory machinery to turn on a functionally related
set of genes, but also the capacity to regulate the timing
of their expression. Although little is known about how
these changes are regulated, many of them involve interaction with specific inducers or hormones. Such hormone
effects have provided some of the best tools for characterizing mechanisms of developmental gene regulation. In
some cases the products of target genes that are directly
activated by steroid hormones may in themselves be
involved in regulating the expression of secondary genes
such as those that define a differentiated phenotype. For
example, some of the early genes induced by ecdysone in
drosophila salivary glands appear to be instrumental in
regulating puffing activity of the so-called middle and
late genes (Ashburner, et al., 1973).

We have previously made use of an adipogenic cell
line (TA1) derived from 10T1/2 mouse embryo fibroblasts to
investigate the temporal and coordinated control of gene
expression during adipogenesis (Chapman et al., 1984).
TA1 cells are indistinguishable morphologically from the
parental 10T1/2 cells while they grow at low density.
After reaching confluence, however, TA1 cells express a
functional adipose phenotype characterized by accumulation

of lipid droplets. We have made use of cDNA clones corresponding to mRNAs induced during differentiation of TA1 cells to study the regulation of specific genes expressed during adipogenesis and the control of adipogenic gene expression by glucocorticoid hormones, and other molecules.

Acceleration of the Developmental Program

We have previously shown that treatment of TA1 cells with certain hormones, notably the synthetic glucocorticoid dexamethasone and insulin, leads to an acceleration of the phenotypic changes associated with adipogenesis and to the precocious accumulation of specific mRNAs (Chapman et al., 1984). We show here that dexamethasone alone is

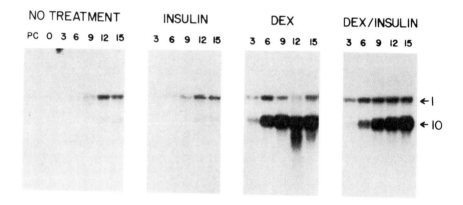

Figure 1. Time course of clone 1 and clone 10 RNA accumulation in control and hormone-treated cells. TA1 preadipocytes were treated at confluence with either 1 μM dexamethasone, 5 mg/ml insulin, or a combination of both. RNA was isolated from cells one day prior to confluence (PC), at confluence (0), and every three days post-confluence with continual hormone treatment (3-15). Ten mg of total RNA were electrophoresed in an agarose formaldehyde gel and transferred to a nitrocellulose filter. This blot was then hybridized to nick translated clone 1 and clone 10 DNA. Clone 1 RNA is 4.3 kb and clone 10 RNA is 2.3 kb.

capable of producing this effect (Fig. 1). For most of the genes examined (see below for an exception), dexamethasone affects the timing of gene expression without altering the eventual steady-state mRNA level. In Figure 1 for example, clone 1 RNA reaches a similar level in the presence or absence of dexamethasone. In order to further delineate the role of glucocorticoids in temporal regulation of the developmental program, we have measured transcription rates for several adipose-inducible genes to examine the role of dexamethasone in the temporal control of these genes.

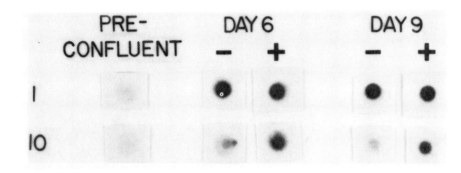

Figure 2. Transcriptional induction of clone 10 by dexamethasone. TAl preadipocytes were grown after confluence in the presence (+) or absence (-) of 1 μM dexamethasone. Nuclei were isolated at the indicated times and ^{32}P-UTP was incorporated into nascent RNA chains. Labeled RNA was then hybridized to 3 mg of clone 1 or clone 10 DNA immobilized on nitrocellulose filters. Exposure time was for 3 days.

The data in Figure 2 demonstrate that the rate of transcription for two adipose-inducible genes is increased dramatically when TAl cells are allowed to differentiate into mature adipocytes. Clone 1 is a cDNA corresponding to an mRNA that is undetectable in pre-adipocytes, but quite abundant in differentiated cells. Clone 10 is unique among these genes in that its expression appears to be directly regulated by glucocorticoids (see below.) Similar results to those seen with clone 1 have been obtained for several other adipose-specific genes (data not shown).

The differentiation of TA1 cells can be accelerated by treatment with the synthetic glucocorticoid dexamethasone. The accelerated morphological differentiation is accompanied by precocious accumulation of adipose-specific mRNAs as documented in Fig. 1, and the earlier transcriptional activation of the corresponding genes in the presence of dexamethasone (data not shown). Although transcription is activated earlier when dexamethasone is present, the maximal transcription rates for most adipose-specific genes are similar with or without dexamethasone (for example, see Fig. 1 Clone 1). This result is unlike the higher maximal transcription rates seen in typical glucocorticoid induced genes (for review see Ringold,

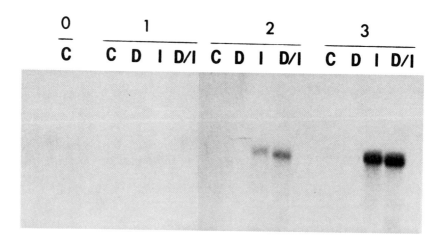

Figure 3. Acceleration of clone 1 RNA accumulation by indomethacin. TA1 cells were grown to confluence (day 0) and treated with 1 μM dexamethasone (D), 125 μM indomethacin (I), or both (D/I). Untreated control cells (C) were also included in this experiment. Cells were harvested at 0, 1, 2, or 3 days after confluence, total RNA was extracted and subjected to electrophoresis on an agarose-formaldehyde gel. The RNA was transferred to nitrocellulose and the filter was probed with nick-translated clone 1 cDNA and analyzed by autoradiography.

1985), suggesting that the hormone affects the triggering mechanisms which orchestrate the transcriptional induction of adipose genes rather than superimposing a second mode of regulation upon the genes directly.

Dexamethasone is known to limit production of arachidonic acid metabolites such as prostaglandins by inducing an inhibitor of Phospholipase A_2, a key enzyme of that pathway (for review see Schleimer, 1985). To investigate whether this pathway is indeed involved in regulating adipogenesis, we added indomethacin, an inhibitor of the cyclooxygenase in the arachidonic acid pathway, to differentiating TAl cells. Figure 3 demonstrates that indomethacin also accelerates the accumulation of clone 1 RNA compared to untreated control cells. In fact, the effect is even more pronounced with indomethacin than with dexamethasone.

Because dexamethasone and indomethacin accelerate TAl cell differentiation, and both compounds are known to inhibit production of arachidonic acid metabolites, one model for the regulation of adipose genes supposes a product of the arachidonic acid pathway, perhaps a prostaglandin-like molecule, may be responsible for maintenance of the pre-adipose state. Sometime after cell confluence, production of this putative regulator may be inhibited, allowing expression of the adipose developmental program. Dexamethasone and indomethacin may prematurely limit production of the regulator, leading to an acceleration of adipogenesis. Characterization of glucocorticoid induced gene products present shortly after cells have reached confluence and identification of the precise metabolic pathway through which indomethacin exerts its effect on TAl cells (which may of course be unrelated to the arachidonic acid cascade) might provide insight into the nature of this developmental switch.

Negative Regulation of Adipogenesis by Cachectin

In contrast to the acceleration of differentiation by glucocorticoids and indomethacin in TAl cells, we have observed suppression of differentiation by a factor produced by endotoxin-stimulated macrophages. Termed cachectin by Cerami and colleagues, this factor was previously shown to inhibit the expression of certain enzymes involved in lipid metabolism (Kawakami et al., 1982; Pekala, et al., 1983). When added to TAl preadipocytes, we find that cachectin inhibits lipid accumulation after cell conflu-ence. Figure 4 shows that cachectin also dramatically reduces the amount of detectable mRNA for several develop-mentally regulated adipose genes. We have seen a similar cachectin-mediated reduction in mRNA levels for all the adipose-specific genes we have studied. In this experi-ment, β-actin (Gunning et al., 1983) is included as a con-trol to show that cachectin does not indiscriminately inhibit mRNA synthesis. Using nuclear transcription assays, we have shown that the reduced mRNA levels follow-

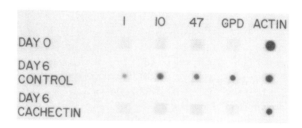

Figure 4. TAl cells were grown with 1 μM dexametha-sone present in the media for the first three days after confluence, and 5 mg/ml bovine insulin for the first 6 days after confluence. Conditioned media from the macro-phage cell line RAW 264 treated with endotoxin (24 hr at 10 mg/ml in serum-free medium) (cachectin) was first added to preadipocyte cultures two days prior to confluence at a concentration of 10 μl/ml. Cells were fed with resupple-mentation of hormones at day 0 (confluence) and day 3. Cells were harvested at day 6. Total RNA was isolated and applied to nitrocellulose in a dot blot apparatus (BRL). Nick translated cDNA clones of genes whose expression is seen only in differentiated TAl adipocytes (clones 1, 10, 47, and glycerophosphate dehydrogenase), as well as a β-actin cDNA clone were used to probe these filters. Filters were washed, then exposed to XAR5 film at $-70°C$ with an intensifying screen.

ing cachectin treatment are due to a lack of gene transcription (Torti, et al., 1985). Cachectin, therefore,
appears to act by preventing the transcriptional activation of adipose genes.

We have also observed that cachectin has the capacity
to deplete adipocytes of lipid and to inhibit the expression of previously activated adipose genes. Figure 5
shows that when cachectin is added to fully differentiated
TA1 cells, the amount of mRNA for two developmentally activated adipose genes is reduced to low levels quite rapidly. Nuclear transcription assays reveal that the transcription of these genes is shut off after cachectin
administration (data not shown).

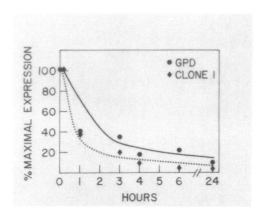

Figure 5. Ten μl/ml of cachectin was added to day 6
adipocyte cultures differentiated as described in
Figure 4. Total RNA was isolated from cells at the indicated times after cachectin exposure and applied to nitrocellulose. Filters were probed with the indicated cDNAs,
washed, autoradiographed, and scanned using a Hoeffer
GS300 densitometer attached to a reporting integrator
(Hewlett-Packard). Points shown were normalized for differences in amount of applied RNA using a cDNA probe made
to total cellular RNA. The levels of β-actin mRNA were
also determined and found not to be altered by treatment
of cells with cachectin.

Cachectin thus appears to be able to prevent TA1 differentiation, and possibly to revert the cells, at least morphologically, to a fibroblast-like state. The exact nature of the macrophage factor(s) responsible for this response is still undefined. The experiments described here were carried out with crude conditioned media of endotoxin stimulated macrophages. A purified macrophage factor, interleukin-1, (mouse recombinant IL-1), does not inhibit adipocyte differentiation. However, Beutler et al. have recently purified to homogeneity a protein which has similar effects on lipoprotein lipase activity and synthesis to those of cachectin. Interestingly, this protein has a high degree of sequence homology to human tumor necrosis factor (TNF), another macrophage secretory product (Beutler et al.). Preliminary experiments with recombinant human TNF show similar morphologic effects on adipocyte differentiation and lipid mobilization to those of cachectin (Torti, data not shown). In addition, TNF rapidly diminishes the levels of adipose-specific mRNAs and the transcription of their cognate genes (Torti et al., data not shown). Further characterization of cachectin and its receptor will help to clarify the nature of signal transduction to the cell nucleus and the mechanism by which cachectin regulates the adipose developmental program.

Clone 10 - A Glucocorticoid Inducible Gene

When characterizing the hormonal acceleration of gene induction by dexamethasone and insulin, we found that clone 10 RNA, unlike the other RNAs studied, did not reach similar plateau levels in treated and control cells. Recent analysis of the DNA sequence of clone 10 indicates that it belongs to the family of cytochrome P-450 genes (Knight, unpublished). Figure 1 shows an autoradiograph of a nitrocellulose blot containing RNA samples from TA1 cells treated with various hormone regimens which had been hybridized to nick translated clone 1 and clone 10 DNA. Whereas clone 1 RNA reaches similar levels by 12 days after confluence in treated and control cells, clone 10 RNA reaches much higher levels (approximately 25-fold) in cells treated with dexamethasone or dexamethasone and insulin than that found in control or insulin treated cells.

The behavior of the clone 10 gene is most easily explained if in addition to being activated during adipocyte differentiation, it is specifically responsive to glucocorticoid hormones. This hypothesis is borne out by the observation that clone 10 mRNA is inducible by dexamethasone in fully differentiated adipocytes that had never been exposed to hormone (data not shown). None of the other adipose induced clones studied to date has shown this induction by dexamethasone once differentiation is complete. Thus dexamethasone's action in inducing clone 10 RNA seems to be separate and in addition to its effect on accelerating adipocyte differentiation.

The specific inducibility of clone 10 mRNA by dexamethasone appears to be restricted to differentiated cells; clone 10 RNA is undetectable in control or dexamethasone-treated 10T1/2 cells. Although TA1 preadipocytes do show a small amount of clone 10 RNA in dexamethasone treated cells, we estimate that the level of clone 10 RNA expression in these cells is approximately 9,000-fold lower than that seen in mature hormone-treated TA1 adipocytes. We believe that these low levels of clone 10 RNA most likely reflect dexamethasone mediated induction in a small number of differentiating adipocytes in the preadipocyte population. The lack of clone 10 inducibility in 10T1/2 on TA1 preadipocytes is not due to a lack of glucocordicoid receptor; both cell types contain similar levels of functional receptor (data not shown). Thus, the hormone inducibility of clone 10 RNA appears to be dependent on its prior developmental activation.

Transcriptional Induction of Clone 10 mRNA Synthesis

Relative transcription rates of the clone 10 and clone 1 genes were measured using a nuclear transcription assay. Although no transcription of the clone 1 gene can be detected in preadipocytes (Figure 2), by six days after confluence, transcription has reached a plateau level reflecting its activation during adipocyte differentiation. In dexamethasone treated cells, a similar plateau level of clone 1 transcription is reached. Although clone 10 gene transcription is also not detectable in preadipocytes and reaches a plateau transcription rate in both treated and control cells, a significantly higher level is found in dexamethasone treated cells. Thus dexamethasone's specific induction of clone 10 RNA is in large part, if not completely, transcriptional.

Recent studies on MMTV have revealed a correlation between gene activity and hormonal inducibility which is reflected in an altered chromatin DNAase sensitivity (Zaret, et al., 1984). Studies of the chicken vitellogenin (VTG II) gene have revealed DNAase hypersensitive sites which exist prior to estrogen mediated expression and which correlate in tissue distribution with VTGII hormone inducibility (Burch and Weintraub, 1983). It has not yet been possible, though, to observe and study the generation of such sites that mark future hormone inducibility during differentiation. TA1 cells may offer an advantage in characterizing such changes since the precursor cells in which clone 10 RNA is not inducible are readily available. Analysis of clone 10 chromatin structure is underway in an attempt to find changes which correlate with transcriptional activity, potential hormone inducibility, and hormone induction itself. If the induction of clone 10 transcription is indeed a primary glucocorticoid response it will be particularly interesting to identify DNA binding sites for the glucocorticoid-receptor complex and analyze the factors that affect their chromatin structure during differentiation.

We have explored three instances in which the expression of developmentally regulated genes is modulated by hormones. The effects produced by exogenously added molecules provide a useful way to investigate molecular mechanisms of developmental gene regulation.

ACKNOWLEDGEMENTS

This work was supported by grants from the National Institutes of Health (GM25821), the March of Dimes, and Cetus Corporation. D. Knight is a recipient of an NIH postdoctoral fellowship, A. Chapman is supported by an NIH medical scientist training program grant, and G. Ringold is an Established Investigator of the American Heart Association. F. M. Torti was supported by a grant from the Veterans Administration.

REFERENCES

Ashburner M, Chihara C, Meltzer P, Richards G (1973). Temporal control of puffing activity in polytene chromosomes. Cold Spring Harbor Symp Quant Biol 38:655-662.

Beutler B, Greenwald D, Hulmes JD, Chang M., Pan Y-CE, Mathison J, Ulevitch R, and Cerami A (1985). Identity of tumor necrosis factor and the macrophage-secreted factor cachectin. Nature 316:552-554.

Burch JBE, Weintraub H (1983). Temporal order of chromatin structural changes associated with activation of the major chicken vitellogenin gene. Cell 33:65-76.

Chapman AB, Knight DM, Dieckmann B, Ringold GM (1984). Analysis of gene expression during differentiation of adipogenic cells in culture and hormonal control of the developmental program. J Biol Chem 259:15548-1555.

Gunning P, Ponte P, Okayama J, Engel J, Blau HM, Kedes L (1983). Isolation and characterization of full-length cDNA clones for human α-, β-, on γ-actin mRNAs: Skeletal but not cytoplasmic action have an amino-terminal cysteine that is subsequently removed. Mol Cell Biol 3:787-795.

Kawakami M, Pekala P, Lang MD, Cerami A (1982). Lipoprotein lipase suppression in 3T3-L1 cells by an endotoxin-induced mediator from exudate cells. Proc Nat Acad Sci USA 79:912-916.

Pekala P, Kawakami M, Angus CW, Lang MD, Cerami A (1983). Selective inhibition of synthesis of enzymes for de novo fatty acid biosynthesis by an endotoxin-induced mediator from exudate cells. Proc Nat Acad Sci USA 80:2743-2747.

Ringold GM (1985). Steroid hormone regulation of gene expression. Annu Rev Pharmacol 25:529-566.

Schleimer RP (1985). The mechanisms of anti-inflammatory steroid action in allergic diseases. Ann Rev Pharmacol Toxicol 25:381-412.

Torti FM, Dieckmann B, Beutler B, Cerami A, Ringold GM (1985). A macrophage factor inhibits adipocyte gene expression: an in vitro model of cachexia. Science, in press.

Zaret KS, Yamamoto KR (1984). Reversible and persistent changes in the chromatin structure accompany activation of a glucocorticoid-dependent enhancer element. Cell 38:29-38.

Cellular Endocrinology: Hormonal Control of Embryonic
and Cellular Differentiation, pages 445–454
© 1986 Alan R. Liss, Inc.

REGULATION OF GENE EXPRESSION DURING THE DIFFERENTIATION OF
3T3-ADIPOCYTES

Bruce M. Spiegelman, Kathleen S. Cook and
Clayton R. Hunt
Dana-Farber Cancer Institute and Department of
Pharmacology, Harvard Medical School, Boston,
Massachusetts   02115

INTRODUCTION

The differentiation of 3T3-adipocytes in culture
closely resembles the development of fat cells in vivo
(Green and Kehinde, 1974, 1976, reviewed in Green, 1979).
During this process, the cells develop enzyme activities
related to fatty acid and triglyceride synthesis, exhibit
changes in morphology and acquire sensitivity to particular
hormones. Adipocytes also begin to secrete factors related
to angiogenesis (Castellot et al., 1980, 1982). These
changes are part of a program in which the composition of
cellular protein is extensively revised (Sidhu, 1979;
Spiegelman and Green, 1980) through changes in mRNA content
(Spiegelman and Green, 1980; Spiegelman and Farmer, 1981;
Spiegelman et al., 1983; Bernlohr et al., 1984; Chapman et
al., 1984).

We have been studying the differentiation of 3T3-F442A
preadipocytes with 2 major goals: 1) to use these cells as
a model system for the regulation of gene control during
mammalian cell differentiation, and 2) to improve our understanding of how the adipocyte carries out its major role in
vivo as a homeostatic regulator of serum glucose and lipids.
We have approached these problems by cloning mRNA sequences
which are specific to the adipocyte form of 3T3 cells. Subsequently, we have identified several encoded products and
studied how the production of these mRNAs is controlled.

RESULTS

Several approaches were used to isolate developmen-
tally-regulated sequences from an adipocyte cDNA library
(Spiegelman et al., 1983). To isolate a clone for glycerophosphate dehydrogenase (GPD), a key lipogenic enzyme, a
radioactive cDNA probe was synthesized from a partially
purified GPD mRNA and was used to screen the library. For
a more general selection of differentiation-dependent
clones, duplicate sets of the library filters were screened
by hybridizing cDNA probes prepared from adipocyte and preadipocyte mRNA. Twenty-two clones corresponding to mRNAs
expressed preferentially in adipocytes were isolated. A
clone for adipocyte β-actin was identified by screening the
adipocyte library with a chicken β-actin probe (Cleveland
et al., 1980).

Table 1 summarizes the properties of the 4 clones we
have studied most extensively. A more complete description
is published (Spiegelman et al., 1983). pGPD hybridizes to
an adipocyte mRNA of 3,500 bases, which is much larger than
the 900 bases required to encode GPD (34K). This mRNA
cannot be detected in the preadipocyte and we estimate that
the increase during differentiation must be at least 200-
fold. Actin mRNA decreases 2-4 fold, as noted earlier
(Spiegelman and Farmer, 1982). Two clones isolated by pre-
ferential hybridization to adipocyte cDNA select by hybridization mRNAs which direct translation of polypeptides of
13K and 28K. Both mRNAs are very abundant and strongly
differentiation-dependent, but unlike GPD and actin, the
identity of the encoded proteins was not immediately
apparent.

Very little is known about the cell-specific proteins
of adipocytes which are not directly related to lipid synthesis or hydrolysis. In order to understand the significance of their physiological role and regulation, the iden-
tities of mRNA sequences encoding the 13K and 28K proteins
were investigated by sequencing these cDNA clones. Figure
1 illustrates that the 13K protein has close homology
(≥ 70%) to rabbit myelin protein P2. Much less striking
homology (25%) is observed between 13K and rat intestinal
fatty acid binding protein. P2-like proteins were not
known to exist in any tissue other than myelin until reported in 3T3-adipocytes (Bernlohr et al., 1984; Cook et
al., 1985). These proteins have been shown to have signif-

TABLE 1. Characterization of Differentiation-Dependent cDNA
Clones

Clone	Insert Size (bp)	mRNA Size (bases)	Translation Product Size (Kd)	Fold Change of mRNAs
pGPD	350	3500	34 (GPD)	>200↑
pAct-1	1200	2100	42 (Actin)	2-4↓
pAd-5	400	650	13	150↑
pAd-20	940	1050	28	>200↑

icant homology to several lipid binding proteins at their
N-termini (Takahashi et al., 1982). We consider it likely
that this protein serves as a lipid carrier in adipocytes.

The 28K protein has homology to the family of serine
proteases, which includes trypsin, chymotrypsin and
elastase, (Figure 2A). Homology between 28K protein and
the proteases listed above is about 30% overall, but 64%
when only those residues generally conserved in the serine
protease family are considered. This degree of similarity
is sufficient to consider this protein to be a member of
the serine protease family, but it does not appear to be
very closely related to any one member of this family in
particular. The presence of His (66), Asp (115) and Ser
(209) residues in the same location as those comprising the
charge relay system in other serine proteases, indicates
that this protein is likely to be catalytically active.
The presence of an Asp residue at position 203 suggests
that the 28K protein will cleave peptide bonds after
arginine or lysine residues in substrate molecules.

Sequence encoding the amino terminus of this protein
(Fig. 2B) was generated by primer extension of adipocyte
mRNA and sequencing the cDNA product. Two forms of 28K
mRNA differing in length by 3 bases are present, and probably arise by alternative splicing of the same primary
transcript (Cook et al., 1985b). The 28K protein is synthesized with a signal sequence, and is presumably targeted
toward membrane insertion or secretion. The protein encoded by the shorter 28K mRNA is missing one alanine residue (20) which would occur at the carboxyl end of the signal peptide upon cleavage of the longer 28K protein at the
site predicted using the method of von Heijne (1983). In
addition a cleavage peptide for activation of the serine

```
              10                  20                  30
P2      S N K F L G T W K L V S S E N F D D Y M K A L G V G L A T R
              : : : : : : : : : : :        : : :      : : :
13K           L V S S E N F D D Y M K E V G V G F A T R
              : :            :            : :
FABP    M A F D G T W K V Y R N E N Y E K F M E K M G I N V V K R


              40                  50                  60
P2      K L G N L A K P N V I I S K K G D I I T I R T E S T F K N T
        :        : : : :      : : :      : :      : : : : : : :
13K     K V A G M A K P N M I I S V N G D L V T I R S E S T F K N T
        :              :        :        :        : :    : :
FABP    K L G A H D N L K L T I T Q E G N K F T V K E S S N F R N I


              70                  80                  90
P2      E I S F K L G Q E F E Q T T A D N R K T K S T I T L E R G A
        : : : : : : : :    : :        : : :    : :    : : :      : :
13K     E I S F K L G V E F D E I T A D D R K V K S I I T L D G G A
        :      : : :    :          : :                    :    :
FABP    D V V F E L G V D F A Y S L A D G T E L T G T L T M E G N K


              100                 110                 120
P2      L N Q V Q K W N - - G K E T T I K R K L V D G K M V V E C K M K
        :    : : : : :        : :    : : : : : :      : : : : :    : :
13K     L V Q V Q K W D - - G K S T T I K R K R D G D K L V V E C V M K
        : :      :        : :        : :                    :    :
FABP    L V G K F K R V D N G K E L I A V R E I S C N E L I Q T Y T Y E


              130
P2      G V V C T R I Y E K V
        : :      : :      : :
13K     G V T S T R V Y E R A
        : :            :
FABP    G V E A K R I F K K E
```

Figure 1. Amino Acid Sequence Predicted from 13K mRNA Aligned with those of Rabbit Myelin P2 and Rat Intestinal Fatty Acid Binding Protein. (Complete nucleotide sequence is in Cook et al., 1985a).

protease zymogen is also present.

The role of transcriptional alterations in the regulation of specific mRNAs was investigated in isolated preadipocytes and adipocyte nuclei by the "run-on" technique. RNA synthesized in adipocyte and preadipocyte nuclei was hybridized to cDNA under conditions where the autoradiographic signals were proportional to input of radioactive nuclear RNA (Cook et al., 1985a). Clear increases in transcription of the GPD and 13K genes could be observed while actin transcription was decreased (Fig. 3). Surprisingly, transcription of the 28K gene could not be detected in preadipocyte or adipocyte nuclei despite the abundance of this mRNA in fat cells. Quantitatively, GPD and 13K transcription are increased a minimum of 6 and 11-fold, respectively (Table 2); these figures are undoubtedly limited by the sensitivity of this assay. Actin transcription is decreased 1.7-fold.

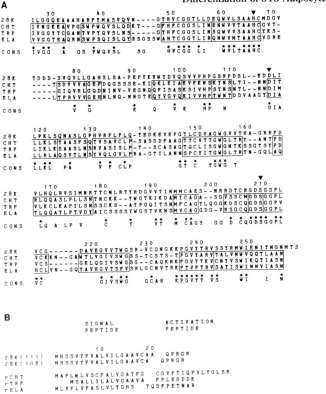

Figure 2. Amino Acid Sequence Predicted from 28K mRNA Aligned with Bovine Trypsin (TRP), Chymotrypsin (CHT) and Elastase (ELA). CONS indicates residue conserved in serine proteases (Young et al., 1978). (Complete nucleotide sequence is in Cook et al., 1985b). A. Residues 26-259; B. Residues 1-25, including signal and activation peptides.

The discrepancy between the abundance of 28K mRNA and its transcription is clear when comparing the ratios of these two measures estimated from the same cell populations (Table 2). Actin, GPD and two clones that show little developmental regulation (pC1 and pC2) all have a very similar ratio of transcription to mRNA abundance (2.3-4.7) in adipocytes. The ratio for 28K is <0.06, while for 13K it is 0.23. In both cases this ratio appears to reflect low levels of transcription relative to the abundance of the mRNAs. These results suggest that other levels of regula-

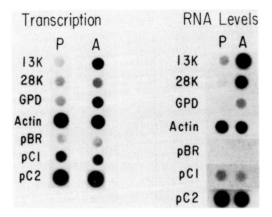

Figure 3. Transcription and RNA Levels During Differentiation. P - preadipose; A - adipose.

tion may contribute to the accumulation of these mRNAs in
fat cells. Preliminary experiments examining turnover of
all of these RNAs in the presence of an inhibitor of RNA
polymerase II, 5,6-dichloro-1-β-ribofuranosyl benzimidazole,
suggest that the 13K and 28K RNAs are very stable in the
adipocyte cytoplasm, compared to other sequences examined
(Cook et al., 1985a).

DISCUSSION

     The ability to study adipocyte differentiation in iso-
lated cell culture began in 1974 when Green and Kehinde described 3T3-adipocytes (Green and Kehinde, 1974). Subsequently, other preadipocyte lines or primary cultures suitable for biochemical studies have been developed (e.g.
Serrero and Khoo, 1982; Forest et al., 1983; Chapman et al.,
1984). Differentiation of adipocytes from preadipocytes results in a striking change in cell form and function, and
it was demonstrated that many changes occur in specific protein biosynthesis during this process (Sidhu, 1979;
Spiegelman and Green, 1980). We (Spiegelman et al., 1983)
and others (Bernlohr et al., 1984; Chapman et al., 1984)
isolated and characterized fat cell specific cDNA clones
from adipocyte libraries.

     The adipocyte is a cell which specializes in fatty acid
and triglyceride metabolism. This is reflected by the
great increase we observe in mRNA for GPD, a key lipogenic

TABLE 2. Nuclear Transcription and Cytoplasmic RNA Levels
During Adipocyte Differentiation

Probe	Fold Changes in Nuclear Transcription	Fold Changes in RNA Levels	Adipocyte Transcription/ RNA Level
13K	> 11↑	4↑	0.23
28K	Undectable	115↑	> 0.06
GPD	> 6↑	> 17↑	4.7
Actin	1.7↓	1.8↓	4.6
pC1	2.3↓	1.4↓	4.8
pC2	1.2↓	1.4↓	2.3

In vitro nuclear transcription and cytoplasmic RNA dot blots
were carried out and quantitated as described (Cook et al.,
1985a). Both sets of data were derived from the same set
of cells using the same probes and were not corrected for
probe length. Ratio of transcription to RNA level in adipocytes was obtained by dividing radioactivity hybridizing
in these two assays.

enzyme. However, the multitude of new proteins which
appear during adipocyte differentiation (Sidhu, 1979;
Spiegelman and Green, 1980) suggests that new gene products
may be made in the adipocyte in addition to the well known
enzymes which comprise the pathways of triglyceride synthesis and breakdown. We have described cDNA clones encoding
two such proteins here. One protein having a molecular
weight of 13K, also described by Bernlohr et al. (1984),
encodes a close homologue of rabbit myelin P2. This level of
sequence homology suggests that the mRNA expressed in 3T3-
adipocytes is a product of the same gene as that expressed
in myelin, but proof of this must await characterization of
the mouse myelin gene product. The precise role of this
P2-like protein in the adipocyte is not clear, but the
homology at the amino   terminus between the P2 proteins and
several other well characterized lipid binding proteins
(Takahashi et al., 1982) suggests some role in the transport of adipocyte lipids. Since adipocytes synthesize and
secrete large quantities of fatty acids, molecules known to
be deleterious to membrane integrity, it seems plausible
that this protein may serve to buffer cellular membranes
from high levels of free fatty acids.

There have been no reports of increased protease activ-

ity in differentiating adipocytes, so the expression of a
novel protease-like protein during adipocyte differentiation was not anticipated. While a role in the processing
of lipid metabolizing enzymes is possible, the extensive
changes in cell shape and in the profile of extracellular
matrix components that occur during differentiation (Green
and Kehinde, 1974; Spiegelman and Farmer, 1982;
Kuri-Harcuch et al., 1984) may require the degradation of
some intra- or extracellular structural elements. The adipocyte serine-protease homologue we have described could be
involved in this process. Interestingly, two forms of this
protein arise by removal of a single codon, via alternative
splicing (Cook et al., 1985b). The shorter protein is
missing a single amino acid near the predicted signal peptide cleavage site, suggesting the possibility that cellular localization or some other process is controlled via
this alternative splice.

Understanding the mechanisms of gene control during
adipocyte development is a major goal of our lab. We have
demonstrated, for the first time, regulation of specific
gene transcription during adipocyte differentiation. Increased gene transcription is observed for GPD and the 13K
(myelin P2-like) protein. The changes appear to be large,
although the nuclear transcription assay is not sensitive
enough to allow us to directly compare the magnitude of
mRNA induction with transcriptional increases. Increased
transcription of the gene for 13K during differentiation
has also been observed by Bernlohr et al. (1985). Surprisingly, we have found transcription of the gene encoding
the 28K serine protease homologue to be too low to detect
in both preadipocytes and adipocytes. Quantitative compar-
isons of the levels of transcription to RNA abundance in
adipocytes suggests that other levels of control contribute
substantially to the abundance of the 28K mRNA and, to a
lesser extent, 13K mRNA. Consistent with these results,
preliminary experiments employing an RNA synthesis inhibitor suggests that these two RNAs are more stable in adipocytes than the other RNAs examined (Cook et al., 1985b).
Of course, since these RNAs cannot be readily detected in
preadipocytes we do not know whether their apparent stability is differentiation-dependent or merely reflects an intrinsic property of these sequences. While it is likely
that the induction of GPD mRNA is mainly transcriptional,
more work is needed to clarify the contribution that non-
transcriptional mechanisms make to the differentiation-

dependent induction of 28K and 13K RNAs.

REFERENCES

Bernlohr DA, Angus CW, Lane MD, Bolanowski MA, Kelly TS
(1984). Expression of specific mRNAs during adipose differentiation: identification of an mRNA encoding a homologue of myelin P2 protein. Proc Natl Acad Sci USA 81:
5468-5472.
Bernlohr DA, Bolanowski MA, Kelly TJ, Lane MD (1985).
Evidence of an increase in transcription of specific
mRNAs during differentiation of 3T3-L1 preadipocytes.
J Biol Chem 260: 5563-5567.
Castellot JJ, Karnovsky MJ, Spiegelman BM (1980). Potent
stimulation of vascular endothelial cell growth by differentiated 3T3-adipocytes. Proc Natl Acad Sci USA 77:
6007-6011.
Castellot JJ, Karnovsky MJ, Spiegelman (1982). Differentiation-dependent stimulation of neovascularization and
endothelial cell chemotaxis by 3T3-adipocytes. Proc Natl
Acad Sci USA 79: 5597-5601.
Chapman AB, Knight DM, Dieckmann BS, Ringold GM (1984).
Analysis of gene expression during differentiation of adipogenic cells in culture and hormonal control of the developmental program. J Biol Chem 259: 15,548-15,555.
Cleveland DW, Lopata MA, MacDonald RJ, Cowan NJ, Rutter WJ,
Kirschner MW (1980). Number and evolutionary conservation
of α - and β -tubulin and cytoplasmic β - and γ -actin genes
using specific cloned cDNA probes. Cell 20: 95-105.
Cook KS, Hunt CR, Spiegelman BM (1985). Developmentally
regulated mRNAs in 3T3-adipocytes: analysis of transcriptional control. J Cell Biol 100: 514-520.
Cook KS, Groves DL, Min HY, Spiegelman BM (1985). A developmentally regulated mRNA from 3T3 adipocytes encodes a
novel serine protease homologue. Proc Natl Acad Sci USA
(in press).
Forest C, Grimaldi P, Czerucka D, Negrel R, Ailhaud G
(1983). Establishment of a preadipocyte cell line from
the epididymal fat pad of the lean C57BL/6J mouse. In
Vitro 19: 344-354.
Green H, Kehinde O (1979). Formation of normally differentiated subcutaneous fat pads by an established preadipose
cell line. J Cell Physiol 101: 109-172.
Green H, Kehinde O (1974). Sublines of mouse 3T3 cells that
accumulate lipid. Cell 1: 113-116.

Green H, Kehinde O (1976). Spontaneous heritable changes
leading to increased adipose conversion in 3T3 cells.
Cell 7: 105–113.

Kuri-Harcuch W, Arguello C, Marsh-Moreno M (1984). Extracellular matrix production by mouse 3T3-F442A cells during adipose differentiation in culture. Differentiation
28: 173–178.

Serrero G, Khoo JC (1982). An in vitro model to study adipose differentiation in serum-free medium. Anal Biochem
120: 351.

Sidhu RS (1979). Two-dimensional electrophoretic analysis
of proteins synthesized during differentiation of 3T3-L1
preadipocytes. J Biol Chem 254: 11111–11118.

Spiegelman BM, Farmer S (1982). Decrease in tubulin and
actin gene expression prior to morphological differentiation of 3T3-adipocytes. Cell 29: 53–60.

Spiegelman BM, Frank M, Green H (1983). Molecular cloning
of mRNA from 3T3-adipocytes: regulation of mRNA content
for glycerophosphate dehydrogenase and other differentiation-dependent proteins during adipocyte development.
J Biol Chem 258: 10083–10089.

Spiegelman BM, Green H (1980). Control of specific protein
biosynthesis during adipose conversion of 3T3 cells. J
Biol Chem 255: 8811–8818.

Takahashi K, Odani S, Ono T (1982). A close structural
relationship of rat liver Z-protein to cellular retinoid
binding proteins and peripheral nerve myelin P2 protein.
Biochem Biophys Res Commun 106: 1099–1105.

von Heijne G (1983). Patterns of amino acids near signal-
sequence cleavage sites. Eur J Biochem 133: 17–21.

Young CL, Barker WC, Tomaselli CM, Dayhoff MO (1978). In
Atlas of Protein Sequence and Structure, ed. Dayhoff MO
(National Biomedical Research Foundation, Silver Spring,
MD), Vol 5, Suppl 3, pp 73–93.

The authors thank Douglas Groves for technical assistance and Adah Levens for help in preparation of this manuscript. This work was supported by NIH grants AM31405 and
AM34605.

Cellular Endocrinology: Hormonal Control of Embryonic
and Cellular Differentiation, pages 455–465
© 1986 Alan R. Liss, Inc.

CLONING OF MUSCLE REGULATORY FACTORS

Woodring E. Wright

Department of Cell Biology, University of Texas
Southwestern Medical School, Dallas, Texas 75235

INTRODUCTION

Most laboratories investigating the molecular mechanisms regulating gene expression have focussed on isolating differentiated structural genes, then analyzing the
flanking sequences in order to discover important control
regions. The identification of factors that bind to these
sequences would then allow one to proceed "upstream" to
the earlier stages in the differentiation sequence. We
have developed a novel strategy that should permit the
direct cloning of the upstream molecules regulating the
initial decision of myogenic cells to differentiate. One
way in which hormones might regulate cell differentiation
is by influencing the production of the molecules that
interact with the DNA and change the expression of the
genetic program. The cloning of the molecules regulating
the decision to differentiate should thus provide the
appropriate materials for studying the mechanisms by which
hormones influence the initiation of terminal myogenic
differentiation.

The strategy for isolating the factors controlling
myogenesis consisted of first producing a myoblast line in
which the expression of the factors had been amplified,
and then enriching a cDNA for the messages for these
factors by removing all of the sequences that were also
expressed in a differentiation defective myogenic line.
The enriched cDNA was then cloned and analyzed. This
chapter will describe the theoretical background for a
protocol for producing such an amplified line, its produc-

tion and characterization, and the preparation of probes enriched for the sequences regulating the decision to differentiate, and their cloning.

THEORETICAL BACKGROUND

The proceedure for isolating a myoblast cell line that had amplified the expression of the factors regulating the decision to differentiated evolved from two sets of somatic cell hybridization experiments. In the first, we examined the regulation of differentiation in hybrids between differentiation defective and competent myoblasts (1). As is the case for most cultured models of cell differentiation, the ability of L6 rat myoblasts to differentiate is gradually lost after several months of continuous cultivation. It is thus very easy to isolate differentiation defective variants simply by cloning an "old" culture. Three sets of hybrids were constructed: competent x competent, competent x defective and defective x defective. They were then analyzed for their ability to form cells that stained with an antimyosin antibody following a prolonged stimulus to differentiate. Whereas 65% of the cells in competent x competent hybrids differentiated, only 0.05% of the defective x defective cells became myosin-positive. The competent x defective cells exhibited an intermediate behavior, in which 2-8% of the cells differentiated. We developed the following model to explain these results. The dashed vertical line in Figure 1 represents a threshold concentration of a regulatory factor that must be produced in response to a stimulus to differentiate before an all-or-none decision to differentiate is made. If the mean concentration of factor produced in a population of myoblasts is 0.36 standard deviations greater than this threshold, then 65% of the cells will exceed threshold and differentiate. If the mean concentration is 3.71 standard deviations below threshold, then only the tail end of the distribution exceeds threshold and only 0.05% of the cells differentiate. Finally, if the production of this factor is regulated in cis so that each genome in a cell hybrid continues to express its own initial level of the factor, then the cell hybrid will express an arithmetic average of the two extremes and will differentiate with a frequency of 7%.

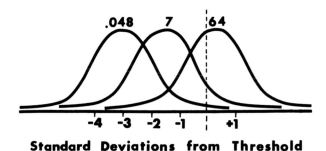

Standard Deviations from Threshold

Figure 1. Molecular model for the mechanism regulating the probability of differentiation. (Reproduced from ref. 1 with the permission of the Rockefeller University Press.)

This model implies that differentiation defective myoblasts are underproducing a critical factor involved in the decision to differentiate. Since differentiation defective variants arise with a very high frequency, this suggests that underproducers are generated with a high frequency. Unless there is some directionality involved, this in turn implies that overproducers should also be generated with a high frequency. Such overproducers would normally be rapidly lost from the culture, since they might produce threshold amounts of the factor even in the absence of a stimulus to differentiate and would thus make the decision to differentiate and become postmitotic. This would explain the tendency of cultures to lose the capacity to differentiate upon prolonged cultivation: the retention of underproducing variants and the loss of overproducing variants would result in a progressive shift of the mean towards a decreased production of the critical factor(s). A method for avoiding the loss of overproducers was suggested by a second series of cell hybridization experiments.

5-bromodeoxyuridine (BUdR) is a thymidine analogue that inhibits cell differentiation in a wide variety of experimental systems including myogenesis. We had demonstrated that differentiated chick skeletal myocytes contained factors capable of inducing rat myosin light chain synthesis in the initial fusion product (heterokaryons) formed by fusing mononucleated chick myocytes to undifferentiated rat myoblasts. In order to investigate the mechanism by which BUdR inhibited cell differentiation (did it block the production of regulatory factors or the action of regulatory factors?), we first grew L6 myoblasts in the presence of BUdR, and then fused them to already differentiated mononucleated chick myocytes (2). Under these circumstances, although chick myosin light chain synthesis continued, the induction of rat myosin light chain synthesis was blocked. A variety of evidence suggested that the chick factors were present in limiting quantities. We reasoned that if BUdR altered the efficiency with which regulatory molecules bound to DNA, and if these factors were present in limiting quantities, then BUdR might cause their effective concentration to fall below threshold and thus block their action. We tested this hypothesis by exploring gene dosage effects. Chick myoblasts were grown in cytochalasin B for the last cell division before they differentiated. Since cytochalasin B blocks cytokinesis as well as myotube formation, this resulted in a population of mostly binucleated differentiated chick myocytes. Increased amounts of chick regulatory factors were then provided by fusing these binucleated myocytes to BUdR-blocked L6 rat myoblasts. The ability to induce rat myosin light chain synthesis was recovered in these heterokaryons. The interpretation of these experiments was that increased amounts of regulatory factors could overcome the inhibition of differentiation produced by BUdR.

THE PRODUCTION OF AMPLIFIED MYOBLASTS

The first set of cell hybridization experiments described above suggested that cells overproducing the factor(s) involved in the decision to differentiate should be generated with a high frequency. The second set of experiments suggested the following strategy for isolating these overproducers. L6 myoblasts could be cloned in a partially inhibitory concentration of BUdR. Those clones derived from overproducing variants would contain the highest concentration of the regulatory factors, and would thus be the first to overcome the inhibition by BUdR and exhibit myotube formation. Since cell density is the most important stimulus for differentiation, cells in the center of a clone differentiate first. There would thus be many undifferentiated dividing cells still present in the clones at the time the first myotubes appear. The first dozen clones to differentiate could then be picked, pooled, and then immediately recloned in a slightly higher concentration of BUdR. Successive cycles of this selection in progressively higher concentrations of BUdR should then result in the selection of variants with a progressively amplified expression of the factors regulating the decision to differentiate. Initially, 0.25µM BUdR almost totally inhibited myogenesis under clonal conditions. After 36 cycles of selection, cells were isolated that differentiated well in the presence of 32µM BUdR. Examination of the density shift of the DNA from these cells in cesium chloride gradients indicated that about 70% of the thymidine residues had been replaced by BUdR, demonstrating that the cells were incorporating BUdR and were thus not resistant due to either transport or incorporation defects.

The above strategy for isolating amplified myoblasts relied on two effects of BUdR. The presence of BUdR in the DNA first prevented the overproducing cells from differentiating under growth conditions, and second permitted the greatest overproducers to be identified once the local clonal cell density reached the point where differentiation was stimulated. If this model were valid, it predicted that the continued presence of BUdR would be required to prevent the cells from differentiating under growth conditions. Figure 2 compares the clonal size at which myotube formation began for the parental L6 rat myoblasts and the BUdR-resistant variants. This data is derived from cells after 21 cycles of selection, when the variants were resistant to 2 µM BUdR.

50% of the parental L6 myoblast colonies contained myotubes when the average colony contained about 3000 cells. These parental cells did not form colonies capable of differentiating if they were cloned in 2 µM BUdR. The BUdR-resistant cycle 21 cells, selected for early myotube formation in BUdR, showed differentiation in 50% of its colonies in the presence of 2 µM BUdR when they only contained about 200 cells. When these cycle 21 cells were cloned in the absence of BUdR, microscopic colonies containing 10 nuclei, half of which were already in myotubes, could be seen as early as four days after

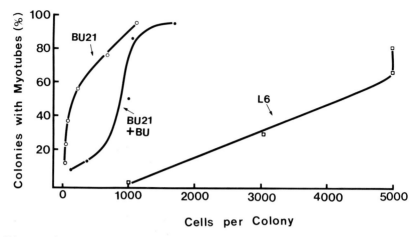

Figure 2. The BUdR-dependence of BUdR-resistant myoblast variants. (Reproduced from ref. 3 with permission of the Rockefeller University Press.)

cloning. Half of the colonies contained myotubes when there were only 50 cells per colony. The cells were thus behaving exactly as predicted by the theoretical model for the mechanism of BUdR resistance.

If the myoblasts have become BUdR-resistant as a result of their ability to overproduce the factors regulating the decision to differentiate, then the molecular model for the regulation of the probability of differentiation (fig. 1) would predict that cell hybrids between these cells and differentiation defective myoblasts should exhibit a high probability of differentiation. The average frequency of differentiation observed in different hybrid clones from BUdR-resistant x differentiation defective combinations was 71% + 2%, compared to only 8% + 2% for the parental L6 x differentiation defective combination (3). The BUdR-resistant cells thus behave as if they have in fact amplified the expression of the factors regulating the decision to differentiate.

MOLECULAR CLONING OF THE REGULATORY FACTORS

Myotubes begin to form and biochemical differentiation can first be detected approximately 40 hours after near confluent monolayers of rat myoblasts are stimulated to differentiate by changing the medium from one containing 20% fetal bovine serum to a mitogenically poor medium containing 1% fetal bovine serum and 5 µg/ml insulin. The molecules regulating the decision to differentiate should be at maximal levels prior to that time. We have somewhat arbitrarily defined the period 24-36 hours after the stimulus to differentiate has been applied as the "mid-decision" phase when these molecules should be at high levels. Figure 3 presents a flow chart for the preparation of a cDNA from cycle 36 BUdR-resistant cells that has been enriched for these molecules by removing sequences that are also expressed in differentiation defective myoblasts.

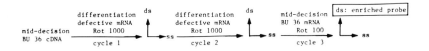

Figure 3. The enrichment of mid-decision cDNA

After each hybridization the cDNA was bound to hydroxyapatite in 0.01M phosphate buffer. Single stranded material was then eluted in 0.075M phosphate buffer, and finally the double-stranded material eluted using 0.175M phosphate buffer. The single-stranded material was then rehybridized to differentiation defective RNA. The single-stranded unbound fraction was then hybridized a final time, but now to homologous mid-decision RNA. Since we assumed that a factor with an abundance of 0.001% would represent the limit of detection of this system, this final cycle was performed at Rot 100 (Rot = RNA concentration at time zero multiplied by time in seconds) where approximately 50% of a message of average size and 0.001% abundance should hybridize. After correcting for losses, we then recovered about 2% of the original cDNA as double-stranded material. When the RNA in this heteroduplex was hydrolyzed and the cDNA subjected to Rot analysis, we found that 50% of the material was now specific for the mid-decision Bu36 cells, while 50% still hybridized to differentiation defective mRNA. The subtraction hybridization protocol was thus successful in producing a probe that was significantly enriched for sequences expressed in the BUdR-resistant mid-decision myoblasts.

After three cycles of subtraction hybidization, 3 ng of cDNA were recovered from about 1.5 µg of starting material. Because of initial difficulties in forming a library from this small amount of cDNA, we adopted the protocol shown in figure 4. A partially enriched cDNA was made by performing one subtraction cycle with differentia-tion defective mRNA, then recovering the hybridizable material with an homologous hybidization. The approxi-mately 45 ng of cDNA that was recovered was then cloned into λ gt10 to yield a 2.5x10⁶ member partially enriched library.

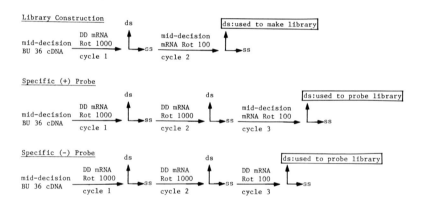

Figure 4. Protocols for the enrichment of cDNAs for library construction and probing.

The Rot analysis described above indicated that half of the material recovered during the third hybridization cycle for the specific (+) probe still hybridized to differentiation defective mRNA. We reasoned that those contaminating sequences could be recovered if the third cycle was performed using differentiation defective rather than BUdR-resistant mRNA. A "specific (-) probe" was thus constructed by using differentiation defective mRNA as the driver for all three cycles of hybridization. A lift from a dish containing 20,000 plaques was then probed with the

specific (+) enriched cDNA (Figure 5, left), autoradiographed, the radioactive probe was washed away, and the
lift then re-probed with the specific (-) enriched probe
(Figure 5, right).

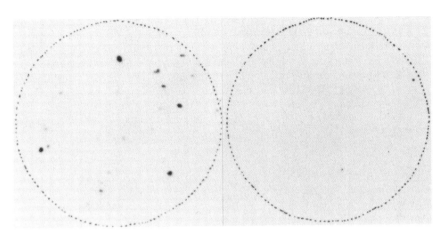

Figure 5. Differential screening of a partially enriched
mid-decision cDNA library.

It is clear that there are many colonies (approximately 1 per 1000 in the library) that react with the
enriched (+) probe that do not react with the enriched (-)
probe. Since the enriched (-) probe should reflect any
non-specific background effects or contaminating sequences
that had not been removed by the subtraction-hybridization
procedure, its failure to bind to the colonies hybridizing
to the enriched (-) probe suggests that they are potentially specific for mid-decision sequences.

The positive colonies are now being screened according to the following four criteria: The levels of message
coded by their insert should be 1) absent or at very low
levels in undifferentiated L6 myoblasts; 2) at near
maximal levels during the phase encompassing the decision
to differentiate; 3) at the same or lower levels in fully
differentiated myotubes (message levels that continued to
rise dramatically would probably represent myogenic structural proteins); and 4) present in higher levels in
mid-decision BUdR-resistant myoblasts than in the parental

L6 myoblasts at a comparable stage. This final criterion is very powerful. There are probably many molecules that transiently appear during the mid-decision phase of myogenesis which reflect the adjustment of the cell's physiology from a dividing to a stationary and finally to a postmitotic state. However, only the regulatory molecules required for differentiation should have had their expression amplified in the BUdR-resistant cells. The fourth criterion should thus allow us to eliminate many of the messages for structural proteins and focus in on those that code for regulatory factors.

CONCLUSION

Cell differentiation probably results from a sequence of regulatory events, of unknown number and complexity. There might be a strictly linear cascade of regulatory interactions, or multiple branch points involving many different factors that coordinate the hundreds of new proteins synthesized in the differentiated cell. Although a great deal of exciting new information is being generated about the regulation of structural gene expression (promoters, enhancers, splicing mechanisms, etc.), very few systems exist for approaching a molecular analysis of the upstream events. The model system presented here should provide such an opportunity. Although the differential expression of the factor(s) during the different stages of cell differentiation will only provide indirect evidence for their regulatory role, more direct proof can be obtained by demonstrating that microinjection of their antisense RNA is capable of blocking myogenesis. Because of the theoretical basis for their isolation, many of the functional characteristics of the isolated factors can be predicted: they should be DNA binding proteins whose affinity for DNA should be altered by BUdR. Footprinting and filter-binding experiments should then permit the identification of the sequences to which they bind and the proteins whose synthesis they control. This approach should thus provide an extremely powerful method for analyzing the sequence of events by which a cell makes and executes the decision to terminally differentiate. The molecular definition of these events will in turn greatly facilitate a detailed analysis of the mechanisms by which hormones influence the process of cell differentiation.

REFERENCES

Wright WE (1984). Control of differentiation in heterokar-
    yons and hybrids involving differentiation-defective
    myoblast variants. J Cell Biol 98:436-443.
Wright WE, Aronoff J (1983). The regulation of rat myosin
    light chain synthesis in heterokaryons between BUdR-
    blocked rat myoblasts and differentiated chick myocytes.
    J Cell Biol 96:1571-1579.
Wright WE (1985). The amplified expression of factors
    regulating myogenesis in L6 myoblasts. J Cell Biol 100:
    311-316.

Index

Date Due